CAMBRIDGE LIBRARY COLLECTION

Books of enduring scholarly value

History of Medicine

It is sobering to realise that as recently as the year in which On the Origin of Species was published, learned opinion was that diseases such as typhus and cholera were spread by a ,Äòmiasma,Äô, and suggestions that doctors should wash their hands before examining patients were greeted with mockery by the profession. The Cambridge Library Collection reissues milestone publications in the history of Western medicine as well as studies of other medical traditions. Its coverage ranges from Galen on anatomical procedures to Florence Nightingale,Äôs common-sense advice to nurses, and includes early research into genetics and mental health, colonial reports on tropical diseases, documents on public health and military medicine, and publications on spa culture and medicinal plants.

A Medical History of Persia and the Eastern Caliphate

Published in 1951, this book presents a continuous history of the art and practice of medicine in Persia (Iran), from the earliest times to the twentieth century. Elgood's prefatory chapter defines the scope of the *History*, and informs the reader of his extensive resources – due to his knowledge of Persian and Arabic, he was able to study original manuscripts of medical historians in the Middle East. He also draws upon his own experiences, having lived and practised in Iran for many years. Packed with medical curiosities and little-known facts, the book describes the impact of Western medicine on Persia from the seventeenth century, and includes discussion of the status and lifestyle of women, and the high status and great influence of Persian doctors. Placing the story of medicine against the background of general Persian history, Elgood demonstrates the important part played by Persia in the world's history of medicine.

Cambridge University Press has long been a pioneer in the reissuing of out-of-print titles from its own backlist, producing digital reprints of books that are still sought after by scholars and students but could not be reprinted economically using traditional technology. The Cambridge Library Collection extends this activity to a wider range of books which are still of importance to researchers and professionals, either for the source material they contain, or as landmarks in the history of their academic discipline.

Drawing from the world-renowned collections in the Cambridge University Library, and guided by the advice of experts in each subject area, Cambridge University Press is using state-of-the-art scanning machines in its own Printing House to capture the content of each book selected for inclusion. The files are processed to give a consistently clear, crisp image, and the books finished to the high quality standard for which the Press is recognised around the world. The latest print-on-demand technology ensures that the books will remain available indefinitely, and that orders for single or multiple copies can quickly be supplied.

The Cambridge Library Collection will bring back to life books of enduring scholarly value (including out-of-copyright works originally issued by other publishers) across a wide range of disciplines in the humanities and social sciences and in science and technology.

A Medical History of Persia and the Eastern Caliphate

From the Earliest Times Until the Year A.D. 1932

CYRIL ELGOOD

CAMBRIDGE
UNIVERSITY PRESS

CAMBRIDGE UNIVERSITY PRESS

Cambridge, New York, Melbourne, Madrid, Cape Town, Singapore,
São Paolo, Delhi, Dubai, Tokyo, Mexico City

Published in the United States of America by Cambridge University Press, New York

www.cambridge.org
Information on this title: www.cambridge.org/9781108015882

This edition first published 1951
This digitally printed version 2010

ISBN 978-1-108-01588-2 Paperback

A MEDICAL HISTORY OF PERSIA AND THE EASTERN CALIPHATE

Shifá'í, poet and court physician, boon companion to Sháh 'Abbás the Great.

The Persian inscription above and below says:

A portrait of the Plato of his time—Ḥakím Shifá'í.

On Saturday 15th Muḥarram 1085 Mu'ín the painter finished this copy. My late Master Riẓá 'Abbásí made the portrait in the year 1044.

Another portrait of this physician exists in the British Museum (OR. 1372 f. 7a) which is possibly the original referred to. This has been reproduced by Prof. Browne in his *Literary History of Persia*, vol. IV, p. 256.

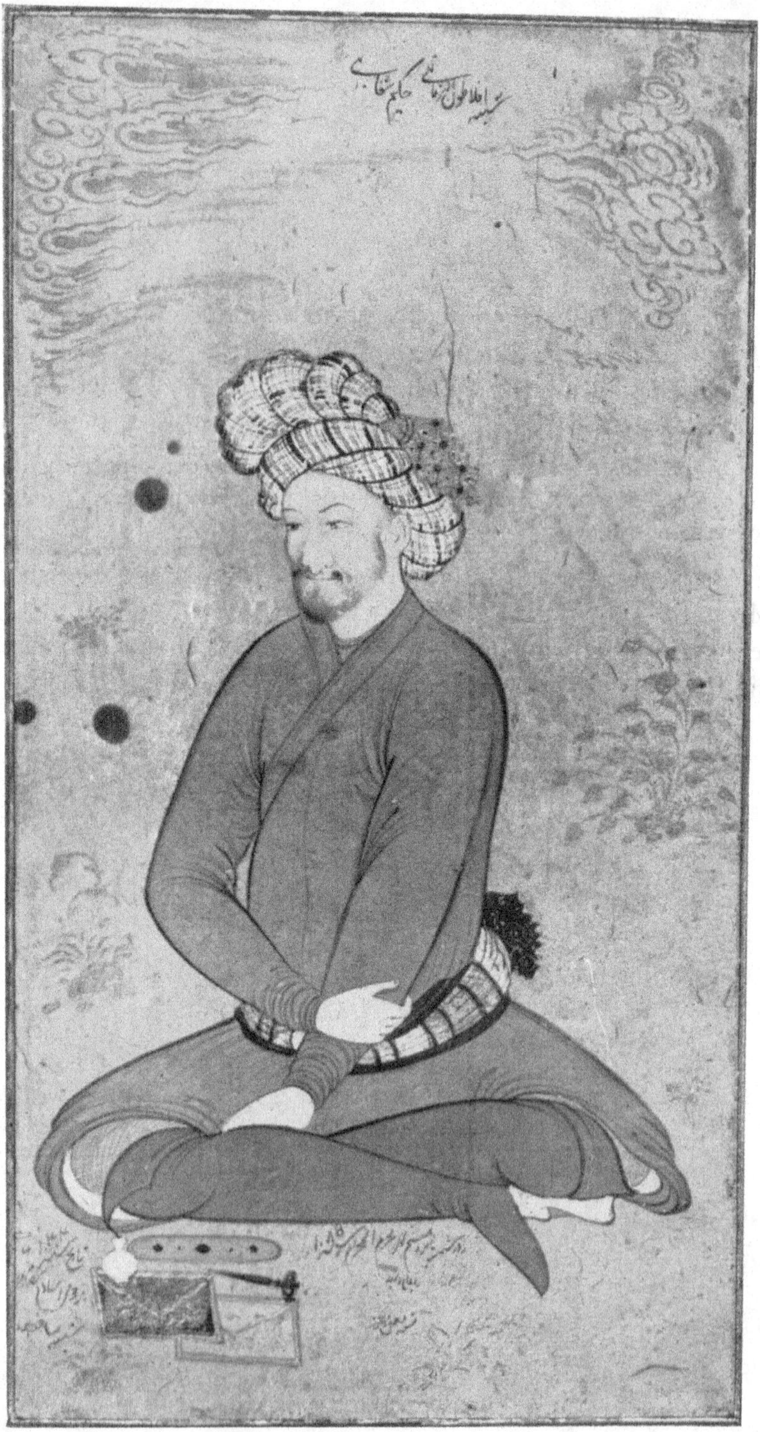

PLATE I. Portrait of a Persian Physician

(See note on back of plate)

A MEDICAL HISTORY OF PERSIA

AND THE

EASTERN CALIPHATE

FROM THE EARLIEST TIMES
UNTIL THE YEAR
A.D. 1932

BY

CYRIL ELGOOD
M.A., M.D., F.R.C.P.
late Physician to H.B.M. Legation,
Teheran, Persia

CAMBRIDGE
AT THE UNIVERSITY PRESS
1951

PUBLISHED BY
THE SYNDICS OF THE CAMBRIDGE UNIVERSITY PRESS

London Office: Bentley House, N.W. 1
American Branch: New York

Agents for Canada, India, and Pakistan: Macmillan

Printed in Great Britain at the University Press, Cambridge
(Brooke Crutchley, University Printer)

PREFACE

NO other country in Europe, Asia or Africa seems to inspire writers as does Iran. Light works of travel and heavy books on more or less obscure subjects are printed and published by the score. Yet no complete history of Medicine in Iran, that part of the Middle East that was formerly called Persia, has up till now been attempted. It is strange, for Persia has played as important a part in the world's history of Medicine as have Persian poetry and Persian miniatures in the world's history of literature and art. Of the three I think Medicine has played the greatest part.

The subject has not, of course, been entirely neglected. Nevertheless, more remains, as Professor Browne pointed out many years ago, to be accomplished in this branch of oriental studies than in any other of equal importance. A few Arabists have dealt with some of the Persian physicians who wrote in Arabic. These are, it is true, the greatest of the Persian School of Medicine. Important though they are, they all flourished about the same time and are representatives of a very short period of medical history. The later physicians who wrote in Persian have been almost entirely neglected. These few modern Arabic scholars, therefore, though they have dealt adequately with Arab or Persian Medicine (for I use the adjective indiscriminately) during the time of the Caliphs of Baghdad, have entirely neglected its history before the coming of Islam and after the invasion of the Mongols. I have here attempted—and I believe that I am breaking virgin soil in so doing—to give a continuous history of the art and practice of Medicine in Persia and the bordering countries from the earliest times until the present day and thus to place the well-known Arab names in the correct historical position and true perspective. For Arab Medicine, even though it may have had a Golden Age, shows a continuous growth in Persia and 'Iraq from the dim ages until a generation ago when the Persian suddenly became Europeanized and Western learning destroyed the very foundations upon which his ancient science was built.

It is easy to see why pre-Islamic Medicine has received so little attention. Very few people can read Pahlavi or the old Persian tongues. Very few, too, of their scientific manuscripts have survived. Possibly none of the people who can read them have sufficient knowledge of Medicine correctly to interpret them. I, too, must admit complete ignorance of any of the languages used in the Middle East before Arabic became the lingua franca of all Mussulmans. I have had to rely for my information on all medical subjects of those times upon Greek writers and on translations and commentaries on the holy books of the Parsees. There are, however, two modern works which contain a lot of information upon pre-Islamic Medicine. These are *Zoroastrian Civilization* by Maneckji Dhalla[1] and *L'Iran sous les Sassanides* by Christensen.[2] I have used very freely both these works. Gibbon, too, is by no means to be despised and I have borrowed liberally from his *Decline and Fall* to give the necessary background to the more purely scientific part of my study of Sassanian Medicine.

With the advent of the Arabs, Arabic became the tongue of all men of learning. It was only towards the end of the period of the Baghdad Caliphs, say in the beginning of the twelfth century, that Persian began to be used as a scientific language. Anyone writing a history of Medicine in the Middle East during the period which extends from the eighth to the thirteenth century, will find plenty of information in contemporary Arab writers. Above all there are the three great medical biographers Ibn abí Uṣaybi'a,[3] al-Qifṭí,[4] and Bar Hebraeus,[5] all of whom wrote in Arabic and all of whose texts have been published in modern editions. These authors I have used as my foundation stones for the strictly Arab period of Persian Medicine. For the years during which the first

1 Maneckji Dhalla, *Zoroastrian Civilization.* New York, 1922.
2 Christensen, *L'Iran sous les Sassanides.* Copenhagen, 1936.
3 Ibn abí Uṣaybi'a, *'Uyún-ul-Inbá' fí Ṭabaqát-il-Aṭibbá.* Cairo, 1882.
4 Al-Qifṭí, *Ta'ríkh-ul-Ḥukama* (Lippert's ed.). Leipzig, 1903.
5 Bar Hebraeus, *Historia Dynastiarum* (Pocock's ed.). Oxford, 1663.

five or six caliphs were ruling in Baghdad, a knowledge of Syriac too might be useful. In my ignorance I must leave research in that language to others.

It is this period of Arabian Medicine which has been most studied by modern writers. Leclerc,[1] in his invaluable history in two volumes (but how it needs an index!), Fonahn,[2] in his excellent catalogue of sources (which, by the way, urgently demands to be brought up to date), and the late Professor Browne's[3,4] various works are the chief modern authors whom I have consulted. There are others, of course, such as Wustenfeld,[5] Garrison,[6] and Campbell[7] whom I ought to mention. But the list of authorities becomes too long. Fonahn himself thirty years ago enumerated 151 works dealing with this period. This number has been considerably increased since then.

Of authorities who have devoted themselves to a study of Medicine in the times of the Caliphs of Baghdad there is one who can rank with any that have ever lived or written. This is the late Dr Max Meyerhof of Cairo. I have quoted from his works so often that it becomes impossible for me to acknowledge my debt to him on each separate occasion. He has helped me by his published works: he has helped me by private letters answering specific points. Whenever I have had a difficulty, I have written to him and invariably I have received the information that I wanted. If I have plagiarized from his articles, if I have made his thoughts to seem to be my own, I apologize. It is only because he has so exactly and so much better expressed just what I have wanted to say.

With the fall of Baghdad before the Mongol invaders in the middle of the thirteenth century Arab Medicine became more

1 Leclerc, *Histoire de la Médicine Arabe*. Paris, 1876.
2 Fonahn, *Zur Quellenkunde der Persischen Medizin*. Leipzig, 1910.
3 Browne, *Chahár Maqála of Nizámí-i-'Arúzí* (Gibb series). London, 1921.
4 Browne, *Arabian Medicine*. Cambridge, 1921.
5 Wustenfeld, *Geschichte der Arabischen Aerzte*. Gottingen, 1840.
6 Garrison, *Introduction to the History of Medicine*. London, 1917.
7 Campbell, *Arabian Medicine*. London, 1926.

truly Persian and the language of the sources of information became almost entirely Persian. Leclerc is here less trustworthy, Browne scarcely touches the period at all, and Meyerhof has published nothing about it. Fonahn is a help. A modern Persian book which I have used extensively is the *Maṭraḥ-ul-Anẓár*,[1] but apparently only the first volume has been published. I hope that the long delay does not mean that the other two contemplated volumes will never be printed. My old friend the S͟háhzáda Lissán-ul-Ḥukamá tells me that he too is writing a book on the history of Medicine in his native land. But when I last inquired of him about it, it was still far from completion.

When the East India Company entered the Persian Gulf, a Factory Diary was kept, recording events in Persia. This is an extremely important contemporary source of information. Scattered throughout are many references to physicians and methods of treatment. These diaries are preserved in the India Office, London, and form 131 volumes. Dr Lockhart tells me that in writing his recent work on Nadir Shah he consulted similar diaries preserved in Paris, written by French merchants, and that these too, contain a certain amount of medical data. These French diaries, I am afraid, I have not read.

For the history of Medicine in Persia during the last fifty years I have relied upon the information supplied me by the Foreign Office, London, and my friends in Persia. To the Foreign Office I would like to express my very grateful thanks and above all to the late Sir Stephen Gaselee for his help. A similar courtesy I received from the Church Missionary Society, whose Secretary showed me all their files which deal with modern medical missions in Iran.

I must add a few words about my system of writing Persian names. Colonel Lawrence gloried in his inconsistency; he hardly ever spelt any name twice in the same way. I, on the contrary, boast of my scrupulous accuracy. Some years ago the Royal Asiatic Society published a system of transliteration of proper

1 Zeylessouf-ed-douleh, *Maṭraḥ-ul-Anẓâr*. Tabriz, 1916.

names written in the Arabic script. No one, not even Professor Browne, seems to have followed out their advice without reserve. Yet it is so highly desirable to be able to recognize at once the original form of the name. It is perhaps the most tiresome of all the habits of modern French orientalists that they follow no system and thus make it very difficult to read any of their works until you have constructed a table of alphabetical equivalents.

Yet even I am obliged to make two exceptions. My first offence is when I use very well-known names which popular usage demands should be spelt in the usual form, not in the form that the system of the Asiatic Society requires. Thus, I write Delhi, not Dihli, and Meshed, not Ma<u>sh</u>had. My second exception is when I use the names of living or recently deceased Persians who were in the habit of writing their own names in a European script. I bow to their wishes and write their names as they wished them to be written, not according to my rules. From Chapter XVIII to the end of the book, therefore, the same name may be found spelt in various ways. It depends upon the caprice of the owner, not upon me.

Briefly, the system recommended for transliterating Persian and Arabic words into English lettering demands that every Arabic letter be represented by a corresponding English letter with the exception of the signs ʿAin and Hamza, which are represented by ʿ and ʾ respectively. For the benefit of those who do not know Arabic I should like to point out that all the written letters need not necessarily be pronounced. Thus, in <u>Kh</u>wárazm, the old Persian name for the modern town of Khiva, the w is silent. Again, when one word ends in a vowel and the next word begins with another vowel, the second vowel (if hamza) is written but not pronounced. Thus, the proper name Abú-ul-Fatḥ is pronounced Abulfat, the final h being just faintly sounded as in the English phrase fat h-errings. Professor Browne would therefore write the name Abu'l Fatḥ. But in the Arabic script both vowels are written. I therefore follow suit and write both, although I am aware that such words will be sadly mispronounced by those ignorant of the language. I feel that the only way of straightening out the present hopeless confusion among oriental writers on this question is to follow exactly the rules which the Asiatic Society has laid down for our guidance.

As for the transliteration of Pahlaví and Zend names I am in the hands of my authorities. If I have failed to make clear to the Pahlaví or Zend scholar the form of the original name, I can only plead ignorance.

C. E.

1948

CONTENTS

LIST OF ILLUSTRATIONS

CHAPTER I

FROM THE EARLIEST TIMES TO THE DEATH OF ALEXANDER

THE source of all medical knowledge in the world was a subject which intrigued the Persian medical biographer of old.[1] There are very few medical writers who do not at some point in their work air their views about the origin of some disease or even of the art of medicine as a whole. Some maintain that medicine is coeval with creation. Others, following Hippocrates and Galen, believe in a partly divine and partly empirical origin. Their view is that theory and doctrines of medicine became known to man by the direct revelation of God: the practice and means of cure were learnt from a variety of sources. In some cases it was a direct revelation from the Almighty: in others it was a matter of observation, just as Cain learnt the trade of grave-digging from a raven.[2] Thus the use of the clyster, says Ghiyáṣ-ul-Dín quoting Galen, was introduced into medical practice by someone who observed a pelican in great distress after having indulged too freely in a shoal of little fishes. To relieve the pain of his stomach, which was manifest upon his face, the bird filled his long beak with water and proceeded to administer to himself a high enema. The result being entirely satisfactory to the bird, the observer used this method on his patients who came to him complaining of gastric disturbances.[3]

The exact spot in the world where medicine was first revealed provoked an even greater divergence of opinion. Some maintained that Egypt was the country to be thus honoured and pointed to the drug *rásen* in proof, claiming that this was the

1 Ibn abí Uṣaybi'a. *Ṭabaqát-ul-Aṭibbá*, vol. 1, p. 5 (referred to hereafter as *I.A.U.*). Bar Hebraeus. *History of the Dynasties*, vol. 1, p. 21 (referred to hereafter as Hist. Dynst.). *Et alii.*

2 Jalál-ul-Dín al-Rúmí. *Masnaví* (Nicholson's translation), bk. iv, v. 1301.

3 Ghiyáṣ-ul-Dín. *Mirát-ul-Saḥḥat*, bk. 1, f. 5.

first drug to be used by physicians and that the word is Egyptian.[1] *Rásen*, as used by the later writers, is the equivalent of helenium. Others named other parts of North Africa as the site of God's revelations: others again preferred Rhodes, Cnidus, or Cos. The divine inspiration was thought to have come by way of dreams. Others, following Galen, claimed that the revelation was direct, like that of the Qur'án, because it was impossible that the human mind should discover for itself such an abstruse and predominant science. Ibn abí Uṣaybi'a, the author of the *'Uyún-ul-Inbá' fí Ṭabaqát- il-Aṭibbá* or Choicest News on the Classes of Physicians (whom I look upon as the greatest of all Persian medical historians), gives as his opinion that this last view is the correct one, for medicine is to be preferred even to philosophy.[2]

Ḥájjí Khalífa in the *Kashf-ul-Ẓanún* in a brief discussion on the origin of medicine quotes the views of Ṣábit (he does not say which Ṣábit) that the source of all medicine was Aesculapius, who handed on this knowledge to his disciples, who then propagated it through the world.[3] He also quotes 'Alí bin Riẓván, a physician of Cairo, who maintained that the art of medicine existed long before Hippocrates, but that the knowledge of it was confined to the descendants of Aesculapius. Aesculapius was himself an angel, whom God sent to teach men. All his teaching was oral. Such books as were written were in cypher and were unintelligible to the uninitiated. This was the state of affairs until the birth of Hippocrates at Cos and Democritus at Abderata. Democritus developed the theoretical side, Hippocrates the practical. Hippocrates had two sons, Thessalus and Draco, and a disciple Polybus, who developed the art and set it out in the form in which the *Masá' il* of Ḥunayn and the *Faṣúl* of Buqráṭ presented it.

Persian mythology ascribes the introduction of medicine into Persia to Jamshíd, the fourth of the early hero kings of Iran. Firdausi refers to this belief in his *Shánnáma*, an epic poem of the end of the ninth century of our era. He says that Jamshíd found

1 Ḥájjí Khalífa, *Kashf-ul-Ẓanún* (ed. Flügel) vol. IV, p. 126.

2 *I.A.U.* vol. I, p 5.

3 Ḥájjí Khalífa, vol. IV, p. 125.

the land rude and barbarous, but that under his wise administration order was introduced, men were taught to build houses and not to be content with caves, to search for the treasures that lie concealed within the earth, and that finally the art and means of healing were made known.

Jamshíd thus spent
Another fifty years and did much good.
He introduced the scents that men enjoy,
As camphor, genuine musk, gum Benjamin,
Sweet aloe, ambergris, and bright rose water.
Next leechcraft and the healing of the sick,
The means of health, the cause of maladies,
Were secrets opened by Jamshíd.[1]

He is also credited with the introduction of alcohol to mankind through the mistake of one of his wives. He had preserved some grapes, which had fermented and were thought to be poisonous. The woman, who was suffering from some painful and incurable disease, drank deeply of this wine juice in the expectation of putting an end to her miserable life. To her astonishment she fell into a comfortable sleep and awaking found herself cured.

To be more scientific and to ponder over the status of medicine among the prehistoric inhabitants of Persia is interesting as a speculation, but valueless as a history. In all probability their views and their methods of advance were the same as those of other primitive people. It would be more profitable, were it within my power and within the scope of this book, to consider at length the knowledge of the early Babylonians and Assyrians, inhabitants of the Mesopotamian plains and Persian foothills. For the Babylonians and the Assyrians, though they may have acquired their knowledge from other sources, must have built upon the foundations laid by the even earlier inhabitants of Syria, Iraq, and Persia. In turn they must have passed on this knowledge, augmented by their own discoveries, to the Medes and Persians, who were their conquerors at the beginning of historical times.

1 *Sháhnáma*, bk. I, p. 133.

The medical evolution of the Babylonians began about 6000 years ago, nearly 4000 years before Greek medicine emerged. The cardinal feature of their system was a polytheism. Certain gods caused illness as a punishment for sin: other gods cured disease as a reward for goodness. The action of the gods upon man was direct; the action of man upon the gods was indirect, the intervention of a priest being required. Like all other primitive peoples, it is probable that the early inhabitants of Iraq and Persia looked to the priests to save them both from sin and disease. But it is notable that the Babylonians, as compared with their contemporary Egyptians, were from a medical point of view in a more advanced stage. Their priests appear to have been less powerful, for they relied less on magic. They were more intellectual and without caste. It was even possible for a foreigner to enter the ranks of the priesthood. Moreover, the separation of spiritual and physical functions, that is between the priest and the doctor, had already appeared among these early Babylonians.

The conquest of the Babylonians by the Assyrians was a gradual process, not a sudden and violent invasion. It is roughly true to say that the Assyrian supremacy over Mesopotamia was complete from 1270 to 538 B.C. Such medical views as the Babylonians had either inherited or evolved became the inheritance of the Assyrians. They, too, believed that health and disease were the gifts of the gods. The three principal evil gods, who were responsible for disease, were the demon of phthisis, the demon of diseases of the liver, and the demon of abortion and infant death. Treatment was largely through prayer and incantation. Had it been entirely so, the Assyrians would deserve to be classed below the Babylonians in the evolutionary scale. But that their methods were by no means confined to spiritual activities and magic is proved by numerous clay tablets, by their use of surgical methods, and by the most important find of all, the Stele of Hammurabi.

A study of the prescriptions of these ancient Assyrians shows that for the most part their physicians chose drugs which were the rarest and most difficult to obtain. Frequently they were revolting and their material disgusting. The theory underlying this choice was that just as the patient was nauseated by the sight and smell of the cure, so the evil spirit, which was the cause of the disease, would be disgusted with what was offered to him and would quit the diseased part. The natural corollary was that the more serious the disease the more nauseating should the remedy be. From this sprang the doctrine that like cures like, an homœopathic theory which underlies all later Persian medicine.

A notable feature of the Code of Hammurabi is that there is here enshrined a code of ethics, which raised the standard of medical men to a very high level, first by fixing the remunerations which they are to receive at a substantial figure, and secondly by punishing them for transgressions due to ignorance. As such transgressions were mainly surgical errors, a by-product of this code was the virtual suppression of surgery. To this high standard the physicians of Persia succeeded and from this high standard they never fell.

Another feature of Assyrian medicine is the beginning of a public-health mentality, produced by a strict code of religious ceremonial laws. A woman after childbirth was considered unclean and she contaminated everything she touched. A similar impurity was attached to those who came in contact with corpses.

These ideas are reflected in the earliest Persian medical works which we know, the surviving books of Zoroaster, and it is clear that the Persians, even before they conquered the Assyrians in 538 B.C., had largely adopted the medical and sanitary ideas of their neighbours on the plains. The exact date of the birth of Zoroaster, or Zarathustra, is uncertain. His mother is said to have been an inhabitant of Ray. He himself was an Iranian, born most probably in the town of Urumiah, a city in the north-west corner of modern Persia. The dates of his birth and death are equally uncertain. Some place him as early as the eleventh century B.C.; more probably he lived about the seventh.

The *Avesta*, or Zoroastrian Bible, as it is known to-day, consists of the *Yasna*, the *Yashts*, the *Vendidad* and the *Bundahishn.*

This is only a fragment of the original scriptures, which are said to have consisted of twenty-one books or a million verses. These were revealed by God to Zoroaster and by Zoroaster to Gushtásp, king of Bactria, the patron of the Faith. Two archetype copies were deposited, one at Samarqand and one at Persepolis. Al-Ṭabarí claims that the original of all the scriptures was deposited at Persepolis, which was in consequence known as *Dizh-i-Nipisht* or 'The Stronghold of Records'. This latter version, and possibly also the version at Samarqand, was destroyed by Alexander the Great.

The underlying principle of such parts of these works as concern medicine is the belief in the war in nature and the law in nature. The war is described as a storm which is always raging. Indra is in battle with the serpent Azi, who has carried off the goddesses and kept them captive in the folds of the clouds. The two principles, the good principle and the bad principle, are continually in opposition. But fortunately for human beings for every disease which the genius of Evil is allowed to set upon the earth there exists also a remedy, which the genius of Good is ready to apply. 'Aryama conquers all sickness and death, just as the evil genii produce them. Rain from heaven produces plants and trees, whose properties are to cure disease and prevent death.' Such an idea finds an echo in the saying of the Prophet Muḥammad: 'Verily for every sickness upon earth which I have created, I have also created a remedy.'[1]

Later the serpent, the most powerful evil spirit created by Angra Mainyu, is said to be killed by Thraetona, who is therefore looked upon as the inventor of medicine. 'To him did Ahura Mazda (the supreme spirit of Good) give ten thousand healing plants.' In another verse he is regarded as one of the priests of Haoma, who was the source of life and death. All disease originated from the serpent Ahi. Thraetona was, therefore, doubly the patron of medicine, both as the killer of the serpent and as the priest of Haoma.

The belief in demoniacal possession as the cause of disease

1 *Ṭibb-ul-Nabbí*, p. 2.

survived into Sassanian times and consequently the most efficacious cure was the recital of sacred spells and invocations for supernatural help. It was therefore the duty of the supreme high priest of the country to direct and control the work of the members of the medical profession. Such possession might also be caused by the magic of an enemy or even by the Evil Eye. In such a case the patient would send for a priest, who would probably recite the verses dedicated to Asha Vahishta or to Aryama or to Haoma. At the same time he waved a white cloth over the patient from head to foot and from time to time called out the name of the demons whom he suspected, and tried to conjure them away. Asha Vahishta was the spiritual source of healing, the priest the earthly medium.

Even in the earliest times such a theory was felt not wholly to explain disease. It was well understood that physical and natural causes also played their part. Cold and heat, stench and dirt, hunger and thirst, anxiety and old age were all recognized as causes of natural disease. Intemperance and bad habits also contributed. The part that the blood played in the dissemination of disease through the body was recognized at any rate in Sassanian days, for the faithful were exhorted to preserve and augment the purity and vitality of the blood, which embellishes the body like an ornament. Infection by means of somites was also recognized as a cause of natural disease, for physicians were warned that they should not move carelessly from case to case lest they become the source of a new epidemic among a previously healthy people.

The natural functions of birth and death provide the greater part of the ceremonial laws of the *Avesta*. In the rules which forbid the producing of abortion theological and scientific views are at one. To destroy life is to destroy the highest form of the creation of Ahura Mazda and therefore the punishment for the procuring of abortion was the same as the punishment for wilful murder. It was fought against both by priests and physicians. Whether in the earliest stages of the pregnancy abortion was forbidden seems uncertain, for the *Avesta* lays down that a foetus receives a soul after four months and ten days of pregnancy. Professional abortionists were mainly women.

A miscarriage, however caused, rendered a woman impure and imposed upon her segregation of at least twenty paces from fire and water. To remedy her loss of health she was given draughts of *madhu*, a sweet, mild wine, which was also prescribed after a normal delivery. A case of miscarriage was also treated with *gomez* or cow's urine, both by the mouth and as a douche 'to wash over the grave in the womb'. The woman was given food but no water. If she had fever, she was allowed on the fourth day a little water, because 'the first thing for her is to have her life saved. Having been allowed by one of the holy men, she shall drink of the strength-giving water.' But the penalty was 400 strokes. If the lochial discharge had not ceased by the tenth day, 200 ants were sacrificed.

The abortefacient properties of certain drugs were well recognized and the severest penalties were enacted for those procuring a criminal abortion. Such drugs mentioned in the *Avesta* are *banga* (hempseed), *shaeta* (gold or possibly some yellow plant or liquid), *ghana* ('that which kills'), and *fraspata* ('that which expels the fruit so that it perishes'), none of which can be identified with certainty. In cases of abortion the man and the girl were equally guilty, as well as the woman who performs the operation or who provides the drugs. Sexual relations with a woman with an issue of blood were also strictly forbidden. 'Whosoever shall lie in sexual intercourse with a woman who has an issue of blood, either out of the ordinary course or at the usual period, does no better deed than if he should burn the corpse of his own son.' Equally forbidden was intercourse with a woman quick with child 'whether the milk has already come to her breasts or has not yet come'.

Equally elaborate were the rules which governed a case of menorrhagia or any vaginal discharge. From these rules it appears that water was of almost equal importance and sanctity as fire in the eyes of the early Iranians. It was said scoffingly that the magi once caused the overthrow of their king for having built bath-houses, because they cared more for the cleanness of water than for their own.

Complementary to the regulations which forbade abortion are the rules for the care of the pregnant who are left without a guardian. Even dogs came in for the same fosterly care. 'It lies with the Faithful to look in the same way after every pregnant female, either two-footed or four-footed, woman or bitch.' The *Avesta* is in fact the only oriental work which is highly complimentary to dogs. In Iranian ritual the presence of a dog was essential in certain ceremonies. Not only was the dog a sacred animal, but his gaze on a polluted object was thought to remove the demon of defilement. Hence in a case of sickness of a dog it was the duty of his master to provide for him the services of a veterinary surgeon and have him properly treated. The Faithful were to care for puppies for six months, just as they cared for children for seven years. For 'Atar, the son of Ahura Mazda, watches as well over a pregnant bitch as he does over a woman'.

Yet dogs could be a source of considerable harm to human beings. Rabies must have been one of the earliest diseases which forced itself upon the attention of mankind. Zoroaster fully realized the danger of infection. 'If there be a mad dog in the house of a worshipper of Ahura Mazda or one that bites without barking, what shall the worshippers of Mazda do? Ahura Mazda answered: They shall put a wooden collar around his neck and they shall tie him to a post....If they shall not do so and the mad dog smite a sheep or wound a man, the dog shall pay for it as for wilful murder.' For the first bite the dog was to lose an ear. At the fifth bite his tail was to be cut off. Whether ultimately he was to be killed is uncertain, and even the Pahlaví commentators could not make up their minds on this point.

It is in the realm of public health that Zoroastrian medicine reached its highest level. The laws which governed ceremonial purity are so blended with those that aim at preventing the spread of disease that it is impossible to separate them. Fire, earth, water, and vegetation were not to be defiled. It is unfortunate that fire was included among the four holy principles, for it was thus forbidden to utilize the great sterilizing power of heat. The greatest of all ceremonial contaminations was death. The touching of a dead body rendered a person unclean and required a major purification, known as the *Barashnum-i-Nu Shaba* or the 'Ablution of the Nine Nights'. Defilement began even before death. The lips of a dying man were washed with *gomez*. After death had occurred, *gomez* was poured over the whole body and it was washed by an assistant priest wearing a glove of fleece. Burial in the earth was forbidden. To bury the corpse of a man or a dog in the earth and to leave it there for six months could only be atoned by 1000 stripes. To leave a corpse in the earth for a year demanded 2000 stripes, to leave it there for two years or more was an inexpiable sin.

For the reception of dead bodies special towers were constructed, known as *dakhma* or 'Towers of Silence'. Here the body was deposited and secured to the roof by brass or stones so that no animal should carry away any particle and by thus defiling water or vegetation spread further disease. The construction of these towers was carefully regulated so that neither should the human body be desecrated nor fire nor water dishonoured. 'They are to be built of stones, mortar and earth, out of reach of dog, fox and wolf, and where rain water cannot stay.'

Putrefaction was a process which defiled air, earth and water, and was therefore triply accursed. Putrefying matter, mixed with water, spreads through the atmosphere and breeds infectious diseases. It was therefore the duty of a ruler to prevent by law such contamination. Dirt was to be removed from the poultry yard: cattle were to be stabled far from the house. The common house fly was execrated as the most injurious of all noxious creatures and was recognized as the source of contagion and death among the living.

To throw upon the ground the bones of a dead dog or man 'from which the grease or marrow flows' demanded a punishment depending upon the size of the bone. A bone the size of the top joint of the little finger called for a penalty of only 30 strokes. The maximum was reached if the whole body was thrown on to the ground. In this case the earth must be kept fallow for a whole year. The degree of defilement therefore depended partly upon the size of the offending article and partly upon the liquid or solid state of the object defiled. Sassanian writers on sanitation considerably enlarged the list of such defilable objects, both animate and inanimate, and carefully pointed out that some things, owing to their liquid or porous character, could never be properly cleansed.

Water was as easily contaminated as earth. To touch a corpse and then touch water before the ceremonial lustration was completed was a very serious crime. The Achaemenian kings always drank water from the river which flowed past the town of Susa and even when travelling would drink no other water. To insure its purity this water was boiled and stored in silver flagons and conveyed along the road for their use on four-wheeled waggons, drawn by mules. Although frequent washing of the body and of clothes was enjoined, special care had to be taken to keep the water clean. Quite how these two commands were to be reconciled, I am not quite sure. Even the accidental death of an animal was sufficient to cause serious defilement both of water and of its container. Professor Jackson in his book on Persia relates that his cook in Yezd was a Zoroastrian. He once purchased an earthenware jar to store his wine. In order to clean it he left it filled with water all night. A mouse accidentally fell into the jar and was drowned. At once the jar became unclean in the eyes of the cook, because it had been polluted by dead matter.

The carrying out of all medical and quasi-medical matters was in the hands of a special body of men. Conformably with Assyrian practice the divorce between medicine and theology continued. Physicians, however, were still drawn from the priestly class, the highest of the four Iranian classes, the others being the soldiers, the farmers, and the artisans. Occasionally persons from the agricultural class, if especially experienced in the medicinal qualities of herbs and plants, might rise superior to their birth and enter the ranks of the medical profession. This priestly class made a special study both of theology and medicine. After their course of study was completed, each man devoted himself primarily to medicine or to theology according to his personal taste. Those whose duties were mainly priestly were known as Magi, those whose duties were mainly therapeutic were called Athravans. The survival of this double training into the days of Islam is worth noting. Most of the great physicians in the days of the caliphs were also trained theologians and most theologians also were not ignorant of medicine.

Medical training must have taken place in many centres. The largest schools were probably those at Ray, Hamadan, and Persepolis. At these three cities there must also have been hospitals, for it was held to be the duty of rulers to found hospitals in important centres and to provide them with drugs and physicians. The training included a study of the theory of medicine and a practical apprenticeship, and continued for several years. Three kinds of practitioner issued from the schools, healers with holiness, healers with the law, and healers with the knife. The first were the most highly trained. 'If several healers present themselves, O Spitama Zarathustra, namely one who heals with the knife, one who heals with herbs, and one who heals with the holy word, it is this last one who will best drive away sickness from the body of the Faithful.'

The second of these three categories, those who heal with herbs, were the *Athravans* or Protectors of the Fire. Among them too there was a certain amount of specialization. Some were mere exorcists. Others applied themselves to the treatment of natural disease. Of these there were two classes. One, named *Durustpat* or 'Master of Health', aimed at removing the causes which gave rise to disease. The other, known as *Tan Beshazak* or 'Healer of the Body', treated disease after it had appeared. It was considered highly objectionable not to employ one of these three classes and to call in instead an uncertified physician. The priest-physicians were, in fact, the official physicians of the country; they alone were on the Register, so to speak; all others were quacks and charlatans. In addition to them the healers with the knife were also recognized as official practitioners, but they belonged to the fourth or artisan class, were subordinate to the priest-physicians, and were of no social standing. It would even seem that each surgeon was attached to a regular physician as his assistant or even servant.

Physicians being of the noblest families of the land, it was highly desirable that the prestige of the office should be untarnished by professional misconduct. To this end the sacred text enlarges upon the ideal to which all priest-physicians should aim. This ideal is admirably summed up by Maneckji Nusservanji Dhalla in his book on Zoroastrian civilization. The first indispensable qualification of a physician, he writes, was that he should have studied well the science of medicine. He should be a man who has read much, and remembers much, of medical subjects, who has great experience of his profession, who hears the case of his patient with calmness, who is painstaking in diagnosing the disease of his patient, who knows the various bodily organs and understands their functions, who treats his patient conscientiously, who is sweet-tongued, gentle, friendly, zealous of the honour of his profession, averse to protracting the disease for greed of money, and who is Godfearing. An ideal healer heals for the sake of healing; he is the best among healers. The second in rank in the profession is he who practises his art, actuated by the desire for reward and renown in this world. The third in point of honour works both for the sake of merit and for money, but gives preference to the first. The fourth in position of nobility in his profession is the physician who rates money higher than merit. The lowest in the scale is the greedy and heartless physician, who dishonours his noble profession. The duty of a conscientious physician is to watch carefully the effect of the medicine that he prescribes to his patient from day to day, to change and try a still better drug than the one he has already given, to visit the invalid daily at a fixed hour, to labour zealously to cure him, and to combat the disease of his patient, as if it were his own enemy.

The office of *Durustpat* or 'Master of Health' was no sinecure. The possibilities of contamination and of consequent disease were many. The *Durustpat* was therefore promised a reward in heaven in return for his labours on earth. All creation rejoices, says the *Vendidad*, in his work of arresting the spread of contagion. Seeing that this work carried great responsibilities, the fees were fixed correspondingly high. The lord of a province, who had incurred defilement, was compelled to pay to his cleanser a camel of high value. Lower grades of men, women, children and servants had to pay respectively a stallion, a bull, a cow or a lamb.

In addition to the purely religious methods of purification, there were embodied in the ceremonies methods and ideas which lie at the root of all antiseptic and prophylactic methods of to-day. The sun was recognized as the first great cleansing power, which in Iran is available on almost every day of the year for rich and poor alike. The light of the sun, says one of the *Yashts*, brings purification to the entire creation. For this reason it was forbidden to carry a corpse to the Tower of Silence during the hours of night. For the carrying of a corpse, when the sun's rays can no longer exert their influence, exposes the bearers and those who follow in the funeral procession to an unnecessary risk of infection. Similarly, the ossuary, in which the bones were collected after the carrion vultures had picked them clean, were so constructed that the rays of the sun could reach its interior. Garments, too, which have been polluted by blood or vomited matter, had to be exposed to the sun for three months if made of leather, for six months if made of cloth.

In certain cases actual destruction of the contaminated material seemed to the Iranians to be the only way to guarantee that it should not give rise to fresh disease. Thus, clothes which had been worn by a person suffering from an infectious disease were ordered to be utterly destroyed, and anyone privily selling such clothes committed a crime against the general health of mankind and was liable to heavy punishment. A certain portion of corn and fodder, which had been defiled, was to be discarded, and milk drawn from a cow that had eaten dead matter, and had thereby become unclean, was to be spilled upon the ground and never drunk. Similarly, the carcass of such a cow was not held to be fit for consumption.

In the majority of cases washing with *gomez*, or bull's urine, was considered the most satisfactory method of purification. The use of urine in this connection is not to be looked upon as a mere religious rite. It is true that the modern Parsee washes his body once a year with *gomez* for ceremonial purposes. In ancient times, and indeed in the present also, urine was looked upon as having a definitely antiseptic action. The urine of a boy, according to Ghiyáṣ-ul-Dín, a fifteenth-century writer, cures erysipelas, scabies, leprosy, and other skin complaints. Camel's urine is of value, he says, both internally and externally.[1] To this day, I believe, the Mohammedan tribesmen of the plateau soak their wool in *gomez* before weaving it into carpets.

According to the *Vendidad* washing in *gomez* is sufficient to disinfect the clothes of a person who has died of a non-contagious sickness, to cleanse garments which have been contaminated by vomitus, blood or matter of the dead, and to render suitable for use again the garments worn by a woman who has brought forth a still-born child. Vessels, too, provided they are not made of earth, wood or clay, can be similarly purified. The hair and bodies of corpse-bearers were also to be washed in *gomez* and water, and *gomez* plays a large part in the cleansing of all contacts with corpses.

The prevention of disease caused by the contamination of water produced another series of most minute rules. The purity of water was to be maintained by allowing no filth to be thrown into it and by not allowing it to be deprived of its natural purity. More than this, it was the duty of every man to remove from it any impurity that he might see in water, even though the impurity was caused by another. The *Vendidad* discusses in detail

1 Ghiyáṣ-ul-Dín, *Mirát-ul-Saḥḥat*, bk. II, ff. I, II.

the extent to which water is affected by contamination with dead matter. As long as a corpse lies in a river, pond or well, that water is unfit for any use whatsoever. To render a pond or well potable again it is necessary first to remove the corpse and then to remove up to half the total quantity of water. The remainder then becomes potable. The water of a running stream is unusable within an area bounded by three steps downstream, nine steps upstream, and six steps across the spot where the corpse lay before its removal. It is strange that the Iranians held that contamination travelled further upstream than downstream.

As for the *Tan Beshazak* or 'Healer of the Body', the sacred texts frequently refer to the existence of rules for testing the skill of candidates before they were allowed to begin to practise. What these rules were in the case of physicians, there is no means of judging. In the case of surgeons, they had to undergo a very severe trial before they were allowed to operate. 'If a worshipper of Mazda desire to practise the art of healing, on who shall he first prove his skill? On a worshipper of Mazda or on a worshipper of the Daevas? And Ahura Mazda answered: On worshippers of the Daevas. If he shall ever attend any worshipper of Mazda, if he shall ever treat with the knife any worshipper of Mazda and wound him with a knife, he shall pay for it the same penalty as is paid for wilful murder.' The same regulations require the young surgeon to perform his first three operations on non-Zoroastrians. If these are unsuccessful, he is disqualified from any further practice. But if they are successful, he can then practise also on the Faithful without fear of incurring any penalty if a case goes wrong. In this rule the Code of Zoroaster is so close to the Code of Hammurabi that it is clear that the Iranians modelled their medical rules and ethics upon those of the Assyrians. This rule also makes it clear that Zoroastrians were free to practise among non-Zoroastrians. But the converse is not true. The Faithful were bound to seek out and employ a physician of their own faith, if possible, and were only to consult a non-Iranian practitioner if unsuccessful.

The priest-physician on the conclusion of his training did not remain in the place where he was taught, nor did he even settle in his native town and try to build up a practice. Apparently it was the custom for all to travel from town to town and to treat any who applied for his services. The *Avesta* always speaks of 'wandering priest-physicians', never of physicians with a fixed abode. I think that the custom of practising as itinerant doctors must have continued among the Zoroastrians into Islamic times, when Islam was supreme and the faith of Zoroaster despised. This would account for the fact that such wandering physicians, whatever their faith and whatever their capabilities, were despised and looked upon as the dregs of the profession.

The equipment which these priest-physicians carried with them was not extensive. The most important article was a utensil for preparing *haoma*. This was a holy plant which had certain healing powers. It appears also in Hindu mythology, there being deified and given the name *soma* or 'Pressed Juice'. Probably it acted as an intoxicant and made the sick worshipper feel nearer to God. In the later days of Zoroastrian supremacy another preparation of *haoma*, white in colour, as opposed to the early yellow *haoma*, is mentioned in the religious literature of the period. This is to be used only on the Day of Judgement when it will give new life to corpses.

His next article of equipment was a small whip, which he used for offences against religious hygiene, for exorcizing, and for driving out the demons of disease. He also carried a rod or knife for the destruction of harmful insects or snakes. When officiating at religio-medical ceremonies he wore over his head a shawl or cloth, not so much to protect himself, as to guard fire and food from the contaminating effects of his breath. The cloth covered him from the bridge of his nose to well below the chin and was tied with strings at the back of the head. It must have been very similar to the face mask of a modern surgeon.

Although free from any irksome test before starting to practise the conduct of the priest-physician and the fee which he might exact were defined by law. His investigation of the patient was to be thorough and a definite diagnosis was always to precede treatment. He was to attend and make his physical examination within a few hours of being called to a case. If the 'harm' had occurred in the afternoon, he was to attend to the case before nightfall; if it had occurred in the evening, he was to deal with it that night; but if the patient fell sick during the night, he apparently need not attend until the following morning. He was saved the curse of modern practice—the night call.

Sometimes the physician received his fee when the case was finished. Often he demanded it before he started treatment. When Aspasia, the wife of Cyrus the Younger, had a tumour on her face, her father's physician refused to commence treatment before he had received his fee, saying that otherwise he could not buy the necessary drugs.[1] The *Dinkard* states that a good physician should be provided with an income that would enable him to live in a house situated in a prominent locality and furnished with the necessary furniture. Excessive charges, however, were forbidden, for corn and medicine were among the necessities of life and hence inflation of the price of either was a sin. He should have wholesome food, sufficient dress, and swift horses. At least one swift horse is indispensable for him, for without it he cannot visit his patients who live far from his home. Similarly, he should be well equipped with a sufficient quantity of drugs and surgical instruments.

The amount of the fee to be paid by each patient depended not upon the difficulty of the case or the status of the physician, but upon the status of the patient. The chief of a province was compelled to pay four oxen, the lord of a town one domestic animal of the first grade, a camel for example; whereas a householder satisfied his debt by an animal of less value. The cure of the son of a labourer demanded the same fee as the cure of the son of a lord. Another sign of this democratic spirit in ancient Iran is the fact that although a servant was placed in a lower category than

1 Aelian, *Var. Hist.* vol. XII, p. 1.

the master or mistress, the fee which a physician could demand from a slave was higher than that which he could demand for treating the child of the slave's master. Priests paid by giving only their blessing. The wife of one possessing a house gave an ass, the wife of a master of a village a mare, and the wife of a chief of a province a female camel. The patient, moreover, was expected to pay these fees without unnecessary delay.

The status of medicine, therefore, in primitive Persia, judging from such fragmentary knowledge as has survived, was more advanced than that of Assyria. It is not too bold to go even further and claim that the Persians taught the Greeks the elements of that system of medicine, which has been known ever since as Greek medicine. In 700 B.C. the Greeks showed no sign of culture, much less of science. Yet 200 years later so developed were their sciences that Hippocrates was able to write medical treatises that gained for him the title of Father of Medicine. It is hardly possible that the Greeks should have evolved for themselves the system which is now known as the Hippocratic system in those two centuries. Besides, the vocabulary of Hippocrates gives every evidence of being newly made. There are no signs of dialectic decay. Structures are called after every-day objects. Parts of the body are in many cases given a name of Indo-European origin. Other names are frankly Babylonian. Even the Greeks themselves recognized their humoral theory to be an exotic product and in the fashion of the time labelled it Persian. Though by this they only meant foreign.

Historians have turned to Egypt, Babylon, and Phoenicia to furnish a background for this sudden outburst of civilization in the fifth and sixth centuries. The claims of Crete have their supporters. But, even if these claims are granted, yet it was surely not from these countries alone that Cos and Cnidus drew their inspiration. The so-called Greek views had been taught long before on the banks of the Euphrates and even before that in India. The doctrine of the humours is taught in unmistakable terms in the holy books of the Hindus, which were composed prior to

2000 B.C. From India the theory seems to have spread to Persia, and the Persians, who seem in matters scientific always to be torch-bearers rather than torch-lighters, carried the doctrine on, modifying it and expanding it, no doubt, until it reached a nation that was able to express it in a dogmatic and concise form and to give it an independent existence.

If Iran may thus have shared in building up the humoral theory, she had an even greater share in the production of the theory of the microcosm, the basic theory from which the humoral is but an offshoot. According to this second theory man produces in miniature all the features of the universe. Now, there is a chapter in the *Bundahism*, a part of the Zoroastrian Bible, as I have already remarked, but of unknown date. One chapter is called 'On the Human Body: an Image of the World'. Each part of the human body is there likened to some part of the earth. 'The Back is the Sky, the Tissues are like the Soil, the Bones like the Mountains, the Veins like the Rivers, the Blood in the body like the Water in the oceans, the Liver like the Vegetation, the places where the Hair grows profusely like a Thicket, and the Marrow of the body is like liquid Metal within the earth.'

Among the *Corpus Hippocraticum* there is a book entitled *Peri Hebdomadon*, which is so closely akin to this Persian work that an independent formation of the same views by the Persians on the one side and by the Greeks on the other cannot be considered. Which is the original and which the plagiarism? The date of neither text is known with certainty. Plato knew the Greek version. The *Bundahism* in its present form is not pre-Islamic. But on philological grounds there is every reason to suppose that it is a later version of the Sassanian *Avestà*, which itself is a version of a much earlier work.

The Greek rendering of the phrase in the *Bundahism* that 'the marrow of the body is like liquid metal within the earth' makes it probable that the Persian version is the earlier. For the Hippocratic version of the same phrase reads 'the marrow is hot and damp', which is by no means a parallel to the preceding clauses.

Now the word 'damp' may have been rendered originally by the Greek word ὑγρόν, which also means liquid. The Middle Persian and Avestic word for 'metal' could easily be read as the word that means 'hot'. On the supposition that the Greeks borrowed from the Persians, misunderstood the text, and were put right by later copyists, it is easy to see how this divergence of phraseology occurred. No other theory is so simple.[1]

To the Iranians, then, can probably be given the credit of introducing to the world a philosophical concept upon which the Greek systems of anatomy, physiology, and pathology were ultimately based.

It is with the Achaemenian kings, a dynasty founded about 650 B.C., that Persian history, as opposed to legend, begins. Of this line the most famous were Cyrus the Great, the second of the line, and Darius, the ninth. Both these monarchs, in spite of the highly organized native system of medicine, chose their medical advisers outside their own country. 'His adviser was a physician', says Herodotus, 'whom Amasis, when Cyrus had requested that he would send him the most skilful of all the Egyptian eye doctors, singled out as the best from the whole number.' And again: 'Darius had at his court certain Egyptians whom he reckoned the best skilled physicians in all the world.'[2]

By the time that Darius died the Persian Empire had been extended to include within its frontiers three non-Persian civilizations, Egypt, India, and Thrace. The campaign of Cambyses in 525 B.C. added Egypt to the empire. The attempt to push the frontier further south led to his unsuccessful campaigns against Nubia and the Ammon oasis. Cambyses had from childhood suffered from epileptic fits and these two failures completely unhinged his mind and he committed suicide. A legend exists that he wounded himself in the thigh when mounting his horse, but the manner of his death is clearly stated by Darius in

1 Gotze, *Pers. Weisheit in griech. Gewande Zeits. f. Indol. u. Iran*, vol. II, pp. 60–98, 167–77. Leipzig.

2 Herodotus, *Hist.* bk. III, ch. I, 133.

the Behistun inscription. The death of Cambyses was followed by the attempt of a Magian usurper to gain the throne. His reign was very brief. He was soon recognized as an impostor and slain, and Darius ascended the throne. An organized massacre of the magi followed what was perhaps an attempt by the priestly caste to regain ascendancy. It was therefore with no very great love for the magi in his heart that Darius began to rule. The pro-Egyptian policy may thus be ascribed to a religious bias. Although he took the greatest interest in Egyptian medicine, there is no evidence that he made any attempt to foster the scientific studies of the Zoroastrian priest-physicians. He visited Egypt in person, he set to work to win over their priesthood to his side. He re-established the medical school at Sais, which had fallen into decay. And he replaced as far as possible all the books and appliances that it had formerly possessed.

The second distant triumph was the successful invasion of India. Of this campaign very little is known.

The third non-Persian civilization which submitted to the rule of Darius, was that of Scythia, Thrace and Macedonia. These were the fruits of the great expedition of 512 B.C. The ultimate importance of this campaign lies in the fact that it made the frontiers of Greece and Persia coterminous. It also introduced Greek medicine into Persia. For it chanced that Darius, as he leapt from his horse during the chase, sprained his foot. The sprain was of no common severity, for the ankle bone was forced quite out of the socket. The Egyptian physicians twisted the foot so clumsily and used such violence that they only made the mischief greater. For seven days and seven nights the king lay without sleep, so grievous was the pain that he suffered. On the eighth day of his indisposition one who had heard before leaving Sardis of the skill of Democedes, the Crotoniat, told Darius, who commanded that he should be brought with all speed into his presence. When, therefore, they found him among the slaves, quite uncared for by anyone, they brought him just as he was, clanking his fetters and all clothed in rags, before the king.

As soon as he entered into the presence, Darius asked him if he knew any medicine; to which he answered 'No'. For he feared that if he made himself known, he would lose all chance of ever again beholding Greece. Darius, however, perceiving that he had dealt deceitfully and really understood the art, bade those that brought him to the presence, go fetch the scourges and the pricking irons. Upon this Democedes made confession, but at the same time said that he had no thorough knowledge of medicine—he had but lived some time with a physician, and in this way had gained a slight smattering of the art. However, Darius put himself under his care, and Democedes by using the remedies customary among the Greeks and exchanging the violent treatment of the Egyptians for milder means, first enabled him to get some sleep, and then in a very little time restored him altogether, after he had quite lost hope of ever having the use of his foot again.

Democedes at once became the royal favourite. The eunuchs were bidden to conduct him through the female apartments and to proclaim to the women that this was the man who had saved the king's life. Each of the wives is said to have dipped with a saucer into a chest of gold and to have given such good measure to Democedes that the slave who followed him gathered up a great heap of gold which had been let fall from the saucers.

Democedes was now promoted to the post of physician to the king. He was given a palace as his residence and he ate daily at the king's table. The Egyptian physicians, whom he had replaced, were sentenced to be impaled, but he pleaded for them and their lives were spared. In spite of this privileged position, he longed for freedom; he desired above all to see again his native Crotona. This he accomplished by guile. It chanced that Atossa, a daughter of Cyrus and a wife of Darius, had a boil upon her breast. For a long time she hid it. When concealment became impossible, she sent for Democedes to cure her. This he promised to do on condition that she should persuade Darius to make an expedition against Greece and appoint Democedes to be one of the advance party to spy out the land. All went as planned. Democedes cured the boil, Darius decided upon the invasion, and the advance party was sent off. Democedes left all his wealth behind him, promising to return.

At Tarentum the king of the Tarentines in friendship for Democedes removed the rudders from the Persian ships and detained the crews as spies. In the meantime Democedes escaped to Crotona, which lay only 150 miles along the shore above Tarentum. The rudders were then restored to the Persians, who hastened to Crotona and found Democedes in the market place. They laid violent hands upon him with the intention of dragging him back to the ship. But the Crotoniats refused to give him up. They rough-handled the Persian envoys and even stripped them of their cloaks. The Persians were thankful to regain their ships, and with this report they returned to Darius.[1]

The broken faith of Democedes was an additional spur to the Persian king and the first invasion of Greece was launched. The defeat at Marathon must have been at the least a very regrettable check to the ambitions of Darius. Five years after the battle he died and Xerxes, his son by Atossa, ascended the throne. Had Democedes stayed at the court of Darius, the history of the world might have been very different. As the medical adviser of his mother, Xerxes must have known him very well.

In the fourth year of his reign Xerxes began the second invasion of Greece. Thermopylae held up the Persian forces for a short time. Treachery gave them the victory and the city of Athens fell into Persian hands. The battles of Salamis and Platea, however, cancelled the Persian victories and Xerxes retreated hurriedly to the coast of Asia Minor. Here he devoted himself to debauchery until he was murdered in 466 B.C. by the captain of his own bodyguard.

His successor was Artaxerxes I, known to history as Longimanus. At the beginning of his reign he continued to war against the Greeks, but though successful he failed to push home his

1 Herodotus, *Hist.* bk. III, ch. I, 133.

victories. His successors reversed this warlike policy and found that Persian gold was a more successful means of gaining their ends than Persian spears. The policy of Greece, too, became considerably less virtuous. Whereas in the olden days it was the habit of all the Greek states to unite against the Persians, their common enemy, it now became usual to seek his assistance to secure some domestic triumph. Sparta, Athens and Thebes all made treaties in turn with Persia to secure her aid in the overthrow of home rivals. Finally, even the Persian military spirit was sapped by their commerce with the Greeks. Corruption in high places and too much prosperity completed the work. Persian governors found it easier and more profitable to hire Greek mercenaries to fight their battles than to fight them for themselves. Thus, by the end of the century, when Cyrus the Younger disputed with his brother Artaxerxes II for the throne, his army consisted largely of Greeks, whose leaders were allowed to fill the highest commands both by land and sea. It is to one of these leaders, Xenophon, that we owe an account, though perhaps a not very trustworthy one, of how Cyrus was brought up.

The real ruler of Persia after the death of Artaxerxes I was Parysatis, his daughter. Married to her half-brother Ochus, she secured the murder of Soghdanus, her elder half-brother, and then of Roxana, her half-sister. She then secured the vice-royalty of Asia Minor for her favourite son, Cyrus, which gave him a virtually independent command, while she stayed at court to work for the overthrow of his brother Artaxerxes Mnemon, who had been declared king under the title of Artaxerxes II. During the ceremony of the coronation Cyrus attempted to murder him. Parysatis screened her son from his vengeance and secured permission for him to return to Asia Minor. Here he at once began to plot for the removal of his brother from the throne by force of arms.

Three years later the decisive battle was fought. Artaxerxes was accompanied on the field by the Greek physician who usually attended Parysatis, a tribute to the honesty of the physician. This was Ctesias, the son of Ktesiochus. He had been taken prisoner during the fighting between the Greeks and the Persians in 417 B.C. and, like Democedes and Appollonides, had been appointed a court physician. The battle was fought at Cunaxa, not far from Babylon. In the course of the fight Cyrus and Artaxerxes met face to face. Ctesias himself has left an account of this part of the battle. Artaxerxes got in the first blow, but his lance altogether missed his brother. Then Cyrus drove at Artaxerxes and pierced his breast-plate so that the king fell from his horse. His attendants, thinking him dead, abandoned him. Ctesias remained to assist him and finding him only concussed, helped him to make his way to a little hill near at hand where the two rested. In the meantime Cyrus had been unable to check his horse after the charge and was carried out of the fight and lost in the evening mist. His helmet fell from his head and he bore no other sign of his high rank. It was therefore mere chance that a young Persian struck him in the eye with an arrow as he passed. Swooning and senseless Cyrus fell from his horse. The eunuchs who accompanied him, tried in vain to remount him, but he could not sit in the saddle.

At this point again chance interfered, for some camp followers of Artaxerxes joined this little party by mistake, believing that they were their friends. As soon as they discovered their error, one of them, quite ignorant of whom he was attacking, smote Cyrus from behind and severed his popliteal artery. Cyrus again fell and this time bled to death.

His death left the Greeks without an objective. In spite of the efforts of Ctesias to persuade them to surrender, they decided to abandon the revolt and return to Greece. All that Ctesias could do was to persuade the victorious side to give better treatment to the captured Greek generals. The ten thousand Greek mercenaries under Clearchus and Xenophon made their famous retreat to the sea. The empire of Persia, much to its misfortune, continued under the influence of Parysatis and her eunuch advisers.

Ctesias remained at the court for another three years. He then returned to Cnidus and finally to Sparta. Though he wrote several books, most unfortunately none of his works is now complete. The largest surviving fragments are those of his *Persica.* This dealt with the history of Assyria and Media in the first six volumes and with Persia up to the date of his leaving the country in the remaining seventeen volumes. Even more unfortunately his *Commentarii Medici*, which would have been of the utmost interest to the historian of medicine, survives only in name and in a few quotations by other writers.

The failure of Cyrus the Younger to obtain the throne of Persia meant a temporary check to Greek influence there. His backing had been largely Greek and the hellenizing party was naturally suspect. Artaxerxes' efforts were now directed against the Spartans who had taken upon themselves to be the champions of Greece. By a wise distribution of bribes the Spartans were compelled to end prematurely their Asiatic campaign. It was remarked with bitter sarcasm that Artaxerxes had driven them out of Asia with 30,000 archers, for an archer was stamped upon the Persian coins. Conon, the Athenian admiral, was also quite willing to sell his services to the Persian cause. To convey his offer he suborned Zeno, a Cretan dancing master, and Polycritus, a Mendaean physician. His letter fell into the hands of Ctesias, who after interpolating a further request that he should himself be sent to work with Conon, passed it on to the king. Artaxerxes readily accepted the offer and with this added help utterly defeated the Spartans both by land and by sea. All the Greek cities in Asia Minor and all the islands adjacent thus became subject and tributaries to the Persian king.

The declining years of Artaxerxes were saddened by the rivalry of his sons. Worn out with fighting and pleasures he died at last at the age, it is said, of ninety-four. Of his hundred sons Ochus, the child of a Greek lady succeeded him under the title of Artaxerxes III. His murder in 338 B.C. made way for Darius Codomanus, who by no means the least illustrious of the

Achaemenian kings, had the misfortune to be ruling at the time when the greatest conqueror that the world has ever known set out to conquer the known world.

It was in 331 B.C. that Alexander, who had already subdued Greece, Egypt and Asia Minor, reached the Euphrates and by the battle of Arbela defeated the great king with such thoroughness that in the five centuries that lay between the Achaemenians and the rise of the Sassanian dynasty, historical facts are so meagre that Firdausi dismisses them in five pages and modern historians can scarcely fill a chapter.

Of the medical details of Alexander's life during his brief stay in Persia not much is known. He was accompanied on his expedition by his old friend and physician Philippus of Acarnania 'whose practice it was commonly to make use of desperate medicines'.[1] Once, when his exertions, or bathing when overheated, had brought on a fever and when Philip was about to administer a draught, he was warned that Darius had bribed the physician to poison him. Alexander, whose confidence in his friend was unshakable, handed Philip the letter to read while he drank off the medicine. Philip read it and merely remarked that he would recover provided he followed his advice.

Although he took with him in his army physicians from Greece, Egypt and Chaldea, Alexander appears to have completely neglected the native practitioners of Persia. He was wounded nine times in the final campaign which began with the battle of Granicus in 334 and ended with his death in 323 B.C. Besides these, he suffered from malaria and dysentery. The first four wounds he received before he crossed the Tigris, the remainder he received while fighting in the extreme eastern limit of his empire. The most serious of all these wounds, with the possible exception of a blow on the back of the head from a stone hurled by a catapult which may have fractured his skull, was a thrust from a barbed spear that he received in the Indian campaign. The spear pierced his clothes, close to the right nipple, and

1 Diodorus Siculus, XVI, 3.

the tip actually entered the chest cavity. He was treated by Critobulus of Cos. But all the skill of Greek surgery was unable to prevent the formation of a chronic fistula, leading from the chest wall down to the lung.

It was fortunate for Alexander that the spear was not previously treated with poison. In Persia the number of deaths in the Macedonian forces was comparatively small; in India the losses were enormous. This difference must be ascribed to the poisons which the Indians employed. Ptolemy, his general, in a fight near Harmatelia, was wounded by a spear dipped in serpent's venom and came near to death. Legend relates that Alexander saw in a dream a plant which was an antidote for these poisonous weapons. He roused himself, described the place and plant that he had seen, and had it gathered in time to save Ptolemy. It is not at all improbable that he did, in fact, know of some herb which was valuable for infected or even poisoned wounds. This knowledge he may have acquired from Indian doctors, who may well have known an antidote for viper's venom and may have passed on the knowledge to the king. The secret Alexander seems to have kept to himself and to have treated personally all cases of poisoning. According to Plutarch he had in his youth learnt the rudiments of medicine from Aristotle, but not content with the theory he was also in the habit of practising upon his friends to whom he was wont to prescribe a dietary and rules of hygiene.[1]

When his friend Hephaestion fell ill at Hamadan, it was again a Greek who undertook the treatment. What the illness was it is impossible to say. Hephaestion, a young man of thirty-two, was struck down with a fever and in seven days was dead. Alexander was overwhelmed with grief. He had the physician crucified; he had the sacred fire of the magi extinguished throughout the land; and he gave orders for sacrifices to be offered to Hephaestion as a god.

It is quite possible that the cause of the death of Hephaestion was one or both of the diseases from which Alexander himself

1 Plutarch, *Lives*: *Alexander*, bk. viii, 25.

suffered. A bathe in the river Cidnus early in the campaign gave him his first attack of malaria. During the retreat from India dysentery broke out among the troops and almost certainly Alexander became infected while in Beluchistan. It has been suggested that he was already infected with amoebic dysentery and that his flux in the autumn of 329 B.C. was a return of the trouble. Chronic malaria, chronic dysentery, and a chronic empyema proved too much for him. By the time he reached Babylon on his homeward journey his strength was gone. Here he received the alarming intelligence from the magicians that the omens were inauspicious for him for the liver of the sacrificial sheep possessed no gall bladder. He also unwittingly fulfilled the prophecy of the astrologer who had said that he would die when his throne was iron and his sky was gold. For, one day when tired out his nose began to bleed and a general who was near unlaced his own armour and spread it for Alexander to sit on. At the same time he held his golden shield over his head to protect him from the sun. Alexander recognized the situation and hurried home. His temperature rose; two days after this he died at sunset. This was 13 June 323 B.C. He was not yet 33 years old and had reigned 12½ years.

In Persia his life is supposed to have been saved by the perspicacity of Aristotle. He received from an Indian raja four gifts: a girl, a philosopher, a magic cup, and a physician. Of the physician Firdausi has written that he was:

> A youthful leech who diagnoseth
> Disease by making an uroscopy.
> So long as he is at the Court, the Shah
> Will never ail.[1]

The girl according to oriental tradition was a 'poison-maiden'. Aristotle in his old age wrote a series of letters to Alexander on the subject of the preservation of his health. These were collected into one volume and translated into Arabic by Abú Zakariyyá Yaḥya ibn al-Baṭríq. The Latin translation enjoyed an enormous

1 *Shâhnâma*, bk. xx, p. 8.

reputation in the Middle Ages. In these letters Aristotle warned Alexander to beware of deadly poisons. He bade him never accept medicine from a single doctor, but to employ many and only to act on their unanimous advice. He adds:

> Remember what happened when the king of India sent thee rich gifts, and among them that beautiful maiden whom they had fed on poison until she was of the nature of a snake. Had I not perceived it because of my fear, for I feared the clever men of those countries and their craft, and had I not found by proof that she would be killing thee by her embrace and by her perspiration, she would surely have killed thee.

It was the belief of many peoples that it was possible to feed a girl on poisons and thus make her so venomous that a kiss or act of sexual intercourse would prove fatal to her lover. Avicenna speaks of a girl who was so dosed with poison that the noxious insects which bit her were themselves poisoned.[1] Al-Jurjání states that it was the habit of potentates to get rid of their rivals by presenting them with a beautiful slave-girl whose diet had long consisted of poisonous herbs.[2] There is, too, al-Qazvíní's remark:

> Among the wonders of India may be mentioned the plant *al-bish*, which is found only in India, and which is a deadly poison. The Indian kings, we are told, when they want to conquer an enemy ruler, take a new-born girl and strew the plant first for some time under her cradle, then under her mattress, and then under her clothes. Finally they give it her to drink in her milk until the growing girl begins to eat it without hurt. This girl they send with presents to the king whom they wish to destroy. When he has intercourse with her, he dies.

Sir Thomas Browne is on the side of the modern pharmacologists, when he says: 'For my part, although the design were true, I should have doubted the success.' And adds: 'For the stork that eateth the snake and the stare (starling) that feedeth upon hemlock, these, though not commendable aliments, are not destructive poisons.' The whole subject is treated at great length

1 *Canon*, bk. IV, 6. I. I.

2 Al-Jurjání, *Thesaurus*, bk. ix, 2.

in the third appendix to *The Ocean of Story*, vol. II, by Mr N. M. Penzer.

Firdausi, no doubt voicing the tradition of his days, says that the death of Alexander was caused by a disease which he names *azar*, which would appear to be some sort of ulceration. Syriac versions of his life relate that he was poisoned by his Greek cup-bearer. Some have tried to reconcile these three statements, the poison, the ulceration, and the lady, and have claimed that he was the victim of syphilis. Apart from the fact that it would seem that syphilis was unknown in those parts and in those days, the earliness of his death and the clinical picture which other writers give make this diagnosis highly improbable.

Among the Persians Alexander has joined the demigods; he ranks with Solomon and Jamshid. Strange stories circulate among them about the origin of his name. They say that his mother was named Halai. When great with child, she became offensive to her husband on account of an unpleasant body odour. The doctors called in to remedy it prescribed baths of infusion of the Persian sandar tree. In consequence the child which was born was called Halai-Sandarus or al-Iskandar. The curious mistake of Muslim historians, who attributed the Quranic phrase *Zi-ul-Qarnayn* or 'Two-Horned One' to Alexander, whereas clearly Muḥammad must have been referring to Darius as king of Media and king of Persia, has lead to the belief, which has survived until to-day, that all the descendants of Alexander are horned. A friend of mine, a Persian nobleman, used to have a man-servant who claimed descent from Alexander and who could never be persuaded upon any pretext to remove the covering from his head. He claimed, and his fellow-servants believed him, that he had two immature horns just above where the hair started to grow over the forehead.

It is usual to consider that the invasion of Alexander did nothing but harm to Persia. He destroyed Achaemenian culture, laid waste the palaces of Persepolis, and reduced to ashes almost the whole of Zoroastrian literature. Yet such a summary is probably unjust, although the criticism is evidently well founded. In the first place it was due to Alexander the Great that Western civilization penetrated into central Asia. Even if much of the actual work was done by his successors, he blazed the trail. Without his first efforts, they could not have succeeded. He was trained from his youth up by Aristotle and from him must have imbibed an interest in natural science. It was his constant desire to introduce into the East the culture of Greece into which he had been so skilfully initiated. His making of Greek the official language of the empire was by no means the smallest aid which he gave to the spread of Greek scientific ideas. The magistrates now used Greek in their proclamations. This meant that the educated upper classes of orientals could read Greek manuscripts if they so desired. The Persian School of Medicine, which later developed at Jundí Shápúr and later still at Baghdad, was mainly built upon Greek foundations. I often wonder to what extent Alexander was in reality responsible for that great corpus of scientific knowledge which is the glory of Eastern Islam.

CHAPTER II

FROM THE DEATH OF ALEXANDER TO THE FOUNDATION OF ISLAM

WITH the death of Alexander another stage of Persian history came to an end and Persia entered into what may well be called the stagnation period. In the midst of this period, this lull, as it were, at least from the point of view of a medical historian, there was born at Bethlehem a baby at whose birth three Persian priest-physicians assisted. Christian and Zoroastrian tradition alike make the Three Wise Men to have come from Persia. The Bible gives them the official Zoroastrian title of Magus. The majority of the Fathers of the early Church agree in regarding Persia as their native country. Odoric says that Kashan was the city of the Three Kings. According to Marco Polo two of the 'kings' came from villages situated in the neighbourhood of the modern Teheran; the third came from a village about three days' journey away. To-day at Urumiah a church is still known where one, if not two, of the Wise Men are buried. The prominence given to this Persian influence in the Gospel story suggests that the Persians had already begun to play their role as the scientific teachers of the world and that the Jews had already begun to modify their medical views in the light of Persian teaching.

The medicine of the Gospels and the Acts shows three different beliefs as to the cause of disease. The most advanced is the belief that all disease comes direct from God as a punishment for sin. 'Behold, thou art made whole: sin no more, lest some worse thing happen to thee' (John v. 14). And again: 'Rabbi, who hath sinned, this man or his parents, that he should be born blind?' (John ix. 2). In the second place there is the view that disease is due to the indwelling of an evil spirit. 'There met Him a certain man, who had a devil now a very long time' (Luke viii. 27).

And: 'They brought to Him a dumb man possessed of the devil' (Matt. ix. 32). It is hardly possible to read into the many accounts of possession a description of lunacy and to hold that all the possessed of the New Testament were maniacs. That would constitute far too high a percentage of the small population of Palestine. It seems clear that one view of the pathology of disease in general was that the Evil Force of Nature had for the time being taken up his dwelling within the body of a human subject. As illustrating a third type of belief, many of the medical stories savour of pure magic. 'They brought forth the sick into the streets that, when Peter came, his shadow at least might overshadow many of them and they might be delivered from their infirmities' (Acts v. 15).

Now, these views are alien to the views of orthodox Jewry and the views of the Old Testament. The nearest approach is the description of the sufferings of Job. But even here there is no suggestion that he is being punished for his sins, none that he is possessed, and his treatment is certainly not magical. The sole instance of possession in the Old Testament is the case of Saul (I Kings xvi. 14). Magic, of course, there was throughout the land of Egypt and the adjacent countries. But the strict monotheistic and hygienic doctrines of Moses prevented the superstitions of the Jews from even approximating to those of their neighbours.

If these doctrines were not inherited from their forefathers, whence did they come? They certainly did not come from Greece or Rome. As regards Greek civilization the Homeric period, as well as the classical period, are strikingly empty of demoniacal manifestations. Similarly, in Rome before the advent of Christianity there is no trace of dualism. In Egypt, it is true, and in Syria possession was a well-known phenomenon. But in other respects Egyptian theories of disease differed radically from the views that were current in Palestine in those days. In Mesopotamia the resemblance is closer; for in that land all forms of sickness were regarded as the work of evil spirits. Still, in

Babylonian texts no proof has yet been found that possession was an accepted doctrine among that people. It was sickness, rather than possession, that was exorcized. But in Persia, dualism, magic and possession are all found. It would, of course, be idle to claim that the sole source of the medicine of the Talmud and the New Testament is Persia. But it would seem highly probable that Persian lore, modified by its passage through Mesopotamia and linked to superstitions brought up from Egypt, was the chief source of the views of sickness and death that prevailed in Palestine in the year in which Jesus Christ was born.

The debt of Judaism to Persia was soon repaid. Even in the first century A.D. Christian missionaries made frequent journeys to Persia, and Christianity was established as a flourishing faith throughout the south before the end of the second century. In the meantime the House of Seleucus, sprung from Iranian and Macedonian stock, the heirs of Alexander's empire in the east, had fallen before the nomadic tribes of Parthia. Of their achievements the most important was the part they played in securing the continuity of Greek tradition in Persia. The Seleucids were influenced by Greek opinion, continued to use the Greek tongue, and modelled their training and education upon Greek ideals. In consequence, Greek civilization was so alive in Persia that when about 150 B.C. Mithridates of Parthia suddenly invaded Media and forced the submission of Fars and Hyrcania, even the rude Parthians could not remain unaffected by Seleucid culture.

No dynasty in historical times has bestowed less upon posterity than did the Parthians. As for literature they possessed and produced none. In religion they were at first apparently without a creed. Then they began to worship Arsaces, the founder of their empire. Later they became persianized and adopted Iranian names and adored Zoroastrian angels. Assuming at the same time a veneer of Greek civilization, they termed themselves Philhellenics. They retained in their political offices the Seleucid officials and in their religious duties the Zoroastrian magi. Thanks to their adaptability and to their innate virility, of which success never deprived them, their empire remained unmoved even by the attacks of imperial Rome.

Their deadening hand was at last removed by a young soldier, named Ardeshir, a son of Papak, the vassal king of Persia. His birth was obscure. Scandal said that he was the illegitimate offspring of a tanner's wife and a common soldier; flattery said he was an impoverished descendant of the ancient kings of Persia. More certain is it that in the year A.D. 226 by his success in the battle of Hormuz he broke the power of Ardawan, the Parthian monarch, and freed Persia from the yoke under which she had groaned for nearly 400 years. In Balkh he was solemnly acknowledged as King of Kings and thus was founded a dynasty which ruled over a happy and contented people for over four centuries.[1]

One of his first actions was the reform of the Zoroastrian religion. Under the Parthians, it is true, Zoroastrianism had been the national faith. But it was polluted with a mixture of foreign idolatry. To suppress the idolaters, reunite the schismatics and confute the unbelievers Ardeshir summoned the magi from all parts of his new dominions. It is said that 80,000 obeyed the summons. One of these, says Gibbon, named Arda-viraf, a young but holy prelate, received from the hands of his brethren three cups of soperiferous wine. He drank them off and instantly fell into a long and profound sleep. As soon as he waked, he related to the king and to the believing multitudes his journey to heaven and his intimate conferences with the Deity. Every doubt was silenced by this supernatural evidence; and the articles of the faith of Zoroaster were fixed with equal authority and precision.

From now on the administration of Ardeshir was largely directed by the counsels of the Zoroastrian priesthood whose dignity, either from policy or devotion, he restored to its ancient splendour. It was presumably by their counsels that persecution broke out in the land. All worship, except that of the Zoroastrian faith, was forbidden. The temples of the Parthians were thrown down: the sword of Aristotle (as the polytheism and philosophy

1 Gibbon, *Decline and Fall*, pp. 78 et seqq.

of the Greeks was called) was broken: and before long even the Jews and Christians felt the hand of oppression hard upon them.

At the height of his power the kingdom of Ardeshir was bounded by the Euphrates, the Tigris, the Araxes, the Oxus, the Indus, the Caspian Sea and the Persian Gulf. If the empire of the Sassanids is compared with that of the Safavids, the political influence of the magi with that of the mujtahids, the advantage is all for the Sassanids. The number of cities, villages and inhabitants, even allowing for ancient and oriental exaggeration, was not less. Their culture was purer: their genius more marked. It is noteworthy that during the past few years the modern Persian is aiming at a return to the spirit and culture of the Sassanian kings. The times of Sh̲ápúr and Núsh̲írván, no longer that of Sh̲áh 'Abbás, are looked upon as the most glorious period of Persian history.

Within a few years of his assumption of royal power Ardeshir felt himself strong enough to attack the imperial forces of Rome. A haughty embassy, which claimed the whole of Asia as part of the Persian Empire by right, a right which had been suspended but not destroyed since the time of Alexander, was rejected by Severus and war immediately followed. But the result was indecisive and Ardeshir bequeathed his new empire and his ambitions to his successor.

Sh̲ápúr inaugurated his reign by the treacherous murder of Chosroes, king of Armenia. Rome was unable to support with arms the claim of the infant heir Tiridates and Sh̲ápúr, holding this to be a sign of Roman weakness, attacked the garrisons of Carrhae and Nisibis and spread devastation and terror on both sides of the Euphrates. Valerian, who had now succeeded to the imperial throne, set out in person to avenge the insult and crossing the Euphrates encountered Sh̲ápúr near the walls of Edessa. He was defeated and taken prisoner. Europe was humiliated with the spectacle of an aged emperor a prisoner in an Asiatic court and of a puppet emperor, a fugitive of Antioch, stained with every vice, ruling at the will of the Persian monarch.

The treatment of Valerian is well known. It is said that he was constantly exposed to the jeering crowds. Whenever Shápúr rode abroad on horseback, he mounted by means of a foot placed on the neck of the Roman emperor. After his death in captivity his skin was stuffed with straw and formed into the likeness of a human figure and stored in one of the better-known temples of the land. To this day he can be seen, carved in stone, outside Persepolis in an attitude of respect before Shápúr.

Following this crushing defeat of the Romans Iran had peace. Shápúr now set his hand to a very different task. The Avestan language, the original tongue which Zoroaster and the people of his times wrote and spoke, was the language of Iran until the empire of the Medes and Persians replaced it with Pahlevi. The survival of the Avestan text-books of religion was due to the survival of Zoroastrianism through the dark times of the Alexandrine conquest and the blank years that followed. Avestan works on secular subjects, such as medicine, astronomy, geography, and the arts, had for the most part found their way in a scattered condition to India, Greece and other countries. The recollection of these works was now ordered by Shápúr.

Apparently at Rev-Ardeshir, a district in Susiana, there was founded in these times a body of scribes whose duty it was to write down in a special language, possibly a secret code, known as *Gashtagh*, all matters relative to astrology and the secret sciences. These scribes were known as *Gashtagh-Daftaran* or 'Those who keep the Registers in Gashtagh'.[1]

It is clear that medicine formed a very important section of these writings. How large it was and how advanced was their knowledge and to what extent their teaching was coloured by Greek thought, it is impossible to say. For once again the land was overrun by a foreign invader and Zoroastrianism had to submit to the sword of a conquering faith. The Arab, who appeared as the next invader, was not the vandal which the Macedonian

1 Yáqút *Mu'jam-ul-Buldán*, p. 887 of text, p. 271 of translation, quoted in Christensen, *L'Iran sous les Sassanides* (Copenhagen, 1936), p. 413.

had proved. It was left for a later generation to produce a century and a half after the Arab conquest one who would again ruthlessly destroy as much as possible of the indigenous Iranian culture. In the year A.D. 820 there was appointed governor of Khorasan one Ṭáhir, who besides being the founder of the Ṭáhirid dynasty, was also a bigoted tyrant and opponent of Zoroastrianism. A subject with somewhat broader views attempted to reform him and laid before him a copy of the *Andarz-i-Buzurgmihr* or 'Good Counsels of Perzoes'. Perzoes was a prime minister of Núshírván and a Zoroastrian. Ṭáhir was astonished and asked if indeed books of the infidels still survived. When he learnt that they did, he gave orders that every Zoroastrian should bring to him a *maund*, that is about fifteen pounds, of his books that they might be burned, concluding the edict by adding that any one who disobeyed should suffer death.[1]

Thus a second time the scriptures were nearly lost and with them the scanty remains of Iranian science. Fortunately, local governors are not so thorough as world conquerors and many of the writings survived. It is from these few remnants that it is possible to form an estimate of the indigenous medicine of Persia from the earliest times until its replacement by the Graeco-Arab system. Any estimate based upon surviving works represents, of course, the minimum. How much more Zoroaster taught and how later generations of Medes, Persians, Parthians, and Sassanians improved upon it, must remain a matter for speculation until new manuscripts are discovered.

Sh͟ápúr died in A.D. 271 after a successful reign of 30 years. In 283 Varahran or Bahrám III being then on the throne of Persia, the emperor Carus determined to revenge Valerian. The story goes that the Persians, who disbelieved any longer in the might of Rome, became frightened when they found that the approach of the Roman legionaries was now undeniable. An embassy was sent, which entered the Roman camp at sunset about the time of the evening meal. The Persians expressed a desire to be intro-

1 Browne, *Literary History of Persia*, vol. 1, p. 346.

duced at once into the presence of the emperor. They were conducted to a soldier who was seated on the grass eating a piece of stale bacon and a few hard peas. A coarse woollen garment of purple alone showed his dignity. The conference was conducted with the same disregard of courtly elegance. Carus, taking off his cap which he wore to conceal his baldness, assured the ambassadors that, unless their master acknowledged the superiority of Rome, he would speedily render Persia as naked of trees as his own head was destitute of hair. His threats were not in vain. He soon made himself master of Seleucia and Ctesiphon, but a sudden death prevented him from making any headway into the highlands.

In A.D. 335 Shápúr II, then ruler of Persia, renewed the struggle. He was then aged thirty, having already been crowned king nearly 31 years. The story is a strange one. The wife of Hormisdas II, then emperor, was pregnant at the time of her husband's death. His son Hormisdas, the natural heir to the throne, was set aside on account of his inclination towards Hellenic culture. The hopes and ambitions of the nobles were centred upon the unborn, second child. Gibbon's description is most dramatic.

> The apprehensions of civil war were at length removed by the positive assurance of the Magi that the widow of Hormuzz had conceived and would safely produce a son. Obedient to the voice of superstition the Persians performed without delay the ceremony of his coronation. A royal bed, on which the queen lay in state, was exhibited in the midst of the palace; the diadem was placed on the spot which might be supposed to conceal the future heir of Artaxerxes, and the prostrate satraps adored the majesty of their invisible and insensible sovereign.

The cession of the five provinces to Rome, which the Emperor Carus had forced on the defeated Bahrám, acted as a constant spur to young Shápúr when he reached years of understanding; the death of Constantine removed the last obstacle. Constantius, his successor, hastened to the banks of the Euphrates to resist invasion. For the most part the Persians were successful, although in the battle of Singara in A.D. 348 the son of Shápúr, the heir to the throne, was taken captive and after being scourged and tortured was publicly executed by the Romans. In spite of all his endeavours Sh͟ápúr failed to push the frontiers of his empire westward of the Tigris. All vigorous fighting came to an end when the protagonists were recalled to defend the opposite ends of their empires—the Roman to protect the Danube, the Persian the Oxus. In 359 Sh͟ápúr returned to the western front and invaded Mesopotamia, but the prolonged, even though successful, siege of Amida, the modern Diarbekr, wasted so much of the favourable season and of the flower of the Persian troops that Sh͟ápúr was forced to retire with no very decisive success to his credit.

In A.D. 361 Julian, known to posterity as the Apostate, succeeded Constantius and in him Persia found a much more serious rival. He was young, hardy and eager. He remarked that Crassus and Anthony had both felt Persian arrows and that the Romans in 300 years of war had not yet subdued a single province of Mesopotamia or Assyria. He despised the triumphs of a Gothic or Danubian victory. Nothing would please except to meet and defeat the successor of Cyrus and Artaxerxes. Sh͟ápúr II was still on the throne when in the spring of 363 Julian set out from Antioch to cross the great Syrian desert. On 7 April he entered Persian territory and after presenting each soldier with 130 pieces of silver he cut away the bridge over the river Khabur as a sign to them that there must now be no retreat. In May Perishapur, a town only 50 miles distant from the royal residence of Ctesiphon, fell.

Ctesiphon, of which the enormous ruined arch still stands to-day, was in the days of Julian a great and populous city. It lay some 20 miles to the south of Baghdad (which it must be remembered was then only a tiny village), on the eastern bank of the Tigris near its junction with the Euphrates. On the western bank was the city of Seleucia which had been the capital of the Macedonian conquests in Upper Asia. For many years after the fall of the Macedonian Empire Seleucia retained the genuine characteristics of a Grecian colony and no doubt carried on the traditions of Greek learning and formed a continuous source of

Greek scientific practise. The Parthian kings were wont to pitch their tents in the plain between Seleucia and Ctesiphon and, swelled by the followers and hangers-on of the court, the little village of Ctesiphon had developed into a large city. The Roman invasion under Marcus in A.D. 165 proved fatal for Seleucia, whereas Ctesiphon recovered and succeeded Babylon and Seleucia as one of the great capitals of the East. In summer the Sassanid monarchs enjoyed at Ecbatana, the modern Hamadan, the cool breezes of the hills: in the winter the balmy air of the desert made Ctesiphon an ideal residence. It was here that a certain blood-letter used to sit whose name has become proverbial. Al-Qazvíní says that there was once a phlebotomist of Sabas, a village near Ctesiphon. As his practice in his own village was a small one, he used also to attend upon the soldiery of the numerous expeditions into Persia and would doctor them on credit, expecting to be paid on their return. To keep his hand in in-between times he used to scarify his mother. Apparently even so his practice was very small, for his name passed into the proverbs of the Arabs, who used to say: 'More workless even than the surgeon of Sabas'.

It was against Ctesiphon that Julian now directed his attack. The story of the siege is well known. The Roman fleet passed from the Euphrates into an artificial channel and joined the Tigris above the city. The passage of the infantry across was more difficult. The stream was broad and rapid: the ascent steep and difficult: and the banks were securely held. The crossing was effected by night. The first ships to reach the eastern bank were captured and burnt by the Persian sentries. But Julian, seeing the flames, called out to the waiting troops that their fellows were already masters of the bank for the lights were the signal that had been agreed upon. The rest of the army crossed in safety and on the following day utterly routed the Persians, pursuing them to the very gates of Ctesiphon.

Shápúr was in despair. He ate off the ground: he let his hair remain in disorder. But what he could not accomplish in the open field, he effected by treachery. One calling himself a Persian deserter came secretly to Julian and offered to guide him to the summer capital. Mindful of the successes of Alexander, Julian listened and advanced eastwards. The Persian deserter abandoned him: food began to run short. Even now had Julian known the roads, he might have reached Ecbatana or Susa. But wandering unguided and hungry, he decided that it was better to return. Fighting a rearguard action he was himself wounded and soon died, being then only thirty-two and having reigned only 20 months. His successor Jovian gave orders to continue the retreat and, even though he succeeded in recrossing the Tigris, he preferred to make terms with the Persians than to continue the fight. The five ceded provinces and several important towns were restored to Shápúr. This ignominious peace, remarks Gibbon, has justly been considered as a memorable era in the decline and fall of the Roman Empire. Shápúr continued his triumphs, invading and adding Armenia to his empire. But he was now growing old. Peace and moderation began to become for him more pleasant than campaigning and hardship. His death in A.D. 380, at the age of seventy, transformed in a moment the court and councils of Persia. In the first year of the new king an embassy was sent to Constantinople to offer excuses for the unjustifiable measures of the former reign and to offer, as a tribute of friendship or even of respect, a splendid present of gems, silk, and Indian elephants.

For nearly a century there was peace between Rome and Persia when commerce flowed freely and when the art and knowledge of medicine could again develop along normal lines. But besides invasion, commerce and individual adventures there was yet another source through which Greek culture flowed into Persia. This should be considered, perhaps, the main channel and the ultimate reason why to Persia must be given the praise and glory of having transmitted the learning of classical Greece to Europe. I refer to the Nestorians. The Nestorians, now known only as a small sect of Christians which has survived in southern India, were in origin a Semitic or Aramean race. Very early in the history of the world they migrated northwards from out of the Arabian peninsular into Syria and then into Mesopotamia. There for a while they rested. Conquered by Alexander they remained Greek in thought and culture, when the people around had become frankly Asiatic once more.

On the fall of the Seleucid Empire, the area which these Arameans inhabited split up into a number of petty kingdoms. Among them was one which contained the town of Edessa (to use the Latin name), a town founded by Seleucus Nicator in 304 B.C. According to legend Edessa embraced Christianity in A.D. 32. Even if a later date is to be ascribed to its conversion, it was certainly the first town of Mesopotamia to give up paganism. The new faith brought also material success. Situated, as the town was, between Persia and Rome on the east and west, between Greece and Egypt to the north and south, and lying on the main caravan route between China and Europe, its wealth and importance were bound to increase. An astonishing missionary zeal lead its divines to attempt to translate the Christian Scriptures into their own tongue. The existence of two versions of the Old Testament, one in Hebrew and one in Greek, and the Greek writings of the New Testament compelled them to study Greek. In this way, though only as a by-product, they came into touch with Greek scientific writings.

Edessa was at this time no longer independent, but lay within the extreme eastern frontier of the Roman Empire. The defeat of Jovian and his ignominious treaty with Sh͟ápúr II gave Nisibis, a town not very far away, over to Persian suzerainty. Edessa remained within Roman jurisdiction. The result of this treaty was an immediate flight of many of the most learned and richest citizens of Nisibis to Edessa, and the consequent founding in that city of the so-called Persian School of Edessa. In this university the leading faculty was that of theology with medicine as the second. The professors of Edessa, long familiar with Greek and in possession of many manuscripts philosophical, theological, and medical, must have taught a pure Hippocratic and Galenic medicine. Their religious enthusiasm led them to exclude all Babylonian and pagan practises. Probably, therefore, the Persian School of Edessa of the fourth century after Christ was carrying on the Greek traditions of medicine unmodified and without a rival in the world.

A few years before the foundation of this school the General Council of Nicaea had defined the Catholic view of the Trinity and had hoped to put an end for ever to the heretical views of Arius and his followers. A few years after the foundation of the school Nestorius, Patriarch of Constantinople, was deposed from his see for heresy about the Trinity and he and his followers were excommunicated. Most unfortunately the citizens of Edessa threw in their lot with the deposed patriarch, so that from now it is correct to call them Nestorians. The university became the headquarters of the new sect; its theologians became the protagonists of heresy. Papal excommunication cut them off from the rest of the Church. To silence them the Emperor Zeno in A.D. 489 ordered the university to close its gates and teaching in every subject to cease.

The decree was obeyed. The university closed and the great centre of learning abruptly ceased to be. The theologians returned to Nisibis: the medicals for the most part went into a voluntary exile at Jundí Sh͟ápúr, a town well within the Persian frontiers, a town which had been the seat of a Nestorian bishop for several years, and a town which already contained a university. The Persian emperor was well disposed towards the refugees. Any one discontented with Roman rule would naturally receive protection within his frontiers. More especially was Shah Kai Kubád inclined to welcome the students of Edessa because years ago it was the Nestorians who had helped him to escape to the White Huns and to regain his throne.

Jundí Sh͟ápúr was a very different town from Edessa. For whereas Edessa was exclusively Greek, Jundí Sh͟ápúr was markedly cosmopolitan in its tastes. The town itself had a very ancient foundation. A Persian writer states that it was built in the prehistoric days of the Aryan inhabitants, who called it Genta Shapirta, which means 'The Beautiful Garden'. It was refounded by Shápúr I soon after the defeat and capture of the Roman emperor Valerian and after the sack of Antioch. At first it was peopled, according to Firdausi, by Roman and Greek captives.[1] After his marriage with a daughter of Aurelian Shápúr attempted to Romanize the city yet more. Here for the first time in Persia the Hippocratic system of medicine was publicly taught by the Greek physicians who accompanied Caesar's daughter.[2] Shápúr renamed the city Veh-az-Andev-i-Shápúr, a Pahlevi phrase meaning 'Shápúr's Better than Antioch'. The old name and the new name were somewhat similar and the older form remained. The city became known as Gondi Sapor or in the Arabic form Jundí Shápúr.

Under the royal patronage it became the chief city of the district. It was an important centre in the manufacture of perfumery and later of the weaving industry and contained a royal factory. Here was executed Máni, the founder of the heretical sect of the Manichees. Máni was received by Shápúr at first with favour, but was afterwards banished. He returned to Persia in the reign of Urmuzd or Hormisdas, the successor to Shápúr, but in the reign of Bahrám Sháh, who followed, he was sentenced to be flayed alive. Firdausi thus refers to his death:

> This worshipper of pictures is unfit
> To live, so, since he causeth turmoil here,
> Flay him from head to foot, and let his skin
> Be stuffed with hay, and then, that no one else
> May make pretence to like dignities,
> Hang up the skin upon the city-gate
> Or on the wall outside the Hospital.[3]

The gate where the stuffed body was exposed was known thereafter as the Máni Gate.

1 *Sháhnáma*, bk. vi, p. 298.

2 *Hist. Dynst.*, vol. VII, p. 82.

3 *Sháhnáma*, bk. vi, p. 359.

Shápúr II on his accession further enlarged the city and to him is ascribed the founding of the university. The university was probably controlled by the Nestorian church authorities, for medicals as well as divines were compelled to attend a daily service before they settled down each to his own special studies. Native teachers were supplemented by Greeks. The chief of these Greek physicians was Theodosius or Theodorus.[1] So greatly did Shápúr respect him that he caused a church to be built specially for him. His *System of Medicine* is mentioned by the Fihrist as one of the few Persian books on medicine to be translated into Arabic in Islamic times.

The teaching of the university was probably not in the Greek language. The strong ecclesiastical element assured to Syriac the first place. Persian, Arabic and a jargon of their own were also current. Nor probably was the system of medicine taught purely Greek. The political history of the country suggests that medicine was largely dependent upon the predominating political power. The rise of Zoroastrianism under the Sassanids must have brought forward again the doctrine of Dualism which found no place in Hellenistic philosophy. This may well have caused an equal set-back to Greek medicine. In any case the cosmopolitan atmosphere of the place must have assured to other systems a place of almost equal honour.

According to al-Qifṭí the university did in fact develop an eclectic method of its own.

> They made rapid progress [he wrote] in the science, developing new methods in the treatment of disease along pharmacological lines so that their therapy was judged superior to that of the Greeks and the Hindus. Furthermore these physicians adopted the scientific methods of other peoples and modified them by their own discoveries. They elaborated medical laws and recorded the work that they had done.[2]

The arrival of the refugees from Edessa considerably strengthened the Greek influence in the school. This was made still stronger by the reception of the exiles from Athens, when the

1 *I.A.U.* vol. I, p. 308.

2 Al-Qifṭí, p. 133.

school of the Neo-Platonists was closed in A.D. 529. The fame of Núshírván and his university had already excited the Seven Greek Sages to visit a sovereign who, they heard, was putting into practice the ideals of Plato's *Republic*. Their experience of the Persian court did not bear out the high hopes which they had formed and they returned to Athens disappointed. But it is notable that in the treaty of peace made with the Roman authorities Núshírván required that the Seven Sages should be exempted from the penal laws which Justinian had enacted against his pagan subjects.

The medical school was at the height of its glory when the Arab invasion of Persia occurred. Jundí Shápúr surrendered to the Moslem general in A.D. 636 and was left undisturbed. It remained the greatest centre of medical teaching throughout the Islamic world until the growth of the caliphs' capital at Baghdad drained it of its best teachers. Decay then set in. Thanks to its commercial importance the town continued to exist for many years after the university had closed its doors upon its last pupil. A witness in the trial of the *wazír* Ibn ul-Firát was a man of Jundí Shápúr. A little later Ibn Hauqal, a native of Baghdad, writing in the year A.D. 976, says that Jundí Shápúr was in his day a fortified city, abounding in all the necessaries of life, with extensive date plantations and wheat fields, Ya'qúb ibn ul-Lays, the Khárijite general, chose it for his residence on account of its ample resources.[1] Here he died, after having conquered all Khorasan and Fars and when about to attack Baghdad. 'He died of a colic. The doctor told him there was no remedy for it but an enema. This he refused to take and preferred dying. His malady which was a colic accompanied with hiccough, lasted sixteen days.'

The encyclopaedist Yáqút, who died in A.D. 1228, says that he passed the site of the town many times, but that in his day there was no trace of its former grandeur. Yet, as late as A.D. 1340, a town still existed there, for al-Qazvíní says that it was of a medium size and produced much sugar cane.[2] To-day only the ruins, now

1 Ibn Khallikán, vol. IV, p. 321.

2 *Nuzhat-ul-Qulúb*, p. 109.

called Shahabad, which lie eight miles north-west of Shustar, mark the site of the cradle of Persian medicine.

The last official act of the school, that I have discovered, is the publication of a pharmacopoeia by Sábúr bin Sahl in A.D. 869, which was adopted throughout the eastern caliphate and which is probably the first official pharmacopoeia ever to be issued.[1] Al-Jurjání, writing about 1125, speaks of prescriptions which 'used to be employed in the Hospital at Jundí Sh̲ápúr'.[2] Nevertheless, the traditions of the school endured. Al-Anṣárí in his *Ik̲h̲tiyárát-i-Badí'í* repeatedly refers to formulae which he ascribes to al-K̲h̲úzí. In this I see not the name of a man, but the district of Khuzistan, that is, Jundí Sh̲ápúr. In the various Christian terms applied to many of the elaborate pharmacological preparations of later days, such as the Messianic Electuary and the Bishops Electuary, I am inclined to believe that we have a survival of the time when Persian medical education was in the hands of Christian teachers.

From the point of view of medicine the greatest of the Sassanian kings is Núsh̲írván or Anusharwan the Just, also called Chosroes the Great by Western writers and Kisra by the Arabs. He was the third and favourite son of Kai Kubád, an unfortunate sovereign who had been an exile among the enemies of Persia, who had recovered his liberty by prostituting the honour of his wife, and who regained his kingdom by the dangerous and mercenary aid of the barbarians who had slain his father. His eldest brother had already assumed the insignia of royalty, but received only small support. The second was blind in one eye and was therefore ineligible to reign. The third thus entered into his disputed patrimony. To make his position secure he murdered all his brothers and their male offspring. At one time there was just a chance that Núsh̲írván would be adopted by Justinian. But discussions over the method of adoption caused the proposal to be dropped and Kai Kubád felt that he had been personally insulted.

It was in the year A.D. 531 that Núsh̲írván began his long reign,

1 *I.A.U.* vol. I, p. 161.

2 Al-Jurjání, *Thesaurus*, bk. x, 2. 6.

which continued for 47 or 48 years. At once he felt his inability to continue the long war with Rome and in A.D. 533 he made a treaty of peace. Perhaps, too, he was actuated by a more friendly feeling towards the Roman people, for his father had been treated with marked success in a series of illnesses by a Byzantine physician, named Stephen of Edessa. He himself, too, in his youth had been tutored by this same Stephen; and he had chosen as his own physician another Roman named Tribunus. Later in the reign Tribunus returned to Greece, and Núshírván, when negotiating a five-years' truce with Rome, stipulated that Tribunus was to return to his service. Tribunus therefore embarked upon a second term of service in the Persian court. So pleased was Núshírván that at the end of his first year of service he offered to present him with whatever he desired. Instead of asking for money or honours Tribunus asked for the release of 3000 Romans who were held prisoners in Persia.

The government of Núshírván was firm, rigorous and impartial. He enriched the city of Jundí Shápúr and enlarged, if indeed he did not found, the school of medicine there. Astrology was encouraged. By his orders a gigantic work in thirty volumes on poisons was composed, which survived into Islamic times, but which has now disappeared. Though traces of persecution in favour of the magi are to be found during his reign, he allowed himself freely to compare the tenets of the various sects. In such matters he was largely influenced by the philosophical teaching of a Syriac physician named Uranios. In his reign arose the arch-heretic Mazdak, who asserted the community of women and the equality of mankind. Bazanes, his physician and a Christian bishop, was good enough to assist in the murder of the social reformer, and in the following reign the lands and women, which Mazdak had usurped, were restored to their original owners.[1]

His reign was notable for its translations. The most celebrated writers of Greece and India were translated into Persian, notably

1 Niẓám-ul-Mulk, *Siyásatnáma* (Schefer's edition), pp. 161 et seqq. of text; pp. 245 et seqq. of translation.

Plato, Aristotle, and the *Fables of Bidpai*, also known as *Kalíla wa Dimna*. To secure this last the physician Perzoes, or Burzúya in the Pahlaví form of the name or Buzurjmihr in the Persian form, was secretly dispatched to the Ganges with instructions to procure this work at once at any price. Perzoes is the only physician of Sassanian times of whom we have any detailed information. Chance has preserved his autobiography. For Ibn ul-Muqaffa' used it as a preface to his own retranslation of the *Fables of Bidpai*. Al-Bírúní states that it was added to the book of the fables to provoke religious doubts and to gain adherents for Manicheism. On these grounds some have rejected the autobiography as a forgery. But it may well be that al-Bírúní only meant that it existed as a separate work in the days of Ibn ul-Muqaffa' and that he joined it to the fables to form a single work.[1]

This preface has been translated into German by Noeldeke and, as I believe that it is quite unknown to English historians, I think it desirable to retranslate into English the opening paragraphs in order to show the style and matter of the original.

My father [writes Perzoes] belonged to the soldier class: my mother was the daughter of a family of distinguished priests. One of the first favours that God gave to me was that I was the favourite child and that I received a better education than my brothers. My parents sent me when I was seven to an elementary school. As soon as I could write well, I returned thanks to my parents. Then I took up science. The first branch of science that attracted me was Medicine. It interested me so much because I knew how excellent it was. The more I learnt of it, the more I liked it and the more eagerly I studied it. As soon as I had reached such a degree of proficiency that I could think of treating patients, I began to deliberate within myself. For I observed that there were four things to which men aspire. Which of these ought I to aim at—money, prosperity, fame, or a heavenly reward? What decided my choice was the observation that all intelligent persons praise Medicine and that no Religion condemns it. I also used to read in medical books that the best doctor is the one who gives himself over to his profession

1 Gabrieli, 'L' Opera d' Ibnull-Muqaffa'. *Rivi. degli Studi Orient.* t. XIII, p. 203.

and only seeks for a reward in the hereafter. So I determined to follow this lead and to aim at no earthly gain lest I be like a merchant who sells for valueless bauble a ruby by which he might have gained all the riches of the world.

I also read in the works of the ancients that if a physician aspire to gain through his art a reward in the hereafter, he will nevertheless not lose his share of this world's goods. Thus he resembles a sower who carefully scatters his barley grain in his field and for whom there springs up together with the barley all sorts of useful herbs.

So then, with the hope of a reward in the hereafter I set to work to treat the sick. I exerted myself in the treatment of patients whom I expected to cure. And no less did I strive in those cases where I could not hope to effect a cure. In such cases I tried at the least to make their sufferings more bearable. Whenever I could I used to attend in person to my cases. When this was impossible, I would write out for them the necessary prescriptions and give them medicines. From no one whom I treated did I demand any fee or any sort of reward. And none of my colleagues did I envy who equalled me in knowledge and surpassed me in fame or fortune if he was lax in his standards of honesty or in word or deed.[1]

It is said that Perzoes attracted the notice of Núshírván when he was tutor to his son Hormuz. He was then made chief minister of the court and physician to the king himself. According to tradition he was ultimately put to death on account of his Christian views. His writings appear to have been known to Rhazes for he quotes them in his *Continens*. A work by Simeon of Antioch, translated out of Arabic into Greek about 1070, on the *Wisdom of the Indians*, is ascribed to him and may be more of the fruits of his journey to India. There is also in the British Museum a book on divination, written in Persian verse, which is said in the beginning of the poem to be from his pen.[2] Perhaps, too, the formula for some pills found in the *Antidotarium* of Ibn Serapion is to be attributed to him, for they are described in the Latin version as 'Pillulae Barzuiati Sapientis'.

1 Noeldeke, 'Burzoes Einleitung zu dem Buche Kalila wa Dimna'. *Schrift. d. Wis. Ges. in Strassburg*, 1912, pp. 11 et seqq.

2 Brit. Mus. Add. 6591, ff. 122–5.

Like Alexander, his name soon became a mythical one among the Persians, and such wise sayings as were not ascribed to Loqmán (Aesop) were invariably attributed to Perzoes. 'Ministers are like physicians', Sa'dí reports him to have said to the courtiers of Núshírván. 'The physician administers medicine only to the sick. Therefore when I see that your opinions are judicious, it would not be consistent with wisdom for me to obtrude my sentiments. But if I see a blind man in the way of a well, if I keep silence, it is a crime.'[1] His remark: 'To think differently from a king is to wash the hands in one's own blood. If he call the day night, it is prudent to say "Behold the Moon and the Pleiades"' shows that his skill as a physician was equalled by his wisdom as a courtier.[2]

According to some accounts Perzoes brought back with him from India the game of chess and thus gave to Persia the honour of transmitting the game to Europe. According to another version a tributary Indian king sent a set of chess men to Núshírván with a challenge to play one game, chess being at that time unknown to the Persians. The stake was to be the annual tribute. Not only did Perzoes discover how to play the game and defeat the Indian ambassador, but he capped his triumph by inventing a similar game which he sent back to India. The Indian game represented a king, his court, and his army. Perzoes' game represented the heavens, the elements and the virtues. The game proved insoluble to the Indians and thus the Persians triumphed through Perzoes. The ultimate victory, however, rests with the Indians, for chess is still played to-day; the game of Perzoes has perished in all but fable.

A medical fact of some interest is that about the middle of the reign of Núshírván a general meeting of physicians was held by his orders at Jundí Shápúr to discuss the medical problems of the times. The assembly was presided over by the royal physician Jibrá'íl, the Irán Durustpát. Second to him in the gathering was one named al-Tasyufatáí or Sofistáí, which is possibly not the

1 *Gulistán*, vol. 1, p. 38. 2 Ibid. p. 31.

name of an individual but means the representatives of the Sophists. Third in importance was a certain Yúḥanná.[1]

Jibrá'íl owed his position at the court to his successful treatment of Shírín, the favourite wife of Núshírván. Jibrá'íl was a Nestorian Christian by birth who forsook Nestorianism for Monophysism. Shírín, too, was a Christian. He was consulted by her to explain and cure her inability to become pregnant. Jibrá'íl with the supernatural aid, as he claimed, of S. Sergius, cured her sterility and caused her to bear a male child. The king was delighted: Shírín became a convert to Monophysism. After this until the day of his death Jibrá'íl abused his post of physician-in-chief by interfering in ecclesiastical matters. The strife between the Nestorians and the Monophysites was then at its fiercest. Rather than have a Nestorian appointed as Catholicos Jibrá'íl persuaded Núshírván when sees fell vacant to select incompetent prelates or no prelate at all. Among others he had Joseph the Physician appointed Bishop of Seleucia in place of the Nestorian Catholicos. But he only held the post for three years, for he was then deposed for cruelty at the request of the Christians of Seleucia. Any obviously suitable candidate Jibrá'íl accused of being a renegade from Zoroastrianism and had condemned to be crucified.

Upon the death of Núshírván, Hormuz, his son, came to the throne under the name of Hormisdas IV without opposition. His assassination in A.D. 590 left the throne open for the accession of Khosrú Parvíz, known to the west as Chosroes II. The beginning of his reign was as unpropitious as the end. He was defeated by one of his own rebel generals and forced to take refuge with his traditional enemy the Roman Emperor. Maurice, then reigning, placed an army at his disposal and he again took the field. Within a year he was once more reigning at Ctesiphon.

The murder of the whole family of the emperor by a simple centurion called Phocas and his elevation to imperial rank morally compelled Chosroes to show his gratitude by marching against

1 Al-Qifṭí, p. 148.

Constantinople. In this campaign the Persian arms met with success at every turn. First Syria fell, then Palestine, and finally Egypt. The empire of Khosrú Parvíz thus became coterminous with the ancient empire of the Achaemenian sovereigns. In the midst of his triumphs he received a letter from an obscure citizen of Mecca, inviting him to acknowledge Muḥammad as the Prophet of God. He rejected the invitation and tore up the letter. 'It is thus', said Muḥammad, when this reception was announced to him, 'that God will tear up his kingdom and reject his supplication.'

The execution of Phocas and the assumption of the royal purple by Heraclius in A.D. 610 should have caused Chosroes to call an end to his campaign, for his excuse of revenge was no longer valid. But he continued to press on until the Roman Empire was reduced to the walls of Constantinople and a remnant of Greece, Italy and Africa and a few maritime cities. Heraclius was minded to abandon Constantinople, but Sain, a Persian general, offered to conduct an embassy to the Persian king and to secure for him pardon and peace. The embassy utterly failed. 'It was not an embassy', said Chosroes, 'but the person of Heraclius, bound in chains, that should be brought to the foot of my throne. I will never give peace to the Emperor of Rome till he has abjured his crucified God and embraced the worship of the sun.' Sain was flayed alive for his pains and Heraclius consented to pay annually to the Persian court 1000 talents of gold, 1000 talents of silver, 1000 silk robes, 1000 horses and 1000 virgins.

But at the lowest point of despair the fortunes of Heraclius changed. In A.D. 622, 623 and 627 he led successful expeditions against the Persians. The success of the second campaign freed Constantinople from danger and in the third the Roman arms were carried as far as the Tigris. Chosroes fled before him and the Roman Emperor arrived within a few miles of Ctesiphon. The season, the river, or perhaps the reputation of that impregnable city caused him to check. But Chosroes was already in flight. His nation was tired of campaigns, of the pouring out of blood for the whims and ambitions of an old man. To save the throne for his family he voluntarily placed the royal tiara on the head of his son Merdasas, and fled. But the army would have none of this. He was caught, his eighteen sons were massacred before his face, and he was thrown into a dungeon where he died on the fifth day. With him virtually ended the house of Sassan. Within the next four years nine candidates enjoyed the title of king. Henceforth, it is true, Persia had no more to fear from Rome. But a new power had arisen which, building upon the weakness which prolonged wars had brought about in the two great empires of those times, founded a new faith and a new empire. Henceforth the influence of Greece and Rome upon Persia was to come from the written word and not by the sword. Never again did Rome disturb the Persian Empire. For both Rome and Persia were silenced under the common yoke of the Arabian caliph.

CHAPTER III

FROM THE FOUNDATION OF ISLAM TO THE DEATH OF THE CALIPH HĀRŪN-UL-RASHĪD

THE refusal of the Persian court to heed the summons of the Prophet was not left long unnoticed. Not that the first successors of Muḥammad had any intention of founding the empire which they bequeathed to the later caliphs. From the minor tribal warfare which followed upon the death of Muḥammad developed two great wars. For the tribes on the west were supported by the Byzantine emperor and those on the east by the great dynasty of Chosroes. With Abú Bakr's expeditions against Constantinople I am not concerned. With those against the court of Persia I am bound to deal, for they lead directly to the introduction of Arabic culture into the still unfounded city of Baghdad and into all the cities of Persia.

In March of A.D. 633 only twelve years after the flight of Muḥammad from Mecca and within a year of his death, Abú Bakr, the first caliph and immediate successor to the Prophet, dispatched troops into Mesopotamia for the quietening of the Arab tribes there and to secure peace on the eastern borders of the desert. The fertility of the plains of Iraq, watered by the great rivers Euphrates and Tigris, compared so advantageously with the sandy wastes of his native land that Khálid, the Arab general, determined to annex it to the rule of Abú Bakr. With this intention he advanced upon Hafir, the frontier town of the Persian Empire. He was opposed by the Persian governor who, at the so-called Battle of Chains, suffered much to his surprise a severe defeat. A second victory of the Muslim forces, followed by yet another one this same year, completed the discomfiture of the Persian court. The shah fell sick, but persuaded the loyal tribes of the lowlands to unite to drive out the invader. Khálid re-crossed the Euphrates, and for the moment it appeared that Islam was not yet destined to subdue

Persia. In the middle of the battle that followed Khálid is said to have made a vow that, if victory were granted to him, the blood of his foes should flow as a crimson stream. God heard his vow, and at last the Persians broke. Khálid gave orders that no fugitives were to be slain, but that all prisoners and captives were to be brought before him. Then he set to work to fulfil his vow. Enormous numbers were slain in the dry bed of a stream; but the earth soaked up the blood and still the crimson stream did not flow. At last it was suggested that the prisoners should be taken and slaughtered in the water of a running river. There Khálid had the satisfaction of seeing his vow fulfilled. The flour-mills worked by these waters are said to have ground for three whole days the corn for the army with a red stream running through the wheels.

The conquest of the lowlands and the practical overthrow of the Persian kingdom satisfied Abú Bakr. Neither temporal expansion nor spiritual empire at the point of the sword was as yet part of the programme of Islam. Yet many of the conquered Iraqis embraced the faith, although the city of Hira preferred to remain Christian. This policy of non-aggression was followed by 'Umar, the successor of Abú Bakr, in the caliphate. It was an unauthorized minor expedition that brought a further extension of Islamic arms.

The Sassanian monarchy was now so enfeebled that of necessity any strong power could overthrow it. All possible claimants to the throne had been mercilessly massacred by each new monarch, so that at this time the country was ruled by a succession of feeble shahs set up by the royal women who constituted the court. The knowledge of this weakness and the irritation of seeing a hostile and infidel power at such very close range spurred one of the minor Arab generals in Iraq to invade Khuzistan. No doubt he hoped for enormous success and a fame that would rival that of Khálid. At first he met with no resistance and advanced inland and threatened Istakhr, that is, Persepolis. But he soon found that he had neither the fortune nor the genius of Khálid, and he was obliged to send back urgent appeals for help. 'Umar, though furious with this act of disobedience, sent the necessary help and with difficulty extricated him from his position. This defeat to the Arab arms encouraged the Persian satrap Hormuzan of Ahwaz to attack. To check this the second invasion of Khuzistan was officially launched and Ahwaz was occupied by the Arabs.

Again 'Umar called a check to further advance. He bade his Arab soldiery restore regular rule to the lands that they had just conquered, to repair the irrigation channels, and to think more of commercial prosperity than of glory and empire. It was the folly of the Shah Yezdegird and Hormuzan which brought about the final destruction of the House of Sassan and the complete subjugation of the whole of Persia to the caliph of Islam. The continued plotting of these two rendered it impossible for 'Umar to follow his policy, and in the year A.D. 640 he authorized an advance into the hills. The command of the expedition was given to al-No'mán. Hormuzan was soon defeated and captured and sent in chains to Medina. To provide a spectacle for the simple Arab folk of the town the captured Persian was dressed up in his court robes and so made to enter the mosque where 'Umar was sitting. The contrast between a Persian general and the ruler of Islam was so great that Hormuzan failed to recognize 'Umar in the simple, unaffected Arab whom he saw there. 'Umar at once had him stripped of his costly clothes and had him dressed in a garment more fitting for an Arab prisoner. Then he began to question him about Persia and his faithlessness. Hormuzan, expecting from the nature of the examination that this was but a preliminary to a death sentence, quaked with fear and could scarcely speak. At last he asked for a drink of water. When this was given him, he refused to drink it. 'Umar asked him why, and he replied that he feared that it was poisoned or that he would be stabbed in the back while drinking. 'Thy life is safe', said 'Umar, 'until thou hast drunk the water up.' At once Hormuzan poured the contents of the glass to the ground and, though 'Umar would have slain him there and then, the bystanders present interposed and bade him keep his word. Later Hormuzan turned

Muslim and took up his residence in Medina and became the confidential adviser of 'Umar on Persian matters.

In the meantime al-No'mán had not been inactive. He followed up his capture of Hormuzan by laying siege to Sus, the modern Shustar. On its fall the city was treated with respect and a large number of Persians embraced Islam. Next al-No'mán turned to Jundí Shápúr and reduced the city. But, as in the case of Sus, the city was respected and the university and school of medicine were left intact and no interference was allowed with the Christian professors. He now passed on towards Ispahan.

Yezdegird made one more attempt to expel the Arab invaders. He is said to have collected 150,000 men in Hamadan in order to save Ispahan. When this news was brought to 'Umar, he realized at last the impossibility of a proud, though effete, empire resting tranquil while a young and vigorous power pushed upon its frontiers. A reverse in the mountains of Persia might bring defeat in Iraq and consequent loss of the Arab cities of Basra and Kufa. He determined therefore to march himself in support of al-No'mán and, though ultimately the caliph remained in Medina, the Arab forces passed on to the final encounter with the Persians. The army of the unbelievers, some five times as big as the Moslem host, were found to the south-west of Hamadan under the command of Fírúzán. The battle that ensued is known as the battle of Nihavend, and there in the year A.H. 21 or A.D. 642 the Persians were utterly overthrown, the Christian House of Sassan and the faith they professed were driven out, and the way laid open for the introduction of the so-called Arab sciences in place of the Christian Syriac learning. Al-No'mán perished in the battle, and Fírúzán, although he escaped from the field, was killed a few days later. For, flying towards Hamadan, he found the narrow bridle path blocked by a caravan conveying honey. While trying to pass he was overtaken and slain, and hence arose the saying: 'Part of the Lord's host is the honey bee.'

But Yezdegird still refused to yield and the Muslim advance continued. Ray fell in A.D. 643. Yezdegird fled to Ispahan, then to Kerman, and finally to Balkh. At last in the year 652, deserted and helpless, he was murdered. Thus ended the line of Ardeshir and began the period of Arab supremacy and the so-called Arab medicine.

It seems fairly certain that the conquering Arabs contributed next to nothing to the scientific knowledge of the Persians. The sources of information on the subject of the state of medicine in Arabia in the time of the Prophet Muḥammad are extremely scanty. Of true medical literature nothing remains, if indeed it ever existed. Apart from later medical biographies and tradition the only evidence is scattered references in the works of the poets and in the Qur'án itself.

The medical references contained in the Qur'án are most meagre and unsatisfactory. The chapter entitled 'The Elephant' has been eagerly seized upon by medical historians because it is an almost contemporary account of an epidemic of plague or small-pox. It is an early revelation and undoubtedly refers to the Abyssinian invasion of Mecca in the year 570, the year of the Prophet's birth. But it is so short and couched in such poetical terms that it gives no indication of how the Arabs diagnosed and treated this visitation.[1] Resike on the authority of Mas'údí states that small-pox and measles appeared for the first time in Arabia in that year. This is possible, but unlikely. Caussin de Perceval in his history of the Arabs before Islam quotes another case of small-pox, which was noted by the historians of the year 601.[2]

On the subject of personal health the Qur'án contains little more than wise precepts. 'Eat and drink, but not to excess.' It does, however, lay down the unfortunate rule that an infant should be suckled for two years.[3]

Such medical ideas as the early poets of Arabia have left enshrined in their verses have no practical value and give no indication of the state of the medical knowledge of the Arabs themselves. It is to be remembered that there were a considerable

1 Qur'án, ch. 105.
2 Leclerc, *Hist. Méd. Arabe*, vol. 1, p. 22.
3 Qur'án, ch. 2, v. 233.

number of Jews domiciled in the cities of Arabia and that through Jewish and New Testament medical views the Arabian poets may have become acquainted with diseases and pathological ideas which were quite foreign to the native Arabs. Imru'u ul-Qays, who lived in the sixth century A.D., states that he suffered from an alcoholic neuritis and is said to have been poisoned by a cloak which was sent to him by the Emperor Justinian. The poet Labíd bin Rabí'a, a pagan Arab who lived into the days of Islam, refers to his contemporaries as itchy and mangy with their skins dirty and cracked. But this is only a metaphor taken from the camel lines. And al-Nábigha of Zubyán cries to heaven to curse the king with a palsy which will prevent him holding his riding whip.

From a metaphor of the poet Tarfat ibn ul-'Abd, who died seventy years before the birth of Muḥammad, and who likens himself to a camel, coated with tar and turned out into the solitude of the desert, it would seem that at that period the Arabs were accustomed to treat septic wounds and ulcers with disinfectants and that contagious diseases were treated by isolation. Besides tar another treatment for wounds was oil and a gauze drain. For Maymún ibn Qays, known as al-A'shá, likens a hopeless injustice to a mighty wound within which the oil and the drain have disappeared.

Finally, there are the traditional actions and sayings of the Prophet on the subject of health, which have been collected and written down and are still read throughout the Islamic world. Many commentators have set their names to these collections. Their works are usually known as *Ṭibb-ul-Nabbí* or 'Medicine of the Prophet'. Ḥájjí Khalífa in the seventeenth century quotes half a dozen such works. The most popular is that made by Jalál-ul-Dín al-Suyúṭí, which has been translated into French by M. Perron. This was the version which Muḥammad Akbar Arzání translated into Persian for the use of 'Álamgír, the emperor of Delhi.

The *Ṭibb-ul-Nabbí* was of infinitely more importance in the moulding of Persian practices than was the Qur'án. The Traditions are complimentary to the Law and no pious Mussulman would willingly run contrary to either. The Law gave him a few directions about his health: Tradition gave him many. A study of Traditions shows that by far the greater number are concerned with the cure of disease, a few with the prevention of disease. Muḥammad's method of cure was both natural and supernatural. Again and again he insists that God has allowed no disease to exist upon earth for which He has not also created a cure. This was the text which was so eagerly seized upon by the druggists of later years in their attempts to find a specific for every pathological manifestation. Often the Prophet's utterances became poetic. Palms, he says, are blest trees. He bids his followers respect them as they would their parents, remembering that God created the palm tree from the dust which remained over after He had finished creating Adam. And he who in his house possesses honey and olive oil, for him will the angels pray.

Cure, says the Prophet of God, depends upon three things—honey, scarification and the cautery. Headaches and fevers were thus to be treated, though cups were not to be applied to the nape of the neck lest the memory of the patient might fail. For the site of the memory, and here he drops into popular Arab physiology, is the cerebellum. He himself practised a form of faith healing, combined with the power of touch. Ayesha, the daughter of Abú Bakr, says that when anyone was ill, the Prophet used to rub his hands upon the sick person's body, after which he would say, 'O Lord of man, take away this pain and give health; for Thou art the giver of health. There is no health but Thine, even the health which leaveth no sickness.' This was his treatment also for wounds and sores.

Though honey is pre-eminent among drugs, he does not condemn the use of others. Cinders of papyrus grass act as haemostatics; urine taken internally is a cure for dropsy; henna cures gout; and senna appears for the first time in a pharmacopoeia.

His belief in supernatural treatment and cure does not seem to have been so marked as it was in some of the later physicians.

He recommends reading of the Qur'án and above all of the opening chapter. To a magician who asked his advice he replied: 'Go away. Let him who can help his brother do so.'

Among his methods of preventing disease his forbidding to his followers to taste pork or to drink wine is well known. Yet he held that the excessive use of meat was as harmful as wine. The platter kills more than the cup, re-echoes Osler. It was an Arab physician who, when asked how much food a man should eat in a day replied that ten ounces would carry a man, any excess of that the eater would have to carry.[1] Muḥammad forbade the eating of the flesh of lizards and said that the killing of one was equivalent to a hundred good deeds. He also forbade his followers to kill ants, bees, the hoopoe and the shrike.

Quotations from the Traditions are scattered throughout the later Persian writers, more especially among writers of the second class whose aim is not primarily scientific. Al-Qazvíní in particular in his *'Ajá'ib-ul-Makhlúqát* cites them frequently; so does the other Qazvíní in his *Nuzhaṭ-ul-Qulúb*.[2]

The rude health of the Arabs of those days and the consequent lack of need for a complicated system of medicine is also made clear by various stories. The physicians who attended Muḥammad himself were mostly Persians or Arabs trained in Persia. The more menial duties of surgery and phlebotomy were performed by untrained Arabs. One of these, Ibn abí Ramṣia of the tribe of Tamím, is said to have noticed a growth between the shoulders of the Prophet and to have offered to cut it off. Muḥammad refused.[3]

Shaykh Sa'dí, the Persian poet, relates in his *Gulistán* that one of the kings of Persia sent to Muḥammad a learned physician. He remained one or two years in Arabia, but no one approached him or sought his treatment. At last he presented himself to the Prophet and complained: 'I have been sent to treat your Companions; but during all this time no one has asked me to carry

1 *Gulistán*, vol. III, p. 6.
2 *Nuzhaṭ-ul-Qulúb*, pp. 19, 47, 91.
3 *I.A.U.* vol. I, p. 116.

out my duties in any respect whatsoever.' To which the Prophet replied: 'It is the custom of these people not to eat until hunger overcomes them and then to cease eating while there still remains a desire for food.' The physician answered: 'This is the reason for their perfect health', kissed the ground in reverence, and departed.[1]

Such medical knowledge as Muḥammad possessed, he may well have acquired from Ḥáriṣ bin Kalda, an Arab, who is said to have left the desert for a while and gone to Jundí Sh̲ápúr to study medicine. While in Persia he met Núsh̲írván. His reputed conversation with this monarch has been preserved. For the most part they discussed only questions of hygiene and methods for the preservation of health. Ḥáriṣ' main point was the Arab view that excess of diet is the cause of all disease. He also recommended the simplest possible manner of life. Diet should be of the plainest. Water is to be preferred to wine and salt and dried meats to fresh meat. The dietary should include fruit. The hot bath should be taken before meals. As for drugs, he bids the shah leave them all aside as long as the health is good, but as soon as any sign of disease appears, let it be eradicated by every possible means. The remedies which a physician should employ in addition to drugs are enemata and cupping, the latter being administered when the moon is on the wane.[2]

On his return Ḥáriṣ settled in Mecca and became the foremost physician of the Arabs of the desert.[3] Whether he ever embraced Islam is uncertain; but this did not prevent the Prophet from sending his sick friends to consult him. In spite of the unorthodoxy of his views he was reckoned a judge among the Arabs. His strictness for the Law is illustrated by his treatment of his wife. Going into her tent one early morning he found her picking her teeth, upon which he at once sent her a bill of divorcement. When she protested, he justified his conduct by saying that it was too early to pick the teeth. For if she had

1 *Gulistán*, vol. III, p. 5.
2 *I.A.U.* vol. I, p. 110.
3 Ibn K̲h̲allikán, vol. IV, p. 253.

already broken her fast, then she had breakfasted before the regular time and was therefore a glutton; if she had not yet breakfasted, then she must have passed the night with particles of meat between her teeth and was therefore a slut. The divorce stood and the lady was remarried to Yúsuf al-Saqafí.[1]

By this second marriage she had a child whom she named al-Ḥajjáj. He is said to have been born with an imperforate anus. Although an operation relieved the condition, the child refused the breast of its mother or any other woman, so that it seemed likely to die. The mother was at a loss what to do until Satan appeared to her in the form of her late husband, the physician Ḥáriṣ bin Kalda.[2] He asked her to explain the trouble and learning the dilemma, said: 'Kill a black kid and give its blood to the child to drink; the next day do the same thing; on the third day slay a black he-goat and give the child the blood to drink; then kill a snake and make the child swallow the blood and daub his face with some of it. If you do this, the child will take the breast on the fourth day.' They did as he bade them and the child survived.[3]

When al-Ḥajjáj grew up, he became the most cruel of men. This he used to ascribe to his early taste for blood. Among his victims was a certain Sayyid ibn Jubayr, whom he executed for treason. When his head was cut off, a great quantity of blood flowed from the trunk. Al-Ḥajjáj called in his physicians to consult them about the phenomenon and to know why all the other persons whom he had executed bled so very little. To this they made answer: 'When you put this man to death, his soul was still in his body. And blood follows the soul. As for the others, their souls were gone with fright before you killed them and therefore their blood was diminished.'

1 Ibid. vol. 1, p. 357.

2 Persian tradition is fond of making the Devil appear as a physician. Mythology tells how Zohaq, one of the earliest rulers of Persia, was kissed on the back by the Devil which caused serpents to spring forth from the shoulder-blades. The Devil then assumed the garb of a physician and prescribed a diet of human brains to keep the serpents quiet.

3 Ibid. p. 564.

Al-Ḥajjáj is said to have died in the year A.D. 714 of cancer of the stomach. His physician was a Christian named Thiyázúq. When summoned he clinched the diagnosis by tying a piece of meat to a string and passing it down the patient's throat into the stomach. After a short interval it was drawn up again and a swarm of worms was found adhering to it.

Ibn Khallikán says that Ḥáriṣ bin Kalda was impotent and that the sons that he had were only sons by adoption.[1] One of these adopted heirs, named al-Naẓar, was a cousin of the Prophet. Apparently he followed the profession of medicine, like his foster-father, and also travelled to increase his knowledge. It is not at all improbable, therefore, that he too received his medical training at Jundí Shápúr. Avicenna ascribes to the son of Ḥáriṣ certain pills for the cure of vitiligo and rheumatic pains of which the formula had survived to his day.[2] Even more interesting is the tragic end of al-Naẓar. He became the bitter enemy of his celebrated cousin and ridiculed his person and his writings. In A.D. 624 he was found fighting against the Prophet and on the defeated side. He was captured and put to death. His sister lamented his execution in one of the most touching odes which any woman has ever written. Muḥammad reading it was so moved that he is said to have repented of having given way to his desire for revenge.[3]

A period of quiescence in the development of medicine in Persia followed the successful invasion of the Arabs. Of all that happened while the Umayyad caliphs were enthroned in Damascus, while Baghdad was still an unknown village, and while Persian civilization was becoming accustomed to Arab rule, there is a total lack of information. Jundí Shápúr continued to exist and even to flourish. Yet there is not even one name on record to show any activity of the school between the return of that brilliant pupil Ḥáriṣ to Muḥammad and the summoning of that brilliant master Jurjís I to the Caliph al-Manṣúr.

1 Ibn Khallikán, vol. IV, p. 253.
2 *Canon*, bk. V, I. 9.
3 *I.A.U.* vol. I, p. 113.

The rise of the 'Abbásids and the downfall of the Umayyads lay in the plots of a small party in the city of Kufa. Political circumstances had forced the successors of Muḥammad to govern the empire, not from Mecca or Medina, but from Damascus. Here Arab culture first took root and sprung into being. A gradually diminishing virility of the ruling house combined with dissatisfaction in the distant provinces brought about the defeat and flight of Marwán II, the last of the Umayyad caliphs (as the rulers at Damascus were called) in A.D. 750. The 'Abbásid family, the claimants to the caliphate, had in the previous year fled to Kufa. Now seemed the favourable moment to set up the standard of revolt. Abú ul-'Abbás, the head of the house, ascended the pulpit one Friday and under the title of al-Ṣaffáḥ declared himself caliph in place of Marwán. After receiving the homage of the public he retired to al-Háshimíyya, a new residence that he had had built just outside the city, and from there sent out various relatives to replace the officials of the fallen regime. His commands were carried out thoroughly and without mercy; the foundations of the new dynasty were strengthened by massacres such as the history of the world has rarely equalled. To aid him in his daily business al-Ṣaffáḥ instituted the office of *wazír*, a post which was the distinguishing feature of the 'Abbásid system of government. The position was not an enviable one. While in office the *wazír* was second only to the caliph. But he was liable to dismissal at any moment, and impeachment usually followed dismissal. Yet it was a much coveted post. It is characteristic both of this age and of the Persian courts which followed the fall of the 'Abbásid dynasty that the wazirate was frequently held by a physician.

After reigning just short of five years al-Ṣaffáḥ caught small-pox and died in his palace at al-Háshimíyya. Abú Ja'far, his half-brother, older, but a child of a slave girl, was immediately proclaimed caliph in his place and ascended the throne under the title of al-Manṣúr. During his relatively long reign of 21 years, from A.D. 754 to 775, he firmly established the dynasty and gave the impetus towards art and learning which have made the 'Abbásids famous throughout the world.

To al-Manṣúr is to be ascribed the founding of the city of Baghdad. His palace of al-Háshimíyya was too close to the turbulent and rebellious Kufans to be secure. It was too near to the heats of Basra to be pleasant. A search up the valley as far as Mosul showed no place more suitable than the little village of Baghdad. This the caliph determined to enlarge into a city to house himself and his court. So it was planned at first. The city was to be circular so that all the courtiers might be equidistant from the palace in the centre. It was to be surrounded by a wall, pierced by four gates, leading to Khorasan and Persia, to Basra and the south, to Kufa and Arabia, and to Syria and Byzantium. Within the wall were to be the palaces, the government offices, the bazaars, and private dwellings. Even in his own lifetime al-Manṣúr found it desirable to build a palace on the river bank outside. A chance remark by some Greek ambassadors caused him to refound the bazaars also outside the wall. And in a short time offices and private dwellings followed.

The oldest suburb and the first to rise into great importance was that known as Karkh, which lay to the south-west of the original walled city and was approached through the Kufah Gate. Here was built the Bímáristán, which became the Metropolitan Hospital and the cradle of the Baghdad school of medicine. Here lectured, lived, and practised all the great physicians of Baghdad from the time of Bukht Yishú' to that of Rhazes. Known in later times as the Old Hospital, it remained the chief centre of clinical teaching and practice until the foundation of the New Hospital by 'Aẓud-ul-Doula in the tenth century.

The situation of the Old Hospital must have been a delightful one. In front lay the great Karkháya Canal, a branch of the 'Ísá Canal, which joined the waters of the Euphrates to those of the Tigris. The canal above the hospital was still broad enough to be bridged with an arched stone bridge, known as the Qanṭarah-ul-Bímáristán or Hospital Bridge, being the lowest of the great bridges; for opposite the hospital the canal divided into the Canal of Abú Attab and the Amud Canal and neither of these were wide enough to be dignified with a named bridge. Across the waters of the canal lay a collection of houses known as the Quarter of the Men of Wasit. On the northern side of the hospital ran the great Kufah road; on the other side lay the Ẓarabat or House of Female Musicians, then came the mill of a certain Abú ul-Qásim, and then a building called al-Khafqah or 'the Clappers', presumably a house dedicated to some craft or trade carried on by the bank of the stream. The hospital was thus centrally, though perhaps unsuitably, placed.[1]

In the time of Hárún-ul-Rashíd Karkh grew considerably and before long became the commercial centre of western Baghdad. During the reign of the Caliph Wáṣiq a great fire occurred which destroyed many of the buildings. Possibly the hospital too suffered in the fire; but its activities were only interrupted, for the whole of Karkh was promptly rebuilt and new roads were laid out and the general lie of the district improved.

The rise of new suburbs on the eastern bank of the river and the transference of the seat of government there in the ninth century brought about a decay of the old round city of al-Manṣúr. With it the prestige of Karkh also declined, although it continued to remain a centre of active trade and to contain a large population long after the decay of the rest of Baghdad on that side of the Tigris. The founding of the New Hospital at the end of the tenth century removed the medical school from the west side of the round city to the east side. After that date no more is heard of the Old Hospital. Probably it did not altogether disappear, but continued to serve a dwindling and impoverished population. For the suburb of Karkh survived, and to-day the Turkish name Karchiaka is still applied to the more ancient quarter of Baghdad, which stands upon the Arab side of the Tigris.

Apart from the building of the city of Baghdad the most

1 Le Strange, *Baghdád during the Abbasid Caliphate* (Oxford, 1900), pp. 50 et passim.

notable feature about the reign of al-Manṣúr is the infiltration of Persian manners and habits and his toleration of men of unorthodox views. Persian dress with the tall Zoroastrian hat became the fashionable dress at court. With his Persian physicians, mostly Christians or Jews, came other non-Arab men of learning. Magians from Persia brought the philosophy of India and China to the court. Literature, history and astronomy began to be studied. To the last of these al-Manṣúr was particularly partial and possibly some of the responsibility for the withering influence of astrology on medicine is to be attributed to him. Tradition, no longer oral, began to be embodied by the great doctors of the Law in elaborate systems of jurisprudence. Two of the four great founders of the Islamic Schools of Law lived in this reign, Abú Ḥanífa and Málik ibn Anas. Finally, it is to be noted that the Arabs completely lost their pre-eminence. The soldiery of Khorasan replace the Arab body-guard: Persian Christians replace the Arab physician. The revival of Greek learning was welcomed as another blow to Arab prestige. Thus were laid the foundations of the great revival and development of the intellectual life which appeared in the subsequent reigns.

Before passing to a detailed description of the physicians who lived and worked in the days of al-Manṣúr, a word must be said about the system of Arab and Persian proper names. Even in the pre-Islamic days there is a certain amount of difficulty in recognizing the Western forms of oriental names. The Latin name is often so widely removed from the Pahlaví name. But, when the reader enters the period of Islamic medicine, he finds this difficulty a very real one. All the most famous physicians have no less than six names. These names are not single words but may be a phrase or group of words. The first of these six names is their Latin name, which is of course not the true name at all but a barbaro-Latin translation. But because it is the best known to English readers and is also the easiest to pronounce and to remember, I shall invariably employ this name where it exists.

Of the oriental names the first is the man's real name, known technically as the *ism*. This name is never employed unless the user intends to insult the bearer. Next comes his patronymic or *nisba*, which may refer forwards or backwards. A man may thus be described as 'the son of so-and-so', mentioning the father's name, or he may be termed the 'father of so-and-so', mentioning the name of his son. The patronymic too was never used in speech, but was confined to biographies, letters, proclamations and so forth, in which it is necessary to trace a man's exact ancestry to distinguish him from others of the same name.

The remaining three names are all permissible in conversation. The first of these is the title or *laqab*, which may be given by the caliph or shah, by a local ruler, or even by popular usage. The use of many titles came in with the later 'Abbásids. By their lavish distribution the caliphs brought their use into disrepute. Apart from their being a means of distinguishing people of the same name, a further value of the title is that it shows the profession of the holder. Thus a title containing the words *dín* (religion) or *doula* (empire) or Islám, such as Qawám-ul-Dín or the 'Support of Religion' or Sayf-ul-Islám or 'The Sword of Islam', shows that the bearer holds some office of state. Such a title was normally confined to sovereigns, *wazírs*, doctors of law, and *amírs*. Doctors of medicine, who were entitled, usually received some acknowledgement of their art in their title. Thus, Loqmán-ul-Mulk or the 'Aesop of the Country' and Náẓim-ul-Aṭibbá or 'The Director of Physicians', are typical titles granted to physicians. This custom survived the fall of the caliphate. Until recent times in modern Persia every Persian of gentle birth was entitled by a royal *firmán*. Thereafter the holder, even though he might be a mere boy, was known to all, excepting his family, by his title alone. The title was always an Arabic phrase and was more or less suitable to the profession of the holder. Occasionally a touch of ridicule was introduced as when a famous doctor of Teheran was given the title of Lissán-ul-Ḥukamá or 'Tongue of the Wise' in reference to a personal characteristic rather than his public utterances.

Next comes the most important name of all—the *kunya* or nickname. This was invariably a compound name beginning with the word *abú* or 'father of'. But it is not a true patronymic, for it was given to people with no children. The *kunya* was the correct name to use in all conversation with any one. Every host would take great care to learn his guest's *kunya* and to address him by this name alone. Generally a *kunya* was only given to a Moslem, though non-Moslems in imitation adopted a *kunya* for use among themselves. But no Moslem would address a non-Moslem by such a *kunya*. It was looked upon as a mark of signal favour that the Caliph al-Mu'taẓid addressed Ṣábit bin Qurra by his *kunya* Abú Ḥasan at times. But it was remarked that he only did so in private conversation; in public such condescension by the Vicegerent of God to a Sabean heretic would have been severely criticized.

Finally, in case there were two people present with the same *kunya*, it was permissible to add the name of the town from which a man came. For the purposes of Western readers to whom Arabic titles and names are meaningless, it is desirable to use this name when no Latin name has been given, unless it leads to confusion.

All these names are exemplified in the case of Avicenna. Avicenna is his Latin name, the name given to him by the Latin medieval translators of his works, and it is the name by which he is best known throughout Europe to-day. But his fellow-Persians called him Abú 'Alí al-Ḥusayn bin 'Abd-Ulláh bin al-Ḥasan bin 'Alí bin Síná al-Shaykh-ul-Ra'ís al-Balkhí. His *kunya* stands first—Abú 'Alí or father of 'Alí. Then follows his *ism*—the name which is never to be used—al-Ḥusayn. Then comes his *nisba*—the son of 'Abd-Ulláh, the grandson of al-Ḥasan, the great-grandson of 'Alí, the great-great-grandson of Síná. Then comes his *laqab* Shaykh-ul-Ra'ís or Chief of Princes. Actually he had more than one title. And finally comes his birthplace—al-Balkhí, that is, the man of Balkh. Again, Sayyid Abú Ibráhím Isma'íl ibn ul-Ḥasan ibn Muḥammad bin Aḥmad al-Ḥusayní Zayn-ul-Dín al-Jurjání bore the title of Sayyid because he claimed descent from the Prophet; abú Ibráhím is his *kunya*; al-Ḥusayní his *ism*; Zayn-ul-Dín his *laqab*; and al-Jurjání his geographical name. Oriental writers usually refer to him as Sayyid Isma'íl, but I shall endeavour always to call him al-Jurjání, that is, the man from Jurjan, and when that title occurs with no other qualification, the physician Zayn-ul-Dín is always meant.

To revert now to Baghdad and its caliphs. Throughout his life al-Manṣúr suffered from dyspepsia. His personal physician Ibn Allahlaj, who had accompanied him on his pilgrimage to Mecca, and whom Rhazes later esteemed so highly, could do nothing for him. Next he tried in vain the remedies of the doctors around him and finally turned to Jurjís ibn Bukht Yishú' of Jundí Shápúr, whose reputation as a skilled clinician had filtered through the court circles to his ears. The first of this famous family was a certain Bukht Yishú', a Syriac title meaning 'Jesus hath delivered', who was also a physician. Beyond this nothing is known about him. Jurjís, his son, was at this time physician-in-chief of the medical school of Jundí Shápúr. At the caliph's bidding he entrusted the direction of the school to his son and with two of his pupils, Ibráhím and 'Ísá ibn Sahlásá, set out for Baghdad.

On their arrival the party was received with the greatest honour. A few days later the caliph unfolded the story of his unfortunate symptoms and to his great delight Jurjís consented to treat him. His treatment was entirely successful and he was persuaded to stay on as physician-in-chief to the caliph.[1] Thus began the tradition of foreign physicians in the Arab court, for Jurjís was a Persian. He was also a Christian, and apparently a strict one, for he spurned with contempt al-Manṣúr's present to him of three Greek slave girls.

Jurjís remained faithfully in the court of al-Manṣúr until he felt that he had but a short time more in this world. A dying man, he begged for permission to return to his own city of Jundí Shápúr. Before granting him this leave the caliph attempted to convert him to his own faith. But the old man was adamant and

1 *Hist. Dynst.* vol. IX, p. 143.

swore that he would rather burn with his own forefathers than enjoy Paradise with the caliph. The caliph pressed him no further, but asked him if he could not find someone to carry on his court practice. Jurjís therefore named 'Ísá bin Sahlášá, who had been with him all these years. Then al-Manṣúr suffered him to depart.

'Ísá was by no means the equal of his master and proved a very unworthy successor. Abusing his position in the household of the caliph, he began a campaign of blackmail on the Christian clergy. A threatening letter sent to the Metropolitan of Nisibis proved his undoing. For the letter was shown to the caliph, who flew into a violent rage, ordered 'Ísá to be beaten and deprived of his office at court. He then begged Jurjís to return. But he now felt too old to take up the part again and nominated Ibráhím, the other pupil who had accompanied him to Baghdad, to fill the vacant office. Thus, full of honour and in peace among his own, Jurjís died in the year 769, six years before his master, the Caliph al-Manṣúr, and was buried, as he desired, in the vaults of his ancestors.

Besides his fame as a clinician Jurjís is famous for his translations. He is said to have been the first to attempt to render works on medicine into Arabic. Among his pupils were his famous son (whom I always refer to as Bukht Yishú' II), to whom he entrusted the direction of the hospital at Jundí Shápúr during his absence in Baghdad, and 'Ísá bin Ṭáhirbakht, who was also a director of the hospital during the last days of Jurjís.

The short reigns of the next two caliphs form, as it were, a preparation for the great work that Hárún-ul-Rashíd and al-Ma'mún, the two greatest of the line, were to accomplish. Al-Mahdí succeeded his father al-Manṣúr in A.D. 775 and during his ten years on the throne spent his time and his father's treasury on consolidating and civilizing the empire. Mosques were enlarged and beautified; caravanserais were furnished with fountains and other comforts; a postal service was instituted and provided with swift mules and camels. In spite of his father's wishes and plans Baghdad grew enormously. Merchants of every trade settled in the city. Even the unlawful trades in wine and instruments of music were allowed, for the laxity of the court tolerated them.

By a slave girl named al-Khayzurán he had two sons, Músá and Hárún. Músá, now named al-Hádí, was proclaimed heir-apparent. To Hárún was given the additional title of al-Rashíd or 'The Just One'.

Al-Hádí occupied the throne only one year. The cause of his death is uncertain. He was near Mosul at the time. Ibn abí Uṣaybi'a says that a consultation was held in the sick room at which Abú Quraysh 'Ísá, 'Abd-Ulláh al-Ṭayfúrí, and Dá'úd ibn Sarábiyún were present. The investigations and discussions led to no practical result and only annoyed their dying master, who cried out from his sick bed upon them: 'You take my monies and my allowances; but in time of need you sit around and do nothing.' To which Abú Quraysh replied with fitting humility that they could but try and that it was God alone who could give health. This served only to annoy the caliph the more and he demanded that Bukht Yishú' bin Jurjís should be summoned from Jundí Shápúr, where he had been allowed to remain as director of the medical school.

His *wazír*, who was present in the room, suggested that a local practitioner of fame, by name 'Abd Yishú' bin Naṣr of Ṣarṣar, should be summoned in the meantime. Al-Hádí eagerly jumped at the idea and bade them summon him and at the same time cut off the heads of his present attendants. The *wazír* obeyed the first half of his instructions, but considering that the caliph was speaking with a judgement heated by fever passed no orders for the execution of the unsuccessful physicians. Soon 'Abd Yishú' arrived and having inspected the urine and felt his pulse announced to the caliph that the cure required a medicine which would take nine hours to prepare. At the same time he comforted his disgraced colleagues by informing them that the caliph would be dead before the nine hours were passed and that they need have no fear for their lives. The caliph ordered a fee of 10,000 dirhams to be paid to the new doctor and bade him commence at once with his preparation of the remedy. To soothe him 'Abd Yíshu' ordered the druggists to work underneath his window. Thus the last hours of al-Hádí's life were filled with hope by the sound of the clash of pestle upon mortar of those who were struggling to concoct the remedy which would save his life.[1]

Rumour said that the end of al-Hádí was not natural, but that the illness was abruptly terminated by some slave girls, who smothered him at the orders of his mother, who had already prepared letters for the various governors, ordering them to recognize Hárún as his successor.[2] Whatever be the truth, Hárún-ul-Rashíd found himself at the early age of twenty-five ruler of an empire which extended to Constantinople and Tangier in the west and to India in the east. His day of accession was marked by two auspicious events. One was the birth to him on that very day of his favourite son al-Ma'mún and the other was his discovery in the bed of the Tigris of a ring which he had thrown there in a fit of temper several years before.

Bukht Yishú', finding that his services were no longer required and that his position at court was unpleasant on account of the ill-feeling manifested towards him by the mother of the late caliph and by Abú Quraysh, returned to Jundí Shápúr. In the following year, however, he was recalled.[3] Hárún was ill this time. His *wazír*, Yaḥyá bin Khálid the Barmecide, suggested to Hárún that Abú Quraysh had been physician to his father and to his mother and was quite capable of treating his headache. But Hárún would have none of him; the honour that he showed to him was solely on account of his past services, not because he valued him. Yaḥyá then suggested Bukht Yishú'. Hárún, though he knew nothing of him, not even whether he were still alive, preferred to place himself under him if it were possible. So Bukht Yishú' was again summoned to the royal court. On his arrival he presented himself to Hárún. The caliph was unwilling to speak

1 *I.A.U.* vol. I, p. 125.
2 *Hist. Dynst.* vol. IX, p. 152.
3 Ibid.

to him and deputed Yaḥyá to conduct the interview. Yaḥyá, however, did not feel competent to pass judgement on the merits of Bukht Yishú' and summoned Abú Quraysh, al-Ṭayfúrí, and Ibn Sarábiyún. But so great was the fame of Bukht Yishú' that even Abú Quraysh preferred not to pit his wits against his and exclaimed: 'O Commander of the Faithful, there is no one in this company capable of speaking with this man. For he is a master of disputation. He, his father, and his whole family are all of them philosophers.'[1] A striking admission by an unfriendly Mussulman towards a Christian colleague.

So Hárún himself determined to test his skill and calling for the urine of a mule presented it to Bukht Yishú' for a diagnosis. Abú Quraysh swore it was the urine of a favourite slave girl. Bukht Yishú' calmly examined it and exclaimed that in that case the girl was bewitched, for only a mule could pass such urine. When asked what treatment he would give to such a one, he replied that a good feed of barley would be the most suitable. Hárún was delighted, rewarded him with a dress and money, and making him his chief personal physician bade all the others present stand below him.

From that moment Bukht Yishú' resigned his position at Jundí Shápúr and stayed in the service of the caliph. He also attended Ja'far the Barmecide, but a few years later, when Ja'far again fell ill, he excused himself and sent in his place his son, who, he said, knew more than he did and was a physician without equal. He died full of honours in the year 801.

With Jibrá'íl, his son, at the court the family fortunes rose higher than they had ever done before. His successful cure of a favourite slave of the caliph, whom he healed of a hysterical paralysis, led to his appointment as a court physician. The wealth of the Bukht Yishú' family increased; but they were no longer the men of science that they were while they remained at Jundí Shápúr. The characters of Jibrá'íl and the later members of the family do not command the respect that his father and

1 *I.A.U.* vol. 1, p. 126.

Jurjís I must receive from every reader of their biographies. Jibrá'íl lived in a court of splendour, surrounded by intrigue and undignified squabbles. Jibrá'íl entered into this life wholeheartedly. His house and his person equalled in luxury that of the caliph; his intrigues and his quarrels were only matched by those of his colleagues. Gone were those days of scientific isolation which made the director of the school of Jundí Sh͟ápúr the most sought-after physician in Islam. Jibrá'íl could say that the foundation of his medical knowledge were his father's lectures and his father's experience. But no succeeding member of the family could say that. And though a member of the Buk͟ht Yis͟hú' family continued to serve in the court of the caliph until the coming of 'Aẓud-ul-Doula, the scientific pre-eminence of the family departed with the enormous wealth and prestige which Jibrá'íl acquired.

In his capacity as personal physician to Hárún, Jibrá'íl was obliged to accompany him wherever he went and necessarily therefore saw much of the *wazír* Ja'far the Barmecide, who was Hárún's closest companion. The Barmecide family was an old and distinguished one. The first of the line whose name history has preserved was a physician of Balkh. According to Mas'údí, Barmak was not a name, but a title borne by the high priest of the Fire Temple in the city.[1] More probably it was a Buddhist title which Persian pride changed into something more Iranian. As a physician Barmak's claim to fame is the pill, which was named after him, and which was recommended by Avicenna[2] and later writers, and a scent which was widely used by prostitutes.

In the fighting that took place around Balkh in the year 705 the wife of Barmak the physician was captured and given as a slave to 'Abd-Ulláh, the brother of the successful Arab general. When peace was made, the woman was restored to her husband. But the short union with 'Abd-Ulláh produced a son, who was known as K͟hálid the Barmecide. K͟hálid was acknowledged by 'Abd-Ulláh as his natural son, entered the service of the caliph

1 Ibn K͟hallikán, vol. II, p. 460.

2 *Canon*, bk. V, I. 9.

through his assistance, and rapidly rose to the highest rank. In 749 he was a general and becoming known to al-Ṣaffáḥ was given the post of chief of the exchequer.[1] He may thus be considered to be the first to hold the office of *wazír*. He retained this position under al-Manṣúr and was in charge of the building of new Baghdad. Both his personal courage and his taste are proved by his protest against the destruction of Seleucia and Ctesiphon in order to provide materials for the new city.

For some unknown reason Khálid fell into disgrace and was ordered to pay a fine of three million dirhams. His son Yaḥyá begged all round of his friends in order to raise this sum, but was unable to do so. Fortunately at that moment riots broke out in Mosul and Khálid was appointed to the governorship and the fine was forgotten. At the same time Yaḥyá was appointed governor of Azerbaijan. While still at Ray there was born to Yaḥyá a son whom he named al-Faẓal who was born simultaneously with al-Mahdí's son Hárún. So close was the friendship between al-Mahdí and Yaḥyá that the two infants changed mothers. Al-Khayzurán, the wife of the caliph, gave the breast to al-Faẓal and Zubayda, who was a mulatto girl from Medina, gave hers to Hárún. In consequence in after life Hárún always referred to al-Faẓal as his brother.[2]

Khálid was now placed in charge of the young Hárún and accompanied him as tutor in his early campaigns. On his death his place in the royal family was taken by Yaḥyá, who loyally supported the claims of Hárún to succeed al-Hádí, even suffering imprisonment for a short time. Hárún rewarded this loyalty on his accession by installing him as his *wazír* and by granting almost unlimited power to his two sons al-Faẓal and Ja'far. The latter became the favourite of Hárún and the boon companion of his privacy. With Hárún and Masrúr he is the hero of those nightly adventures which form so large a part of the stories of the *Arabian Nights*.

1 Ibn Khallikán, vol. I, p. 305.
2 Ibid. vol. II, p. 459.

As the years passed Yaḥyá resigned his offices into the hands of his two sons. Al-Faẓal became virtual ruler of the empire. Ja'far, although associated with lighter occupations, must nevertheless have been a man in whom the caliph had complete faith, for he gave into his hands the direction of the youthful al-Ma'mún and retained him in the wazirate for 17 years.

Many are the delightful anecdotes which are told to illustrate his wisdom. It is said that a certain Jewish astrologer once predicted to Hárún that he would die within a year. This much distressed Hárún, who firmly believed in the truth of the prophecy. Ja'far promptly sent for the Jew and asked him if it were true that this was his considered opinion. When the Jew replied that it was, he then asked him how long the stars foretold that he himself, that is the Jew, was destined to live. When he replied that he had a great many more years of life Ja'far promptly had him hanged upon the public gibbet in order that Hárún might see how little faith could be placed in his reading of the stars. So fond was Hárún of Ja'far that he had a special cloak made with two separate collars, so that he and Ja'far could both wear it at the same time.

During his service at the court Jibrá'íl bin Bukht Yishú' was also physician to the Barmecides, for it is recorded that he served that family for 13 years. It also fell to his lot to be present on that fatal night when the family fell from power. This was in the year A.D. 802. For several days past Jibrá'íl noticed that Hárún had lost his appetite. Yet he could find no cause for this nor any sign of disease. He recommended a change of air and Hárún moved a little way out of the city. He took with him Ja'far and Jibrá'íl. The change did him no good, but on the contrary he ate even less. One Thursday Jibrá'íl noticed that he ate nothing at all. On the Friday morning Hárún got up early and he and Ja'far rode out together. Jibrá'íl remarked that he kissed Ja'far that morning and held his hand in his for nearly a mile. In the evening Hárún dismissed Jibrá'íl, saying that he wished to be left alone and bade him eat and enjoy himself with Ja'far.

So Ja'far and Jibrá'íl dined together. After dinner Abú Zakár, the blind poet, came in to sing. But there was a strained air over the party: even the songs were dirges rather than carousals. A servant came in and whispered in the ear of Ja'far that the caliph had again not eaten all that day. Of a sudden there entered upon them Masrúr, the chief executioner, Harişima, the sub-executioner, and a company of soldiers. Harişima bade Ja'far arise. Nothing was said to Jibrá'íl and he slipped away to his own quarters. Ja'far could not believe that a command for his death had been given and persuaded Harişima to return to the caliph and report his death. And, he added: 'If he express regret, I shall owe thee my life; and if not, the will of Allah be done.' So saying he followed the slave to hear how the caliph would take the message. To his dismay he heard his master say: 'O slave, if thou answer me another word, I will send thee before him.' And forthwith the slave returned and slew Ja'far. Half an hour later the caliph sent for Jibrá'íl to come to his tent and there he saw to his horror the head of Ja'far upon a plate. Then Hárún explained to him his loss of appetite. 'Reflection about this matter which thou seest here, drove me to the state in which I was. But to-day, O Jibrá'íl, I feel myself like a camel. So bring me food that thou mayest see how wonderfully my appetite has increased beyond what it was. Verily I used to turn from dish to dish lest I might feel heavy and it might make me sick.' 'And then', added Jibrá'íl in his account of this night, 'he called for his food straightway and that evening he did eat a full meal.'[1]

The caliph seems in this affair to have been seized with a momentary madness. For on the one hand he had the unfortunate slave killed because, as he says, he could not bear to look upon the slayer of Ja'far, and on the other hand he continued to show his jealousy by slaughtering the whole of the Barmecide family and giving orders for the exhibition of the head of Ja'far on one side of the Tigris and of the body on the other, after which both were burnt.

1 *I.A.U.* vol. 1, p. 134.

Yaḥyá and al-Faẓal were both kept in prison and their property confiscated. After a time, suspecting that there were still some of the possessions of al-Faẓal which had not yet fallen into his hands, Hárún sent Masrúr to him in prison with orders to give him 200 strokes of the whip unless he confessed to the whereabouts of the remainder of his wealth. Al-Faẓal protested that there were no undisclosed possessions. Upon which Masrúr, disbelieving him, ordered the flogging to commence. So severely did they beat him that he nearly died. A surgeon of the neighbourhood, skilled in treating wounds, was called in. After examining al-Faẓal the surgeon declared that there were not marks of more than 50 strokes on his back and that he must lie down on his back upon a reed mat so that he might tread upon his breast. Al-Faẓal shuddered, but consented. The surgeon then trod upon him and afterwards taking him by the arms dragged him along the mat. By this process a great quantity of flesh was torn from his back. He then dressed the wounds.

Some days later after his examination the surgeon declared that the patient was safe because new flesh was forming. He then said: 'Did I not say that he had received fifty strokes? By Allah, a thousand strokes could not have left more marks. I merely said so that he might take courage and thus aid my efforts to cure him.' Al-Faẓal on his recovery borrowed 10,000 dirhams from a friend and sent them to the surgeon, who returned the money. Thinking that he had offered too little, he borrowed 10,000 more. But the man refused these too, saying that he could not accept a fee for curing the greatest among the generous.

Al-Faẓal died a natural death, but still in prison. When Hárún was informed of his death, he exclaimed: 'My fate is near unto his.' And so it proved, for he died in less than six months after.

The cause of the outburst must for ever remain a mystery. That the house of 'Abbás was prone to sudden violent fits of temper is well known. Writers of that period describe a vein in the forehead, which they say used to swell whenever the caliph was under the influence of any violent emotion. Possibly Hárún was incensed with Ja'far for having consummated the marriage with his sister 'Abbásah whom he had married to him on the condition that she was to remain a virgin. At any rate Hárún in a fit of orthodoxy punished 'Abbásah by burying both her and her child alive. Possibly even he was enraged against a family which was nicknamed Zanádiqa, that is, the 'Students of Zend literature', or in popular meaning, heretic, agnostic. But, as says an almost contemporary writer: 'Of a truth the Barmecides did nothing to deserve al-Rashíd's severity. But the day of their power and prosperity had been long and whatso endureth long waxeth longsome.'[1]

The fall of the Barmecides made no difference to the house of Bukht Yishú': Hárún continued to shower presents upon Jibrá'íl. He even took him with him on the pilgrimage to Mecca and when reproached for taking a Christian to the Holy City, replied that the fortunes of the empire depended upon himself and he himself depended upon Jibrá'íl.

During the last and fatal illness of Hárún the too candid exercise of his profession nearly caused his downfall. A bishop whom the caliph consulted in his place, incited Hárún still further against him, and he was finally condemned to death. His life was spared through the intercession of a *wazír*.

When al-Amín succeeded Hárún-ul-Rashíd, Jibrá'íl was restored to favour and became once more the royal physician. Nothing is related about him during this short reign except that the caliph in a drunken fit compelled him one night to change clothes with the captain of the guard and to march up and down all night.

By the time that al-Ma'mún came to the throne Jibrá'íl was an old man, but not old enough to be passed over by the new ruler who fancied that Jibrá'íl had neglected him in his youth. He was accordingly thrown into prison and it was only because the *wazír* al-Ḥasan bin Sahl required his services that he regained his freedom. Three years later he again fell into disgrace and was succeeded by his son Miká'íl. In 827 al-Ma'mún had again to

1 Ibn Khallikán, vol. 1, p. 309.

send for him as Miká'íl was unable to give advice regarding an illness of the caliph. His cure of the caliph completely restored him to favour. But his character was unchanged. He still sought to increase his wealth and still frequently abused his influence with the caliph. It is said that at this time he wished to build a house at Basra. He demanded for this purpose 500 beams from the governor of the city. Abú ul-Rází, the governor, thought the demand excessive and would allow him only 200, adding that Jibrá'íl was the most contemptuous of creatures that he knew.

Shortly after this al-Ma'mún announced his intention of visiting Basra and Abú ul-Rází put himself to great expense to provide him with a fitting entertainment. To his bitter disappointment Jibrá'íl would not allow al-Ma'mún even to taste any of the exquisite food which was set before him and after a few hours declared that the heat of Basra was too great for the caliph's health to withstand. So the caliph and his train departed, leaving his host much mortified. As the last man passed through the gates, bitterly did Abú ul-Rází exclaim: 'Verily there is no comparison between the difference in cost of 500 and 200 beams of wood and the cost of entertaining the caliph.'[1]

Finally, in the year A.D. 828, when al-Ma'mún was setting out on an expedition against the Greeks Jibrá'íl asked to be excused from accompanying him and sent in his place his son Bukht Yishú'. And so, full of honours he died and was buried in the convent of S. Sergius. His written works include an open letter to al-Ma'mún on Food and Drink, a work on Logic, an epitome of medicine, and one or two similar minor works. He encouraged translations and is said to have patronized Ḥunayn, saying that he could not honour such a man too much and that if he lived, his work would eclipse that of Sergius. His brother Jurjís was also a physician to al-Ma'mún, but an account of his son must be kept to a later chapter.

The success of the Bukht Yishú' family tempted yet another of the staff of the hospital at Jundí Shápúr to seek his fortunes in

1 *I.A.U.* vol. 1, p. 133.

Baghdad. I refer to the pharmacist Másawayh, the father of the two famous physicians, Miká'íl and Yúḥanná. In his case it was not a deliberate choice which made him seek his fortunes in the imperial city, but stern necessity. For 30 years he worked in the dispensary at Jundí Shápúr, an uneducated man, unable either to read or write. At that time Jibrá'íl bin Bukht Yishú' was senior physician to the hospital. Being well pleased with his dispenser he bought for him for the sum of 800 dinars a slave girl who belonged to another physician of the hospital.

A few years later Jibrá'íl succeeded his father at the court of the caliph and his duties at Jundí Shápúr devolved upon others. No doubt there was a certain amount of complaint and perhaps of jealousy among the hospital staff. The words of Másawayh, who had least reason to be envious, were carried to Jibrá'íl's ears. 'This Abú 'Ísá', he is reported to have said, 'has indeed reached the stars. Yet we, we cannot escape from this hospital.'[1]

His wish was fulfilled only too literally as soon as Jibrá'íl heard it. He was immediately expelled and bidden to practise his art elsewhere. In despair Másawayh made his way to Baghdad in order to present his excuses and apologies to Jibrá'íl in person. But Jibrá'íl would not even receive him. In vain Másawayh poured benedictions on his head as he passed; Jibrá'íl took not the least notice of him.

At last, short of money and with no prospect of regaining Jibrá'íl's favour, he betook himself to the Christian quarter of the city and begged for a seat in a monastery porch, thinking that here perhaps something good might turn up for him. A priest, discovering that he knew something of medicine, advised him to practise as a mendicant physician and to take up his stand at the gates of the palace of a certain al-Faẓal bin ul-Rabí', who was then a minister to the caliph.

Chance provided him with his first case. A servant of the minister fell ill with some disease of the eye. The orthodox physicians could do nothing. In despair the servant bade

1 Ibid. p. 171.

Másawayh cure him or clear out. It was just such a chance that Másawayh sought. He exerted his utmost skill; he remembered the various applications which he had dispensed for so many years for the ophthalmologists in Jundí Shápúr; and in a few days the eye of the servant recovered. The servant in due course reported his success to his master and, when the eye of al-Fażal also became affected, Másawayh was called in. In the house of al-Fażal he met once more his old chief. Jibrá'íl was still the haughty physician who despised an ignorant apothecary and refused to pardon a humble colleague, even after 30 years of distinguished service. In Baghdad, however, the scales were more equal than they were in Jundí Shápúr and after a few minutes of undignified wrangling Jibrá'íl left the room, fearing that his discomfiture would be noted. Al-Fażal therefore retained the services of Másawayh as his private physician and bade him summon his wife with her little sons to Baghdad.

The success of Másawayh did not stop here. The Caliph al-Rashíd too fell ill of some disease of the eye and his minister al-Fażal seized the opportunity to relate to him the story of his own case. The caliph bade him send Másawayh to his presence. His luck still held and Másawayh became the ophthalmologist to the caliph. In this capacity he also had the honour of attending the sister of the caliph. Here his prognosis was contrary to that of Jibrá'íl and for his temerity he was thrown into gaol. When time verified him, he was at once released and rewarded by being made the equal both in honour and salary with the haughty Jibrá'íl.

In the meantime his sons had grown up and two of them had become regular and orthodox doctors. One son 'Ísá was afflicted with melancholia, said to have been brought on by excess of study. Another, Miká'íl, is chiefly famous for his die-hard conservative attitude towards all medical thought. He would employ no drug which had not proved its efficacy by at least 200 years of use. He would not even eat a banana because he could find no evidence that the ancients considered it a suitable food. Nevertheless, he became a personal physician to al-Ma'mún, not yet caliph, and his opinion is said to have been preferred to that of Jibrá'íl bin Bukht Yishú' on all medical questions.

The remaining son, Yúḥanná, is by far the most famous of the three and it is because of him that posterity estimates the family of Másawayh above that of the Bukht Yishú's. According to Leo Africanus, Yúḥanná was born in the year A.D. 777. The young man originally chose an ecclesiastical life and had already received minor orders when a taste for science caused him to abandon his monastery. In his later years he was by no means a friend of the Church.

Early in his medical career he was chosen by al-Ma'mún, not yet caliph, to be his personal physician during the time that he was governor of Khorasan. From this task he was recalled by Hárún-ul-Rashíd, who charged him with the duty of translating into Arabic the many Greek medical manuscripts which conquest and treaty had delivered into his hands. Yúḥanná is even said to have gone in person to Greece to search for more material.

In his capacity as a court physician Yúḥanná served four caliphs —al-Ma'mún, al-Mu'taṣim, al-Wáṣiq, and al-Mutawakkil. His reputation as a clinician exceeded that of all the physicians of Baghdad. A contemporary writer states that his consulting room was the most crowded of all in the city and that in his waiting room were to be seen all the leading doctors, theologians and philosophers. His fame as a teacher, too, excelled that of all others in Baghdad. His pupils had the reputation of being the best instructed of all students in logic and in the writings of Galen.[1] The most famous of these pupils was Ḥunayn, whom Yúḥanná with an astonishing lack of judgement held to be incapable of learning medicine and expelled from his classes in disgrace.

With all his success his tongue was terribly sharp and fools he could not suffer gladly. To a patient who consulted him about some illness and who on being recommended to let a little blood replied that he was not accustomed to be bled, he exclaimed:

1 *I.A.U.* vol. 1, p. 175.

'No one is accustomed to being bled while in the bowels of his mother. Neither are you accustomed to your illness. Either grow accustomed to being bled or put up with your disease.' To another patient who came to him complaining of an irritating skin rash and who countered every piece of advice by saying that he had already tried that treatment, he said: 'Then there is nothing left for you but a remedy which neither Hippocrates nor Galen recommend. Take a piece of paper, cut it into a hundred bits, and write upon each "God be merciful upon one afflicted with ill health". Put half the pieces in the western mosque of the city and half in the eastern. Perhaps God will help you by prayer; He will not by medicine.'[1]

Yúḥanná was married to a daughter of al-Ṭayfúrí, a colleague of the court. By her he had a son who most unfortunately died during an illness as the result, according to al-Ṭayfúrí, of an unwise phlebotomy by Yúḥanná. After this the relations between the Ṭayfúrí family and Yúḥanná became somewhat strained. Their two houses were situated in the eastern quarter of Baghdad side by side. Yúḥanná kept a peacock which often sat upon the party-wall. This peacock screeched out during the hot nights and kept the members of the Ṭayfúrí family awake. At last, Daniel, one of the sons of al-Ṭayfúrí, a physician who had become a monk, picking up a hammer hit the peacock on the head and killed it. Yúḥanná did not discover the crime until the following evening, when finding the peacock dead he began to curse the murderer. Daniel admitted the crime and offered to give him several more peacocks to atone for it. But Yúḥanná was not thus to be comforted and roundly abused Daniel as a hunched-back, long-winded monk to whom killing was nothing but from whom admission of the guilt was astonishing. To which Daniel replied that nothing could surprise him in a lay brother who kept many wives and they not above reproach.

Yúḥanná could never resist a cut at his fellow Christians. A certain 'Ísá bin Ibráhím (that is, Jesus, son of Abraham) had

1 *Hist. Dynst.* vol. IX, p. 154.

embraced Islam. On returning home after he had heard the news Yúḥanná exclaimed to the assembled company: 'Go away, for the Messiah has turned Moslem.' To a priest who came to him complaining of the stomach ache, he recommended a series of remedies. At last, when the priest said that they were all useless, he roared out in anger: 'Go away, then. Turn Mussulman. Perhaps Islam will cure your stomach.' Even on his death-bed he bade the praying clergy hold their peace, 'for', said he, 'a few pills will do more good than all your prayers though they go on until the Day of the Resurrection.'

His manners, and perhaps his success, made him many enemies. Besides the Ṭayfúrí family, another colleague named Salmawaíh bin Bunán, a Christian and a much-loved physician of the Caliph al-Mu'taṣim, had neither love for nor confidence in him. When he lay dying he counselled the caliph to consult Yúḥanná as rarely as possible. In any case Yúḥanná would probably have fallen from favour on account of a rude reply to the Caliph al-Wáṯiq. The two were out fishing one day. The caliph could not hook a fish and at last bade Yúḥanná depart as he thought he was bringing him bad luck. 'How can I be unlucky?' said Yúḥanná, 'I am the son of a purchased slave girl; yet I am the friend of caliphs. I will tell you who is the really demented one. That is the man who, though a prince and the son of a prince, yet leaves his palace for a hut by a river and indulges in a sport which is only fit for the lowest of men.'

Yúḥanná died at Sámarra in the year A.D. 857. A wit of the day wrote upon him the following epigram (I borrow Professor Browne's translation):

Verily the physician, with his physic and his drugs,
Cannot avert a summons that hath come.
What ails the physician that he dies of the disease
Which he used to cure in time gone by?
There died alike he who administered the drug and he who took the drug,
And he who imported and sold the drug and he who bought it.[1]

1 Browne, *Arabian Medicine*, p. 8.

He left behind him no children to carry on his name, but instead a large number of written works. The subjects of these range through all branches of medicine—clinical studies, gynaecology, pharmacy, anatomy, and even in a lighter vein. Nearly all these have disappeared. Of the Arabic texts two are preserved in the library at Leyden, one being a tract on diet and the other a brief work on medical curiosities. There are also extant two copies of his *Daghal-ul-'Ayn* or Alterations of the Eye, one at Leningrad and one at Cairo. This work is of particular interest because it is the earliest surviving Arabic ophthalmological treatise that is known to-day. His work is also known through the Latin translations of the Middle Ages. By the medieval translators he was known as Mesue Senior or Janus Damascenus. Nine Latin editions exist to-day in the British Museum. The earliest is dated 1462, the latest 1623. The *Mesue Opera*, printed in Venice in 1603, is illustrated.

Associated with Yúḥanná, at least in his own estimation, was another physician, for he claimed to be the father of Yúḥanná by seducing his mother. He was a Persian, who had deserted Ahwaz for Baghdad, and was named Sahl bin Sábúr al-Kúsaj. Whether he made his claim in jest or because he believed it to be true, is uncertain. Yúḥanná vigorously denied it. Probably it was quite untrue, for at the time of making his will al-Kúsaj named Jibrá'íl as another illegitimate son. He also had a son lawfully begotten, whom he named Sábúr after his grandfather. He too followed the profession of medicine. The young man, however, preferred the quiet life of Jundí Sh̲ápúr to the scandals and rush of Baghdad. So he returned to Ahwaz. He was soon appointed to the staff of the hospital of Jundí Sh̲ápúr and there he composed his *Aqarabádín-i-Kabír* or Great Pharmacopoeia, which became the first pharmacopoeia to receive universal acceptance throughout the caliphate, indeed almost throughout the Islamic world. His big pharmacopoeia consisted of 22 books. For the use of smaller hospitals and for private practitioners he wrote another which he called the Lesser Pharmacopoeia. Both are quoted by Rhazes in his *Continens*. Sábúr bin Sahl died in A.D. 869.[1]

It is important to distinguish Mesue Senior from Mesue Junior. The former is a person of considerable importance in the history of Arabian medicine; the latter is of so little importance that many hold that no such person ever existed. It is suggested that Mesue Junior was a name invented to add Arabian prestige to a commonplace medieval text-book. The sole authority for his existence, apart from the printed books, is Leo Africanus. According to him there was born at Marind on the Euphrates a certain Másawayh, who studied medicine and philosophy in Baghdad, and who died there in 1015. The works of this man were translated into Latin from the original Arabic by a Sicilian Jew who gave to the author the title of Mesue Junior. The original manuscript was then lost, and the world was left with the *Canones Generales*, *Simplicia*, *Antidotarium* and *Grabadin Medicinarum Particularium*, which are said to have come from the pen of Másawayh al-Marindí. These works were among those most widely read by medieval physicians. The *Grabadin* was for centuries the recognized authority on pharmacy throughout Europe and became the basis of later official pharmacopoeias.

The whole question of Mesue Junior is full of mystery. Questions at once arise: Was there such a person at all as Másawayh al-Marindí? When did he live? Who made the Latin translation? What was the authority for the statements which were made by Leo Africanus? According to the Latin text his full name was Joannes filius Mesue filii Hamech filii Abdela regis Damasci. Putting this back into an Arabic form gives the name Yúḥanná bin Másawayh bin Aḥmad bin 'Abd-Ulláh. Rex Damasci may well be merely an honorific title, just as Sábúr bin Sahl is sometimes called by the medieval schoolmen Rex Medorum. It might also be an error of the translator, who read *ḥákim* (governor) for *ḥakím* (doctor). Neuburger says that the work

1 *Hist. Dynst.* vol. IX, pp. 163, 176.

bears the imprint of the Arabian era.[1] Campbell seems to hold very different views and even to disbelieve in the existence of this Mesue. For he always refers to him as the Pseudo-Mesue.[2] In this he agrees with Karl Sudhoff who states dogmatically that Mesue Junior is 'an assumed name under which in the thirteenth-century writings of occidental origin were issued' and holds that the books which bear his name were written in Bologna or Padua and put into their existing form by Peter of Abano and Francis of Piedmont.[3]

The date at which he lived can be more or less determined by the contents of his works. He quotes two authors under the names of Hamech and Ali Senis. These, Leclerc suggests, are Rhazes and Avicenna.[4] Avicenna died in 1034. The year 1015, the date of Mesue's death according to Leo Africanus, is therefore just possible. Some claim to have identified in his works a quotation from Avenzoar, who died in 1162. But the passage is obscure.

It has been suggested that the work is the translation of a genuine Arab composition and that Mesue Senior and Mesue Junior are one and the same person. There is a great deal to be said in favour of this theory. Both wrote pharmacological treatises. The title Janus Damascenus of Mesue Senior at once recalls the title Rex Damasci of Mesue Junior. The argument based on the names Hamech and Ali Senis is not a very strong one. Hamech is a long way from Abú Bakr, although Ali Senis is not bad for Abú 'Alí Síná. But it is difficult to see why the translator did not use the regular medieval Latin forms of the names of these very well-known men. It is strange, too, that Mesue Junior never quotes from his namesake. Alpagus, too, an Italian doctor who spent many years in the East, states: 'Et ego vidi librum arabicum filii mesue antiquioris, sed librum Mesue

1 Neuburger, *Gesch. d. Med.* (trans. Playfair), vol. 1, p. 370.
2 Campbell, *Arabian Medicine*, vol. 1, p. 77.
3 Kremer, *History of Pharmacy*, p. 21.
4 Leclerc, *Hist. Méd. Arabe*, vol. 1, p. 506.

posterioris nullibi in Arabico reperire potui.' For my own part I believe the two Mesues to be identical and refuse to believe that the most popular medieval text-book of pharmacy is a big hoax.

It was an error of prognosis on the part of Jibrá'íl bin Bukht Yishú' that introduced to the notice of Hárún another physician who became later a court physician. It is said that one evening Ibráhím bin Ṣálaḥ, a cousin to al-Rashíd, fell to the ground in a fit. Jibrá'íl was summoned to attend him and being thus engaged failed to appear at the table of the caliph for the evening meal. Hárún refused to start without him and caused a search to be made and sent servants to summon him, but he was not to be found. When at last he did appear, without waiting to hear any excuses Hárún reproached him and abused him for his absence. Jibrá'íl scornfully replied that it was more fitting for the caliph to set about mourning for his cousin Ibráhím than to indulge in abuse of a physician engaged in his work. The caliph was taken aback and inquired what had happened to Ibráhím. Jibrá'íl curtly told him that he was even at that moment taking his last breath.

The caliph was much upset at the news and demanded if another doctor could not be found who might save him. One of the company put forward the name of Ṣálaḥ bin Nahala, an Indian who had lately arrived in Baghdad and who 'was versed in the methods of Indian medicine as was Jibrá'íl in the science of the Greeks'. Hárún straightway summoned him, and Ṣálaḥ went in to examine Ibráhím. To the astonishment of all he emerged from the patient's room saying: 'If Ibráhím dies to-night of this disease, I will give the triple divorce to all my wives.' Hárún was delighted. But the announcement at that very moment of the death of Ibráhím turned his joy to fury and he began to abuse those who had suggested the Indian.

Ṣálaḥ, however, was not satisfied and he bade the company follow him to the supposed corpse. Drawing a lancet from his pocket, he inserted the blade between the nail and the flesh of the thumb. In the sight of all the dead man drew back his hand. Then he applied some pungent drug to his nostrils and soon the dead man sneezed. Ten minutes later he raised himself and recognized the caliph. It is said that later on Ibráhím received the daughter of Hárún in marriage and was created governor of Palestine and Egypt and Ṣálaḥ was rewarded by being appointed a court physician.[1]

The death of Hárún was caused by what was probably a cancer, for he died at the early age of forty-seven. A wealthy lady of Samarqand, whose husband had long been parted from her and was now living at Baghdad, determined to take another. To avoid all difficulties of divorce she abjured the faith of Islam and took her suitor in a second marriage. Her first husband complained to the caliph who was scandalized at the public insult to the Faith. He gave orders that the second husband should at once divorce her and that he should be paraded upon an ass and cast into prison. All these commands were carried out. Unfortunately, the second husband escaped from his prison and returned to Samarqand, where he slew the governor and took both the lady and the city as his own. Hárún sent a general to subdue the rebellious Samarqandis. But in the meantime other people in those parts became restless and so serious did the situation become that Hárún determined to go himself and restore order. In A.D. 808 he took the field, leaving one son al-Amín in charge of Baghdad and taking al-Ma'mún with him. Hárún was already a sick man. Travelling slowly through the hills of Persia, one day he called to his tent his physician and undoing a silk bandage around his waist showed him the fatal disease from which he was suffering. 'But have a care', he said, 'that thou keep it secret. For my sons are watching the hour of my death, as thou mayest see by the shuffling steed upon which they will now mount me, thus adding to my weakness.' And so, having reached as far as Tus, he died.

1 *I.A.U.* vol. II, p. 34; *Hist. Dynst.* vol. IX, p. 154; Táríkh-ul-Tawáríkh, Brit. Mus. Add. 23514, f. 581.

CHAPTER IV

FROM THE ACCESSION OF AL-AMÍN TO THE CALIPHATE TO THE EXTINCTION OF THE QURRA FAMILY

ON the death of Hárún-ul-Rashíd the long suppressed hatred of the Persian for the Arab conqueror appeared on the surface. Unfortunately, Hárún appointed his son, al-Amín, the child of an Arab wife, to succeed to the caliphate instead of the elder son, al-Ma'mún, the son by a Persian slave girl. The prestige of his father's name was sufficient to secure the throne for al-Amín, and al-Ma'mún was forced to content himself with the governorship of the eastern provinces. But al-Amín was only suffered to reign for a little over four years. Going from folly to folly in those four years he attempted to humiliate his half-brother instead of ruling with him as a friend and an ally. The inevitable civil war broke out and Baghdad was forced to stand a long siege after all the rest of the empire had yielded to al-Ma'mún's general. When at last the capital fell, it was too late for al-Amín to save his life. He was murdered while in flight by some pursuing soldiers and al-Ma'mún became caliph. His accession to the throne represents the final overthrow of the Arab supremacy. The caliph's mother was Persian; his general Ṭáhir was a Persian; and the greater part of the army was Persian. Not a vestige of the old Arab intolerance and self-opinionated superiority remained. Christians, Jews and Muslims were equally regarded: merit, whether literary, scientific or purely physical, was the great key which opened the door to the favour of the caliph. It was the direct consequence of this policy that in his days the renaissance of science and literature reached its zenith. Great were the men of his court, but greater still was his influence which secured for the Arabic-speaking world the thoughts and records of a past age upon which Arab science was to be builded.

Arab medicine, to deal only with one side of this question, borrowed from many sources. The biggest debt was to the Greeks. Greek thought and styles had long been current. The debt to Greece was continually growing greater and greater from the time when Darius forced Democedes to display his skill. Yet it would not be true to say that the study of Greek works, as opposed to the utilization of Greek exponents, was first made possible by the Arabs of the 'Abbásid caliphate. For the medicine of Jundí Sháp´ur was also mainly Greek. There must have been Syriac translations in the library of the hospital there long before the Arabs came to Persia. Even less true would it be to claim for al-Ma'mún the glory of initiating the era of translations which now became the fashion and the craze of his capital.

According to Ibn abí Uṣaybi'a the first to translate Greek works into Syriac was Sergius of Rá's-ul-'Ayn, who translated both medical and philosophical works.[1] It was probably he who worked for Chosroes the Great and it was his translations in all probability which were used in Jundí Shápúr.

Of even greater importance in the advancement among the Arabs of Greek medical ideas were the translations made by the order of Khálid bin Yazíd. The author of the *Fihrist* indeed states that Khálid was the first to have works on medicine, astronomy and alchemy made from other languages into Arabic. It is certain that he was devoted to literature, and both in his stormy childhood and in his later peaceful schemes his story bears a striking resemblance to that of al-Ma'mún. The father of Khálid, being the Umayyad caliph in Damascus, died in A.D. 683, a comparatively young man. His son, a brother of Khálid, succeeded to the throne, but only reigned a few months. On his death the name of Khálid was put forward as the new caliph; but he was held to be too young and another was placed on the throne. The new caliph, Marwán by name, to strengthen his position, married the widow of Yazíd, and, declaring Khálid to be a bastard, proposed to give the succession to his own son. He had reigned scarcely a year

1 *I.A.U.* vol. 1, p. 109.

when he was either poisoned or suffocated with pillows by his new wife. Even then Khálid failed to receive the caliphate. In despair he retired to spend the rest of his life in the encouragement of men of learning and in the cultivation of science, more particularly that of alchemy.

The earliest of the known translations of Greek medicine into the Arabic language is that of the *Pandects* of Ahrun by Másarjoyah. Hárún-ul-Qass (or Ahrun the Priest) of Alexandria, was a Syrian who lived about the time of the birth of Islam. Only one book of his has survived and that only in its translation and even that only in fragments. This was entitled *The Medical Pandects* and rapidly became popular among the Arabs. His description of an ulceration of the leg, presumably a varicose ulcer, was considered so excellent that even in al-Jurjání's time, that is some 600 years later, it was still known as an Aaron's ulcer. The *Pandects* according to Bar Hebraeus consisted of 30 chapters. To these Sergius of Rá's-ul-'Ayn added two more. The original work was in Syriac and was translated from this language into Arabic by Másarjoyah.[1] Some authorities believe that the original was in Greek and that the version which Másarjoyah translated was a Syriac version made by Sergius.

Másarjoyah or Másarjawáih was a Jew, born in Basra. Syriac was his mother tongue. Of his ancestry or date of his birth nothing is known. According to some authorities his translation of the *Pandects* was made in the time of the Caliph Merwan. According to others it was written in the days of a later Umayyad caliph, 'Umar bin 'Abd-ul-'Azíz. The later date seems on all grounds the more probable and the translation can thus be dated fairly certainly to the first decades of the eighth century. Másar joyah was therefore born about A.D. 680.[2]

Most Arabic writers speak very highly of the *Pandects* and quote them with evident approval. Alone Haly Abbas refuses to join in the chorus of praise. 'As for modern writers', he says in the

1 *Hist. Dynst.* vol. VIII, p. 99 and vol. IX, p. 127; *I.A.U.* vol. I, p. 109.
2 *Hist. Dynst.* vol. IX, p. 127; *I.A.U.* vol. I, p. 163; al-Qifṭí, p. 324.

opening chapter of the *Liber Regius*, 'Ahrun has composed a book in which he has discussed all diseases, their causes, symptoms, and treatment. But the physiological and pathological sections are too brief; also he omits entirely preventive medicine and surgery. And besides, the translation is rough, crude and filled with obscure remarks, which may sicken the reader unless he happens to have Ḥunayn's translation.'[1]

Of Másarjoyah's other works one is said to be in existence in Istanbul and is called *Kitáb fí Abdál-il-Adviya* or 'Book on the Substitution of Remedies'. Dr Meyerhof after examining it rejects completely the authorship of Másarjoyah and says that it is only a very poor summary of extracts from early Arabic medical books.[2] Three other works are known through quotations. One is On Food, another On Drugs, and a third is On Diseases of the Eyes. Rhazes repeatedly quotes from these, often only referring to the author as al-Yahúdí or the Jew. Hence, in the Latin translations of the *Continens*, *Judaeus* becomes the title which replaces the name Másarjoyah. Later generations were equally enthusiastic, though it is chiefly the authors of books on simples who quote him. Among these must be mentioned al-Gh̲áfiqí of Cordova and Ibn ul-Bayṭár. These quotations show, as Dr Meyerhof points out, that Másarjoyah had not only a thorough knowledge of the drugs and food regimes of the Greeks, but also himself knew and used many remedies which were imported from the Orient and above all from India.

Of Másarjoyah's character a little can be guessed from the anecdotes which have collected around his name. A man who complained of constipation he nearly killed by ordering him to take raw cucumbers on an empty stomach. To another who complained that every few hours his eyes grew dim and that his stomach felt as though dogs were licking it and that he felt no relief except by taking food, Másarjoyah replied unable to control

1 *Lib. Reg.* vol. 1, p. 1.

2 Meyerhof, 'Mediaeval Jewish Physicians in Near East', *Isis* (May 1938), p. 436.

his anger: 'The curse of God upon this illness. Indeed He made a bad choice when He gave it to such a vile creature as you. Verily I would that a like disease befall me and my children. I would give the half of all that I have to be afflicted with it.' When the man said that he did not understand, Másarjoyah calmed down and explained that the patient had a health which he did not deserve, for these pains were nothing else but the pains of a healthy appetite.

Másarjoyah had at least one son who became a doctor, for it is said that 'Ísá bin Másarjoyah wrote a book on colours and another on odours and flavours.[1]

The passion for Greek science, thus stimulated, grew. The fall of the Umayyad caliphate did not check the renaissance of Greek learning. The growth of the 'Abbásid house transferred the centre of intellectual activity to Baghdad. Here Ibn ul-Muqaffa' about A.D. 750, being then in the service of 'Ísá bin 'Alí, the uncle of the Caliph al-Manṣúr, was busy translating works on medicine and logic out of Pahlaví into Arabic. Forty years later Yúḥanná bin Másawayh or Mesue Senior began his translations. Private individuals, whose tastes and means allowed them to do so, were already forming libraries of Greek and foreign texts and then translating these into Arabic. Of such persons the best known is Yaḥyá bin Khálid the Barmecide. He is said to have given orders to Abú Ḥasan and Salmá to revise a translation of the *Almagest* which had already been made for him by an earlier translator.[2] He also employed Mikna (or Manka, for the name can be read either way), the Indian, to translate for him into Arabic Indian medical works.[3] Among these was a book called the *Sarat*, which was known to the author of the *Ṭuḥfat-ul-Mu'manín* and of which a copy is said now to exist in Paris.[4]

Another private family to which the city of Baghdad owed much for their lavish entertainment of scholars and their encouragement of catholic literary tastes was the family of Músá bin Shákir, the

1 *I.A.U.* vol. I, p. 204.
2 Leclerc, *Hist. Méd. Arabe*, vol. I, p. 176.
3 *I.A.U.* vol. II, p. 33.
4 *Bibl. Nat. Cat.* p. 106.

astronomer of al-Ma'mún. Three sons of Músá, named Muḥammad, Aḥmad, and Ḥasan, known collectively as the Baní Músá 'drew translators from distant countries by the offer of ample rewards and thus made evident the marvels of science. Geometry, engineering, the movements of the heavenly bodies, music and astronomy were the principal subjects to which they turned their attention. But this was only a small number of their acquirements.' They have the additional fame of having introduced to the court both Ḥunayn and Ṣábit ibn Qurra. The translators employed by them are said to have been paid at the rate of 500 dinars a month.[1]

The task of stocking the libraries with new manuscripts was made considerably easier by the recent discovery of how to manufacture paper. Paper, as opposed to parchment and vellum, was a discovery of the Chinese. It was introduced to the Moslem world when Samarqand was captured in A.D. 704. Its use spread westward and in A.D. 794 the first Islamic paper factory was established in Baghdad. Other factories were founded in Tabriz and other important towns and soon various kinds of paper were available for the copyists. One such kind was known as Ja'farí after Ja'far the Barmecide; another was called Núhí after Núh bin Naṣr the Sámánid.

Ibn abí Uṣaybi'a at the end of the ninth section of his book gives a list of the private individuals who indulged in the new craze for translating.[2] Some patrons preferred the Greek text to be rendered into Syriac, others into Arabic. It was probably very largely a question of for whom the translation was intended that settled the question of the language. Christians, Jews and students of Jundí Shápúr would probably understand Syriac better than Arabic and hence works intended for them, which must have included a vast amount of scientific material, were probably at first set out in Syriac. On the other hand the Arabs and the people of Basra and Baghdad would find Syriac largely incomprehensible and works intended for them—and they would be mainly philosophical—would be translated direct into Arabic.

1 *I.A.U.* vol. 1, p. 187. 2 Ibid. p. 203.

This is borne out by a study of Ibn abí Uṣaybi'a's list. Heading the list is a certain Shírshú' bin Quṭrub of Jundí Shápúr, who is said to have bought Greek texts at his own expense in order that they might be translated into Syriac. A Christian is to be found in Sádrí al-Usquf, that is Theodore the Bishop, who is said to have 'occupied himself in searching for manuscripts and getting them translated. Many works were dedicated to him by Christian doctors.' Muḥammad bin 'Abdul Malik ul-Zayyát is said to have spent on his professors, copyists and translators more than 2000 pieces of gold every month. In return to him were dedicated works by most of the eminent physicians of the day.[1]

But all these labours, public spirited and valuable to science though they were, are overshadowed by the enterprise of al-Ma'mún, who backed by the will and the wealth of a caliph attracted to himself the greatest of all the translators. According to the *Fihrist*, al-Ma'mún saw in a dream Aristotle seated upon a throne. This he took to be a direct command to utilize the resources of his state to spread a knowledge of Greek culture. He at once opened up negotiations with the Roman emperor, who was at that time Leo the Armenian, and demanded that there should be delivered to him all the scientific manuscripts of the ancient writers which remained, in order that they might be translated into Arabic. He made no request for either poetry or history. The Arabs of that period were either orthodox followers of Muḥammad's teaching on the subject of poets or else they reckoned their own quite sufficient. Of the history of the past, too, they seem to have shown no interest. And very curiously it was only Greek manuscripts which they demanded. There is no record of any Latin scientific work being translated into Arabic. Had Galen written in Latin instead of in Greek, an even larger field would have challenged the Arabs or alternatively the whole history of medicine would have been different. As it is, the Arabs contented themselves with Greek works on philosophy, medicine, mathematics, music, astronomy and kindred subjects.

1 Ibid. p. 205.

When Leo agreed to supply them with what they wanted, al-Ma'mún at once sent al-Hajjáj bin Maṭar, Ibn ul-Baṭríq and Salmá to Greece to go and choose the manuscripts which were suitable for translation. It is said that they chose what they wanted and burnt everything which they thought unsuitable.[1]

With these works as a foundation al-Ma'mún in the year 830 founded a State college of translators, which was known by the Arabic title of *Bayt-ul-Ḥikmat* or 'House of Wisdom'. Within this library worked the most famous of the Arab translators. Ibn abí Uṣaybi'a gives a list of those who were officially attached to the college. Heading the list is Jurjís who, he says, 'was the very first of the translators of medical works into Arabic'. He means presumably Jurjís II, son of Bukht Yishú' II.

This House of Wisdom was in no sense a school of medicine. It was first and foremost a library containing works which dealt with all the sciences cultivated by the Arabs. Certainly these included works on medicine. It was also a centre of research in the sciences. But there is no evidence to show that it was ever a centre of teaching.

It has been asserted by some that most, if not all, the translations of this period passed into Arabic by way of a Syriac version. This would seem to me to be correct although vigorously denied by Leclerc and others. Many works had already been translated into Syriac and these existing versions would certainly have been employed by the early translators of the college of al-Ma'mún. It would even seem not at all improbable that in many cases a Syriac expert in Greek collaborated with an Arabic expert in Syriac and thus between them the Arabic version of the Greek text was produced. This may even have been the normal method, for the author of the *Fihrist* states that Ḥunayn, who no one can deny was proficient in Syriac and Greek and quite capable of translating direct from the Greek into Arabic, mostly 'translated the Greek into Syriac, while Ḥubaysh translated from Syriac into Arabic, the Arabic version being then revised by Ḥunayn,

1 *I.A.U.* vol. I, p. 187.

who, however, sometimes translated direct from Greek into Arabic'.[1]

Little incidents which are recorded casually seem to show that any great knowledge of foreign languages was regarded with surprise, even in the most highly educated. Thus, Jurjís bin Bukht Yishú', the chief physician of Jundí Shápúr, when called upon to attend the Caliph al-Manṣúr, on reaching Baghdad greeted him in Arabic and Persian much to the astonishment of the caliph.[2] It is said that Ḥunayn had to go to Basra to learn Arabic and the story of his journey to Greece to learn Greek is well known. If in Jundí Shápúr, a university town, it was difficult to learn Arabic, how much more difficult would it be to learn Greek in either Khuzistan or Baghdad?

The Sabean translators, Ṣ̈ábit and others, probably knew Greek better than they knew Arabic, for the Sabeans always boasted of their semi-Hellenic culture. It would seem, too, that al-Kindí (who confined himself mainly to mathematics) knew Greek well. But these were exceptions. The only internal evidence that the pro-Greek school can produce is the accuracy of the transliteration of the Greek technical terms in these early translations. But it may well be answered that it is known that Ḥunayn revised many of the translations and this accuracy may be due to the work of the official revisers who would, of course, be men well versed in Greek. It does not necessarily follow that the writers of the Arabic version knew Greek.

Of the many names that have come down to posterity who occupied themselves at this period in translating and were attached to the royal college, no name is more famous than that of Ḥunayn. He was called by his contemporaries Abú Zayd Ḥunayn ibn Isḥáq al-'Ibádí; to the medieval world he was Johannitius Onan and Humainus. He was born at Hira in A.D. 809, and was the son of a druggist. His father belonged to that strange sect of Christian Arabs who had withdrawn

1 Al-Qifṭí, p. 289.
2 *Hist. Dynst.* vol. IX, p. 143.

themselves to a small fortified village near Hira and had received the title of al-'Ibád or 'the Slaves'. Al-S̤alabí in his Commentary on the Qur'án says that these people were called the Slaves because they were subservient to the king of Persia. Ḥunayn was destined to follow his father's footsteps, for he was sent to Jundí Shápúr and later studied under Yúḥanná ibn Másawayh. He was a troublesome pupil though, probably too eager to ask questions and learn. One day, losing his patience Yúḥanná exclaimed: 'What have the people of Hira to do with medicine? Go and change money in the streets.' And he drove him out in tears. Ḥunayn did not lose heart at this rebuff, and determined to put to a good use his enforced exile. He spent it in learning Greek, possibly going to Greece itself. He then went to Basra to learn the intricacies of Arabic grammar. Then he settled down to study clinical medicine. He began by attending the lectures of Jibrá'íl bin Bukht Yishú'.

Here he at once attracted the attention of the lecturer, who always addressed him with very great respect and to the surprise of the onlookers gave him the title of Rabban or Master, being still ignorant of who he was.

His reconciliation with his old and first teacher makes a charming story. Without giving his name he sent him his translation of the *Aphorisms* of Hippocrates. When Yúḥanná bin Másawayh read it, he was filled with astonishment and declared that it must have been written by the inspiration of the Holy Ghost. 'Not at all,' was the answer, 'it is by the pupil whom you drove away some time since.' Then he begged to be reconciled to Ḥunayn and they remained together in harmony and friendship until death parted them.[1]

His two earliest translations were that of Galen's *De Differentiis Febrium* and the *De Typis Febrium*. They were presented to Jibrá'íl bin Bukht Yishú' who was then physician in ordinary to the caliph. Recognizing at once the merit in these works he

1 For Ḥunayn's life, see *Hist. Dynst.* vol. IX, p. 171; Ibn Khallikán, vol. I, p. 478; Meyerhof, *Ten Treatises*, Introduction.

recommended the young man to the caliph and secured for him the post of chief of the house of learning.

Very soon after this appointment Jibrá'íl died and his son Bukht Yishú' III took his place. Within a year the great caliph died also and was succeeded by al-Mu'taṣim. For the moment the Bukht Yishú' family were out of favour; but the new physician to the caliph, Salmawaíh bin Bunán, was equally, if not more, friendly to Ḥunayn than Jibrá'íl had been. In recompense for his kindness Ḥunayn translated for him thirteen of Galen's most important works.

Ḥunayn continued his work, both as a translator and as a practitioner, under the new caliph and under his successor al-Wáṣiq. Ḥunayn himself states that his translating began to improve a great deal after he reached the age of thirty. About this time he took into association with himself his nephew Ḥubaysh, whose fame as a translator was only excelled by that of his uncle.

On the death of al-Wáṣiq a fanatical and intolerantly orthodox caliph succeeded to the throne in the person of al-Mutawakkil. Intrigue, the curse of oriental courts, and the failing of the Bukht Yishú' family now began to shake the position of Ḥunayn. First the caliph bade him prepare a cup of poison for use against his enemies. This is generally taken to have been a test of Ḥunayn's loyalty. But I think it more probable that there was no snare here and that the caliph genuinely wanted the poison for a very practical use and was infuriated by Ḥunayn's refusal. For he threw Ḥunayn into prison and when he again brought him up, threatened him with death. But Ḥunayn answered him calmly: 'I have skill only in what is beneficial. I have studied naught else.' The caliph was moved at the transparent honesty of the man who was still in the full vigour of life and yet threatened with death, and asked him what power had enabled him thus bravely to refuse to fulfil his request. 'Two things', replied Ḥunayn, 'my religion and my profession. My religion commands me to do good to my enemies, how much more to my friends.

My profession is founded for the use of my fellow-men and only for their welfare. It is incumbent upon a physician therefore never to prepare a nocuous drug.'

His second misfortune was due to the intrigues of Bukht Yishú' bin Jibrá'íl or, according to another version, to the plot of a fellow-Christian physician Isrá'íl bin Zakariyyá al-Ṭayfúrí. Bukht Yishú' had a picture painted of the Blessed Virgin Mary. This he showed to al-Mutawakkil who inquired if all the Christians had an equal veneration for such a picture. 'Yes', said Bukht Yishú' 'with the exception of one man', and he named Ḥunayn. Al-Mutawakkil therefore called up Ḥunayn and said to him: 'Do you see this picture? It is a representation of your Lord and His Mother.' 'Heaven preserve me', replied Ḥunayn, 'from believing that it is possible for them to be represented. This is only a simple picture, such as may be seen in our churches and other places.' 'It is a matter of no importance then?' asked the caliph. 'Even as you say, O Prince of the Faithful', replied Ḥunayn. 'If that is all that it is, then you can spit upon it', said the caliph. And Ḥunayn, who had apparently imbibed very Puritan principles, spat upon the picture.

The caliph was astonished at this action and reported him to the Catholicos, the head of the Nestorians of Baghdad. Thereupon the Catholicos had him imprisoned and flogged; the caliph had him fined and deprived of his books. Ḥunayn's own words are remarkably pathetic. 'I lost all the books which I had gradually collected during the course of the whole of my adult life in all the lands in which I had travelled, all of which books I lost at one blow.'

But these trials did not end his life. Four months later he was released from prison in order to attend al-Mutawakkil who had fallen ill, and being successful his books and his money were restored to him. Moreover, his enemies, the two court physicians, were ordered to pay to him 10,000 dirhams each, and very soon after Bukht Yishú' fell into bad odour with the caliph and was banished and died in A.D. 870 without ever regaining the royal favour.

Bar Hebraeus gives a slightly different version of the story and says that he was excommunicated for his sacrilegious act and that the same night he died of poison.

After his restoration to favour, Ḥunayn, by no means yet an old man, settled down with renewed vigour to his work of translating. He was now helped by his son Isḥáq and his nephew Ḥubaysh and a troop of pupils. His body had been ill-treated when he was young and again in middle age he had suffered much. Now he gave himself over to luxury. Every morning he would take a ride on horseback and returning would take a Turkish bath. Here he would sit for a while, drink a cup of wine and eat a cake or two. Then he would sleep a while, then eat the mid-day meal, and then sleep again. Four pints of old wine is said to have been his daily allowance. Leading such a life, unworried and calm, he outlived five more caliphs and finally died in the year A.D. 873 or 877 during the caliphate of al-Mu'tamid. It is said that two months before his death he began a translation of Galen's *De Constitutione Artis Medicae*, but was unable to finish it.

The importance of Ḥunayn can scarcely be over-estimated. At a time when Arab men of science were seeking to assimilate all the best of Greek thought, Ḥunayn was ready with his perfect knowledge of Greek, Syriac and Arabic to offer them that mental pabulum for which they were hungry. At the very moment when the liberality of a caliph offered unlimited means to ensure the scientific pre-eminence of Baghdad there was in Ḥunayn a man to hand who could give to the city that pre-eminence, and that not to Baghdad only but to the whole Islamic world. As Leclerc so justly remarks, even if Ḥunayn did not create the renaissance of learning in the East, certainly there is no one who took a part more active, more sure, or more prolific.[1]

Although Ḥunayn was also a clinician, and his original clinical works must not be forgotten, it is as a translator that his great reputation was made. In the Sophia Mosque Library in Constantinople there were preserved two manuscripts which are a list

1 Leclerc, *Hist. Méd. Arabe*, vol. 1, p. 139.

of Ḥunayn's works drawn up by his pupils after his death. Here it is stated that he translated into Syriac 95 and into Arabic 39 books of Galen. Six more books were rendered into Syriac and 70 more into Arabic by his pupils and were revised by Ḥunayn himself. He also revised the Syriac versions which had been made in a previous age, such as those of Sergius of Rá's-ul-'Ayn and of Ayúb of Edessa. His corrections of another Sergius were so skilful that they converted the translations from being merely mediocre to being first class. All these are considered in detail by Leclerc in his section on Ḥunayn.

Three at least of these translations found their way back to Europe. The *Ars Parva* of Galen was translated from Syriac into Arabic by Ḥunayn and from Arabic into Latin by Gerard of Cremona. A pseudo-Galenic work *De Clysteribus et Colica* went through the same steps and reached a Latin version from the pen of Raphelengius. And his *De Malitia Complexionis Diversae* was translated direct into Arabic by Ḥunayn and into Latin also by Gerard of Cremona.

Of the literary value of Ḥunayn's translations Professor Bergstraesser in his *Hunain ibn Ishak und seine Schule* (Leiden, 1913) cannot speak too highly. Meyerhof quotes the passage in which the translations of Ḥunayn and Ḥubaysh are compared; those of Ḥunayn were adjudged to be the best. 'The correctness is greater; nevertheless one is left with the impression that this is not the result of anxious effort, but of a free and sure mastery of the language. This is seen in the easier adaptation of the Greek original and the striking exactness of expression obtained without verbosity. It is all this that constitutes the famous Fasaha (eloquence) of Ḥunayn.'

Ḥunayn himself declares that his great object was accuracy, that he underwent many difficult journeys in order to find manuscripts for the correction of doubtful texts. For a new manuscript of Galen's *De Demonstratione* he journeyed all over Mesopotamia, Syria, Palestine and Egypt and then only found half of what he wanted at Damascus. Not only did he criticize the faults of his predecessors and those under him, but he was also highly critical of his own past work. Of his own translation of the *De Sectis* he writes:

I translated it, when I was a young man...from a very defective Greek manuscript. Later on, when I was about forty years old, my pupil Ḥubaysh asked me to correct it after having collected a certain number of Greek manuscripts. Thereupon I collated these so as to produce one correct manuscript. This manuscript I compared with the Syriac text and corrected it. I am in the habit of proceeding thus in all my translation work.

He was said by al-Qifṭí to have also translated the Septuagint into Arabic. But if he did so, this version is lost.

Relative to his translations Ḥunayn's original work is unimportant. The most accessible to the ordinary reader is his introduction to the *Ars Parva Galeni*, accessible because translated into Latin, being published at Leipzig in 1497 and at Strassburg in 1534 under the title of *Isagoge Johannitii*. It is a review of the Galenic system of medicine and was used in Europe in the Middle Ages as an introductory medical work.

Among his own countrymen two of his original works were very highly esteemed. One was his *Masá'il fí il-Ṭibb* or 'Questions on Medicine', which was included by Niẓámí among the works with which every student of medicine should be acquainted.[1] This book is a series of questions and answers on general medicine and was left unfinished by Ḥunayn and completed after his death by Ḥubaysh. It became the subject of many commentaries, the first of which is said to have been that of Abú Bakr Muḥammad bin Khalíl al-Raqqí, written when he was in his cups in the year A.D. 941. Ḥunayn's other great original work is his treatise on the eye. This has lately been made available to modern scholars by the publication by Doctor Meyerhof of the text with a translation into English.

This work was apparently well known throughout the Arabic-speaking world. Rhazes quotes from it frequently in his *Continens*.

1 Niẓámí, *Chahár Maqála*, p. 78.

'Alí bin 'Ísá and Zarrín Dast, both of the eleventh century, name this book as the principal source of their extracts. Ibn abí Uṣaybi'a says that Ḥunayn himself wrote:

> For more than thirty years I had been composing various treatises concerning the eye, in which I pursued divergent aims about which I was questioned by several people one after another.... Then Ḥubaysh asked me to collect those treatises—there were nine of them—and to make one book of them. He also asked me to add for him to the nine preceding treatises another one in which I discussed a commentary on the compound remedies composed by the Ancients and laid down in their books for the treatment of eye diseases.[1]

The fascinating story of the discovery by Meyerhof of the Arabic manuscript of the ten treatises, at a time when it was generally believed that the original work had perished, must be read in the introduction to his translation. There is no need to discuss this work more; all details will be found there.

Others of Ḥunayn's original works were written in Syriac. He is said to have composed a Greek-Syriac Dictionary. Professor Budge published in 1913 a work entitled *Syrian Anatomy, Pathology and Therapeutics*, of which the author is reputed to be Ḥunayn. But this is far from being proved. Ibn abí Uṣaybi'a gives a long list of his original Arabic works. Leclerc reproduces the list for the benefit of those who do not read Arabic.

In the story of medicine there have been two great eras of translation with which we are familiar. The first was the period which is here under discussion; the second was the period known as the renaissance of learning in the West. Between the two the art of printing had been discovered. This alone was an inducement which the Arab never had and offered the translators rewards for which the Arab could never hope. The Arabic texts appeared in Europe when the age had just become critical. Greek texts in al-Ma'mún's days were accepted with rapturous joy and a semi-divine reverence. Arabic texts in Tudor days were accepted with

1 *I.A.U.* vol. 1, pp. 198–200.

the respect that 600 years of supremacy must necessarily give to them, but almost from the beginning their authority was challenged. The Florentine painters were the first to refute the Arab anatomists. The English physiologists soon followed.

It is not uninteresting therefore to compare the standard which the two schools of translators reached. All competent judges in the matter give the prize to the Arabs. Nor is this judgement remarkable. In the first place they were more thorough. What European translator wandered into Egypt or the Middle East in order to perfect his Arabic or to collect more perfect manuscripts, as we have seen Ḥunayn to have done? In the second place the college of translators in Baghdad received royal aid and royal encouragement. The European schools of Toledo and Monte Cassino were in comparison mere private adventures. Again, Arabic to Ḥunayn and the others was a spoken language, the language in which they worked, disputed and made love. Latin to Gundisalvi, Constantin and Gerard was a dead language, only of use as a method of conveying scientific ideas or praising God. Ḥunayn could within reason create new words to give the exact rendering of the Greek ideas. For living Arabic is a very flexible language. The medieval translators risked ridicule and certainly misunderstanding if they added to the vocabulary of the Fathers. Finally, it must be owned that the task of the medieval schoolmen was the harder one. In Baghdad Greek manuscripts poured into the college, yielded up by treaties and by discoveries. In Europe manuscripts were rare, scattered through monasteries and university libraries of a dozen different countries. There was no unity between the various European schools of translators, excepting their use of Latin.

It is no wonder then that the European translations fall far short in their style and in their accuracy of those of Baghdad. Unfortunately very few of the early Arabic translations survive which might be compared with the Greek originals. So it is difficult to form a just judgement of their accuracy. On the other hand nearly all the original Arabic versions exist and are easy to compare with the Latin translations. Leclerc considers that the translations from Greek into Arabic was generally effected with much greater skill and knowledge than the later translations from Arabic into Latin. And Browne agreeing with him says that 'it is difficult to resist the conclusion that many passages in the Latin version of the *Qánún* of Avicenna were misunderstood or not understood at all by the translator, and consequently can never have conveyed a clear idea to the reader'.[1]

The system which the Baghdad translators probably used was certainly employed by the European translators, that is to say, the translation was not made direct, but through the medium of a third language. Arabic with its elaborate system of dots to denote letters and dashes to denote vowels gave a far greater opportunity for error than did the simple Greek words. Many of the problems of the meaningless words of the Latin versions can be solved by writing such words in Arabic hand and adding a few extra dots. Thus, the incomprehensible barbarism, which occurs in the heading to chapter III of the first part of book III of the *Canon* of Avicenna, may be solved very simply by one who can write Arabic, 'Sermo Universalis de Karabito qui est Sirsem Calidum' was written in the Venice edition of the *Canon* in 1555. What was the poor student to make of this? A glance at the original Arabic version shows that *karabitus* is the transliteration of *faranitus*, which is a very close rendering of the original Greek word *phrenitos*. But an extra dot over the Arabic letter F converted this into a K, and a dot below the line instead of above changed N into B. Hence the barbarism. As for the word *sirsem*, the transliteration is correct enough, but who without a knowledge of medieval Persian could know that the word means a swelling of the head?

Dozens of examples could be quoted; they occur on every page. Every now and then it is the Arab who trips. His rendering of *peritoneum* by *baritarun*, though just recognizable, is much further away from the original than it need be. But its rendering into

1 Browne, *Arabian Medicine*, pp. 26, 27.

Latin via the Arabic is even further away. For here it becomes *Beritharium*.

Occasionally the Arab was so near to the original that it is difficult to see how or why the medievalist misunderstood him. Thus, there occurs the following passage in the *Canon* of Avicenna: 'And there is seen on the body an excrescence of glandular tissue, similar to the animal which the Greeks called a Satyr.' The Greek word *saturos* is rendered into Arabic *Saturus*, yet the schoolman writes: 'similis animali quod graece nominatur Satos.'[1]

A quite interesting side-issue is raised by a study of these transliterations, for they show firstly how Greek was pronounced in the ninth and tenth centuries, and how Latin was pronounced in the fifteenth and sixteenth.

Of the sons of Ḥunayn Isḥáq is the most famous. As a translator he was the equal of his father, though he devoted his talents to philosophy rather than to medicine. He was as equally skilled as his father in his knowledge of languages and was equally eloquent in the expression of his thoughts. At first he was employed in the service of the caliph, but later he attached himself exclusively to al-Qásim ibn 'Ubayd-Ulláh, *wazír* to the Caliph al-Mu'taẓid. His patron, hearing that Isḥáq had one evening taken a purgative pill, sent him in the morning the following lines. The point of the joke is that the lines are in the style of the love-sick Persian poets, who are for ever writing of their long and tiring journeys to the house of their mistress.

Tell me how you passed the night and in what state you were,
And how often to the solitary room did your camel bear you there.

To which Isḥáq replied:

I write you this to avoid wearing out my shoes by a fatiguing walk.
If you intend to answer me, direct your letter to the closet.[2]

Isḥáq died in the year A.D. 910, having lost the use of his eft side from a stroke.

1 *Canon*, Bk. iv, 3. 3. 2.

2 *I.A.U.* vol. 1, p. 201.

Two other sons are known by name, Dá'úd and Ḥakím. The former was a clinician rather than a translator, the latter is quoted by Rhazes in the *Continens* but is otherwise unknown.[1]

Of his many pupils far the greatest was his nephew Ḥubaysh who on account of the paralysis of one hand was known as al-A'sam. I have already had occasion to mention him several times. Ḥunayn thought so highly of him that he accepted without question any translations made by him. At the same time Ḥubaysh was not without fame as a clinician and was court physician to al-Mutawakkil the caliph and his successors. The date of his death is unknown. His original works, too, are not without importance, for a certain number of drugs appear here for the first time, showing that his studies in therapeutics were not confined to Greek texts, for many of these remedies were unknown to the Greeks.

To enumerate all the translators who worked for al-Ma'mún would be wearisome and valueless. Leclerc briefly describes 101 in the second book of his *History of Arab Medicine*. Some are mere names; but there are a few whose work did more than merely serve as text-books for students. Such a one was Abú Yaḥyá al-Baṭríq, who died about A.D. 800, and his more important son Abú Zakariyyá. Although according to Ḥunayn the son knew more Latin than Greek, yet he made translations of Hippocrates, Galen and Aristotle. Most important of all is his translation of the pseudo-Aristotelian work which now goes by the name of *Secreta Secretorum*. This professes to be a collection of letters which Aristotle wrote in his old age to Alexander the Great. It was lost to the world until al-Ma'mún somehow heard of its existence and ordered a thorough search to be made. In the words of al-Baṭríq: 'he left no temple among the temples where the philosophers deposit the hidden wisdom, unsought.'

The search was rewarded with success and to al-Baṭríq was confided the task of translating the letters into Arabic. All authorities are now agreed, I think, that Aristotle was not the

1 Leclerc, *Hist. Méd. Arabe*, vol. 1, p. 154.

author of the *Secreta Secretorum*. Sarton believes that the original text, though based on early Greek models, was either Arabic or Syriac.[1] In the light of Ḥunayn's scathing remarks about his knowledge of Greek, it is scarcely likely that al-Baṭríq made his version from a Greek manuscript. Nor is it likely that he was the perpetrator of a deliberate fraud. Probably therefore his version is the translation of an even earlier Syriac version. Penzer holds that the background of the book is entirely Eastern.[2] The allusion to chess, the occurrence of Eastern place-names and animals, all these point to an Asiatic, not European origin. It may well be that, like the *Alfiyya Shalfiyya* and the *Kalíla wa Dimna*, it is to India that the original version is to be attributed and that all that al-Baṭríq did was to give to al-Ma'mún a new translation of a book which the Syriac translators of Jundí Shápúr had given to Persia centuries before. Whatever may be the real truth of this matter, the text of al-Baṭríq, which he entitled *Sirr-al-Asrár*, is the earliest extant version of this very interesting work.

Hárún-ul-Rashíd had died at the age of forty-seven; al-Ma'mún only lived one year longer. His death occurred at Tarsus and was due to a fever said to have been brought on by eating too many fresh dates and drinking too much iced water. Seeing his end approaching he nominated his brother Abú Isḥáq his successor under the title of al-Mu'taṣim. Arabic historians, who delight in the bizarre, called him the Caliph of the Eights, for he was the eighth of the dynasty, the eighth child of his father, proclaimed caliph at eighteen, reigned eight years and eight months, had eight sons and eight daughters, was born in the eighth month of the year, and died on the eighteenth day of the month. His short reign from A.D. 833 to 842 was marked by a continuance of the policy of tolerance in all subjects except that of religion. Science and philosophy continued to flourish. To this period is to be ascribed the best works of al-Kindí 'the philosopher of the Arabs'. But al-Mu'taṣim's introduction of thousands of

1 Sarton, *History of Science*, vol. I, pp. 537, 557.
2 Penzer, *Ocean of Story*, vol. II, p. 290.

Mamlukes, or Turkish soldiery, into the capital to serve as his bodyguard and in his army meant no good either for the city or for the throne. Nor did the transference of the seat of government from Baghdad to Sámarra, a new imperial palace which al-Mu'taṣim had constructed 60 miles higher up the river, give any aid to the intellectual movement with which Baghdad was now associated. With his death the glory of the 'Abbásid family and nation expired, as Gibbon said.

He was succeeded by his son al-Wáṯiq, who, though born of a Greek slave girl, inherited his father's Persian proclivities. He died apparently of diabetes, for the historians of the day say that he was seized with a dropsy and an insupportable thirst. His physicians prescribed for him exposure in a hot oven. But the oven was overheated, he caught a chill on emerging, and a few days later he was dead.

Under al-Mutawakkil, his successor, the medical profession suffered severely. For he was an intolerant and orthodox rigorist. The sumptuary laws against the Jews and Christians, which under the preceding reigns had never been enforced, were now reimposed and made even stricter than before. Coloured stripes were ordered to be sewn upon their garments and upon those of their slaves. Horses were forbidden to them: the stirrups upon their mules and asses were to be made of wood. Offices of state were closed to them. A figure of Satan was to be attached to the door posts of their houses. A Christian apothecary, who had embraced Islam but later returned to Christianity and refused to recant, was put to death at the stake.

In the case of his personal physicians al-Mutawakkil apparently made exceptions, for he retained the services of Bukht Yishú', the third of that name. He was already well known at court in the time of al-Mu'taṣim. Nevertheless, on the accession of al-Wáṯiq the tongues of his various detractors had compelled him to retire into temporary exile at Jundí Shápúr. The caliph, when overcome by his last fatal attack of dropsy, sent messengers to summon Bukht Yishú' to return to Baghdad with all speed.

He obeyed, but arrived too late. Al-Wáṣiq was already dead. Al-Mutawakkil, in spite of his Christianity, received him in a friendly spirit and allowed him to enjoy the immense wealth which the family had collected.

But al-Mutawakkil was a waster and a spendthrift and he soon found that his treasury was empty. Vast sums were spent upon a new residence that he built for himself at Sámarra, which had now replaced Baghdad as the seat of the government. To raise money for fresh extravagances the offices of State were put up for sale. An unfortunate entertainment which Bukht Yishú' gave to him, too generous in his loyalty, made the caliph turn eyes of envy upon his wealth. A few days later Bukht Yishú' was dismissed from office, his money seized, and all his goods that were worth anything were transported to the warehouses of the caliph. Even the charcoal and fire-wood, which at first had been overlooked, were later seized and sold and the proceeds paid into the caliph's privy purse. Some of his wealth, even if not all, was ultimately restored to him, for the historians say that he left three daughters after his death and that there was great competition for their hands among the court officials on account of the large dowry which would accompany each.[1]

Among the orthodox court physicians of this reign was Ibráhím bin Ayúb, known as al-Ibrish. His fame rests rather upon his translations from Greek into Syriac and Arabic than upon his clinical acumen, though tales of this are not wanting. He served not only al-Mutawakkil himself, but also his famous wife Qabíḥa the Ugly One, so called on account of her exceeding beauty in order to avert the evil eye. For his cure of Isma'íl, a son by this wife, al-Mutawakkil and Qabíḥa vied in showering rewards upon him. His final present amounted to sixteen large bags of gold.[2]

Of all his physicians al-Mutawakkil's favourite was Isrá'íl bin Zakariyyá, known as al-Ṭayfúrí, whom I have already spoken of as the enemy of Ḥunayn. This man, starting life in a relatively

1 *I.A.U.* vol. 1, p. 141. 2 Ibid. p. 170.

humble department of State, finally became the right-hand man of the caliph. The Ṭayfúrís were a well-known medical family. The first about whom history has anything to relate was named 'Abd-Ulláh. He was a popular physician in the court of the Caliph al-Hádí. The title of al-Ṭayfúrí he acquired by virtue of his services, as personal physician to Ṭayfúr, brother of Khayzurán, the wife of al-Mahdí. From his refusal to accept the verdict of the quack Abú Quraysh in his diagnosis of the sex of Khayzurán's unborn child it is clear that he was an honest and orthodox physician and no charlatan. His interest in science is also shown by his encouragement of Ḥunayn's translations. Later he became physician to al-Hádí himself.

Of his son Zakariyyá nothing is related except an anecdote which is too good to pass over. He is said to have served in the army and to have been charged by the commander in the field to make an investigation into the credentials of the druggists and pharmacists who were accompanying the troops. Knowing that many of them were completely ignorant of their trade and were dishonest enough to take any steps to hide it, he bade the general write out a series of prescriptions, but instead of the name of the drug to insert the name of a little-known food. Some of the druggists replied that they did not keep such a thing; but others sent back some preparation or other rather than admit that they did not know what it was. These last Zakariyyá drove out of the camp and wrote to the caliph, praying him to replace them by more honest and more competent druggists.[1]

The son of Zakariyyá, by name Isrá'íl, gradually worked his way up through the court and finally became personal physician to al-Mutawakkil. Such a hold over the caliph did he obtain that it is said that the caliph would taste no food until Isrá'íl had pronounced it suitable. One historian says that the position of Isrá'íl al-Ṭayfúrí in al-Mutawakkil's court even resembled that of Bukht Yishú' in the court of Hárún-ul-Rashíd. When Isrá'íl

1 The same story is told of Muḥammad bin 'Abd-ul-Andalusí. See *Contes du Cheykh el-Mohdy*, vol. 1, p. 268.

fell ill, the caliph seemed heart-broken and declared that were he to die, his own life too would be ended. It would seem that this affection was genuine. For when Isrá'íl, piqued at some trifling professional slight for which he held al-Mutawakkil responsible, left the court and vowed he would not return, the caliph sent enormous presents after him to try and persuade him to come back.

Early in his reign al-Mutawakkil divided his kingdom between his two sons. The western half he gave to al-Muntaṣir and the eastern to al-Mu'tazz. By degrees he began to show a marked preference for the latter. Al-Mu'tazz was set over the mint and treasury; his name was stamped upon the coins. This was equivalent to naming him the successor. Al-Muntaṣir, being the elder, could bear his humiliating position no longer, and one night being insulted by his father when in his cups, with the aid of Turkish officers assassinated him and took the throne for himself. Isrá'íl bin Z̲akariyyá found himself confirmed in his office. But he could not serve the man who had murdered his master and his friend. He lent a willing ear therefore to a plot that was being hatched within the palace walls. The Turkish officers, fearful that al-Muntaṣir or his brothers would murder them on the excuse of revenging the death of al-Mutawakkil, prevailed upon al-Muntaṣir to disentail his brothers from the succession. This done they decided to murder al-Muntaṣir himself. For this purpose they approached Isrá'íl and persuaded him to make an attempt upon the caliph's life on the pretext of a surgical operation. A lancet was soaked in a deadly poison. The caliph fell ill of a fever. Isrá'íl prescribed venesection as the essential treatment. The poisoned lancet was handed to the phlebotomist. Within a few hours the caliph was dead. Whether this story is true or not is uncertain. Some historians narrating it complete the tale by adding that a few months later Isrá'íl himself had occasion to be bled and by accident the same knife was used. The poison was still potent and the physician went the same way as the master.[1]

1 For the history of the whole Ṭayfúrí family, see *I.A.U.* vol. 1, pp. 153–8.

The Turkish troops, having thus disposed of the caliph whom they feared, now put on the throne a nominee of their own who should be entirely subservient to their wishes. But growing weary of him after a few years they replaced him by al-Mu'tazz, the son whom al-Mutawakkil had originally intended for the throne. Of the policy of al-Mu'tazz both at home and abroad it is not necessary here to speak. Sufficient is it to say that he kept his word to no man, that he did not hesitate to murder any whom he feared or suspected, and that even though he was but 24 years of age when he died, he richly deserved the fate which he met from the hands of the sons of two of the Turkish chiefs whom he had deceived and cheated. These two going to the palace with a clamorous troop of Turcomans called upon the caliph to come forth. He replied that he had taken physic and therefore could not come out; but unsuspecting invited the two young men within. Here they set upon him, beating him and tearing his clothes to pieces. They left him lying in the court-yard beneath a burning sun. Three or four days later he was dead.

The next caliph only reigned one year, when he too was murdered, and al-Mu'tamid in the year A.D. 870 ascended the throne. One of his first actions was to transfer the seat of government from Sámarra back to Baghdad, which removed the person of the caliph from Turkish intrigues to the midst of the Arab populace. In consequence, for three reigns there were no murderous attacks upon the reigning caliph and al-Mu'tamid enjoyed a longer period of power than any caliph since Hárún-ul-Rashíd. Actually the length and success of his reign were due to the vigorous policy of his brother al-Muwaffaq, who when attacked by elephantiasis and feeling that his end was near, secured for his own son, al-Mu'taẓid, the succession to the throne. In the following year, A.D. 892, the caliph drank himself to death and without any difficulty al-Mu'taẓid ascended the throne.

Al-Mu'taẓid was 36 years of age when he succeeded his uncle. His health was already undermined by years of dissipation and the hardships and exertions of campaigning. His temper was not of the best and his physicians often found it impossible to treat him. He refused to follow their directions and refused to take their physic. His physician-in-chief, Abú 'Uṣmán Sa'íd bin Gh̲álib, survived him, but another, named Aḥmad bin ul-Ṭabíb al-Sarak̲h̲sí (not to be confused with 'Abd-ul-Raḥmán al-Sarak̲h̲sí, who lived 200 years later), who was his minister, his companion at table, and a very versatile writer, was condemned to death for the supposed revealing of State secrets. To another, more insistent than the rest, he gave such a kick in the stomach that the wretched man collapsed and died.

His ill-treatment of his physicians is perhaps redeemed by his friendship for Ṣ̈ábit of Harran, the greatest of the Sabean physicians. Abú ul-Ḥasan Ṣ̈ábit bin Qurra bin Marwán bin Ṣ̈ábit bin Karáya bin Ibráhím bin Karáya bin Márínús was originally a tax-collector, living at Harran. Owing to his heretical views he was condemned by his co-religionists and forced to leave Harran. So he took up his residence at Kafratusa, a town not very far from Baghdad. Here he met a certain Muḥammad ibn Músá̲, who was then on his return journey from Greece to Baghdad. Muḥammad, struck with his talents and his eloquence, took him with him to Baghdad and lodged him in his own house. At the first opportunity he presented him to the reigning caliph, then al-Mu'taẓid, who gave him a post among his court astronomers. Here he employed his leisure in the study of the sciences of the ancients, that is logic, philosophy, mathematics and medicine. Of all these he acquired a profound knowledge and soon became employed in the *Bayt-ul-Ḥikmat*, translating Syriac texts into Arabic.

It was mere chance which led to his becoming court physician to al-Mu'taẓid. The latter, not yet caliph, had incurred the anger of his father al-Muwaffaq and for some time languished in prison. Ṣ̈ábit was able to render him certain small services by virtue of his post of physician to the prison. Three times a day, so the record runs, he used to go and comfort him in his anxiety. This sympathy al-Mu'taẓid never forgot. One of his first acts on ascending the throne was to appoint Ṣ̤ábit his personal physician. Not only was Ṣ̤ábit consulted in the matter of the caliph's health, but his opinion was also asked on all important matters of state. He was allowed to sit in the Presence when all others stood. Abú Isḥáq writing about him says: 'One day Ṣ̤ábit the son of Qurra walked with al-Mu'taẓid in Paradise, which was the name of a garden at the seat of the caliphate. Al-Mu'taẓid leaned upon the arm of Ṣ̤ábit. Suddenly he removed his hand remarking that this position was unfitting because that the learned, such as Ṣ̤ábit, should always be the uppermost.'[1]

Ṣ̤ábit died in the year A.D. 901 at the age of seventy-six. Judging from his recorded works, which are many, and his existing works, which are few, it is difficult to say in which branch of learning Ṣ̤ábit excelled. More than a hundred books are ascribed to him. In addition to his medical works, which require a special notice, he is said to have written a correction of the translation of Euclid which Ḥunayn bin Isḥáq had already made into Arabic and to have composed in Syriac treatises on the Sabean religion and some others on music which were never translated into Arabic.

His capabilities as a clinician can be guessed from the many personal observations which are scattered about his great work 'The Treasury' and from the almost miraculous story which is recorded by three medieval biographers, al-Qifṭí, Ibn abí Uṣaybi'a and Niẕámí.

One day he was passing through the sheep-slayers' market. A butcher was skinning a sheep, and from time to time he would thrust his hand into the sheep's belly, take out some of the warm fat, and eat it. Ṣ̤ábit, noticing this, said to the green-grocer opposite him: 'If at any time this butcher should die, inform me of it before they lay him in the grave.' 'Willingly', replied the green-grocer. When five or six months had elapsed, one morning it was rumoured abroad that such-and-such a butcher had died suddenly without any premonitory illness. The green-

1 *I.A.U.* vol. 1, p. 215; Ibn Khallikán, vol. 1, p. 288.

grocer also went to offer his condolences. He found a number of people tearing their garments, while others were consumed with grief, for the dead man was young and had little children.

Then he remembered the words of Ṣábit and hastened to bear the intelligence to him. Said Ṣábit: 'He has been a long time in dying.' Then he took his staff, went to the dead man's house, raised the sheet from the face of the corpse, felt his pulse, and ordered someone to strike the soles of his feet with the staff. After a while he said to him: 'It is enough.' Then he began to apply the remedies for apoplexy, and on the third day the dead man arose, and, though he remained paralytic, he lived for many years, and men were astonished, because that great man had foreseen that the man would be stricken by apoplexy.[1]

The above is Browne's translation of Niẓámí's version of the story. As Niẓámí ascribed the cure to Adíb Isma'íl, I have changed the name in deference to the authority of the other two biographers.

Of the medical books ascribed to Ṣábit a large number are his versions of works by Galen. Among his original writings are treatises whose subject varies from discussions on hygiene and the nobility of the profession of medicine to a monograph on small-pox and measles (and it is a matter for speculation whether in his views he supported or even anticipated Rhazes) and another on the anatomy of certain birds. But of all his works the best known is 'The Treasury' or *Al-Z̲ak̲h̲ira*, which is accessible to all readers of Arabic in the Cairo edition of 1928. It has never been translated, so far as I know, and it is worth while therefore summarizing its contents, for it is a book with a great reputation in the ancient medical world. It is one of the five works which Niẓámí says formed the subject of study for the second-year student of medicine.[2] It was sufficiently popular to call for an answer and in opposition to Ṣábit's views Ibn Karníb wrote a special book.[3] According to al-Qifṭí, Ṣábit II declared 'The Treasury' to be a spurious work to which his grandfather's name had been attached, 'although it was a good book enjoying a wide

1 Niẓámí, *C̲h̲ahár Maqála*, p. 93. 2 Ibid. p. 78.
3 *Maṭraḥ-ul-Anẓár*, pp. 73, 83.

circulation'.[1] But Ibn abí Uṣaybi'a accepted it as genuine, and from internal evidence it would seem probable that the book is from the hand of Ṣ̤ábit I, as is generally believed. It seems to be a sort of composition of extracts from all his medical works, condensed and arranged as a single work for the use of his son Sinán.

After the ordinary invocation of God he writes:

This is the Book of the Treasury which contains everything that needs to be known in the Science of Medicine—in the description of disease and its treatment—in the concisest manner possible according to the experience in the physical sciences of the Master of his Time, Ṣ̤ábit ibn Qurra. He compiled it during his lifetime for the benefit of his son Sinán ibn Ṣ̤ábit ibn Qurra. It contains thirty-one chapters.

Chapter I is a lengthy consideration of prophylaxis and hygiene in general, based mainly upon Galen's works.

Chapter II is a very short discussion on 'hidden' diseases, by which he means asthenia or sub-acute attacks of disease.

Chapter III deals with the hair, its physiology, its pathology, and the treatment of affections of the hair in other parts of the body besides the head.

Chapter IV is of the nature of a treatise on Beauty Treatment. Here he discusses various pigmentary errors, spots, pimples and similar affections. In conclusion there are numerous prescriptions for lotions and applications.

Chapters V–XIX deal with diseases in different parts of the body with one chapter (XVIII) on diseases peculiar to women. These chapters call to mind one of his aphorisms:

Nothing is more harmful to an aged person than to have a clever cook and a beautiful concubine. For the former forces him to abuse food and he falls ill, and the latter entices him to the abuse of sexual intercourse which makes him grow older still. For the comfort of the body depends on the ingestion of small amounts of food and the comfort of the spirit is in the non-commital of sin, and the happiness of the heart is in the lack of worry, and the comfort of the tongue is in the non-abuse of talking.

1 Al-Qifṭí, p. 169.

Chapters xx–xxvi describe a variety of diseases, including guinea-worm infection, diseases of the nails, whitlow and troubles of the feet due to tight sandals (xx), tumours (xxii), poisons (xxv), and fevers (xxvi).

Chapter xxvii is mainly devoted to plague and the climatic conditions which give rise to it.

Chapter xxviii deals with fractures, dislocations, and similar conditions.

Chapters xxix and xxx deal with milk and wine respectively. It is strange how at all times a treatise on wine-drinking was required by a Moslem clientele, theoretically teetotal. Jibrá'íl bin Bukht Yishú' was once asked by that famous poet and toper Abú Nuwás how much wine he ought to take.

> I asked of my brother Abú 'Ísá—and Jibrá'íl is wise—
> Saying to him: 'Wine is agreeable to me.'
> But he replied: 'Excess is fatal.'
> So I begged that he set me a limit;
> And he spoke to me thus in detail:
> 'The nature of man is fourfold
> 'And four are the foundations of his nature.
> 'To each I allow one: to the whole of man therefore four.'

Chapter xxxi is the usual chapter on sexual intercourse which no Arab text-book of medicine ever omits.

The concluding paragraph of the book describes briefly a method of birth control and quotes the opinion of Ḥáriṣ bin Kalda: 'If you do not wish conception to take place, then anoint the glans at the time of intercourse with oil.'

The death of Ṣábit deprived the court of al-Mu'taẓid of a wise counsellor and an honest physician. He left behind him to carry on the tradition two sons and his dearest pupil, 'Ísá bin Asyad, the Christian, who had aided him in his translations. Of one son Ibráhím, called Ibráhím I to distinguish him from Ṣábit's grandchild Ibráhím II, very little is known. But the other, named Sinán, is to be reckoned one of the outstanding characters of this period. Although a Sabean in origin, he was born and bred in

Baghdad and was an enforced convert to Islam in his adult days. He learnt his medicine at his father's knees and rapidly rose to the top of his profession. He is not to be confused with that Sinán who is said to have been one of the leading physicians of Baghdad when 'Aẓud-ul-Doula entered the city; for this Sinán was already dead. But one of his pupils, the unpleasantly garrulous Ibn Kashkaráyá, and his son Ṡábit were both members of the staff of the 'Aẓudí Hospital.

A year after the death of Ṡábit, al-Mu'taẓid also died after a prosperous reign of nearly 10 years. He was succeeded by his son al-Muktafí, who made himself popular by his generosity to the common people and by abolishing the cruel subterranean prisons which his father had so freely filled. During his short reign there flourished a physician named Yúsuf al-Sáhir, also called *al-Qass* or 'The Priest'. From this title it may be inferred that he was a Christian. The name *al-Sáhir* means the 'Wakeful One'. Arab writers suggest that he received this name because he spent the greater part of the night studying medicine. Bar Hebraeus believes, and states that his written works bear out the theory, that he had a growth in the fore-part of the brain and that it was this that kept him awake, not a love of science.[1]

The death of al-Muktafí led to the succession of the decadent al-Muqtadir who, coming to the throne as a boy of thirteen, never escaped from the bonds with which the womenfolk of the palace had secured him. Even the heavens were unpropitious, for during the first year of his reign Baghdad was visited with the rare phenomenon of a heavy fall of snow which destroyed the palm trees and even froze the vinegar and the eggs. He was weak and a bully. Within a year of coming to the throne he promulgated an edict forbidding to Jews and Christians all State functions, except those of physician and banker. He was a wanton and a spendthrift. The treasury was empty through repeated wars. The Greeks were bought off with 120,000 gold pieces. All Persia was in revolt. His drinking bouts became a mere matter of routine.

1 *Hist. Dynst.* vol. IX, p. 186.

'Alí bin 'Ísá declared that five days of sobriety would have shown him to be as wise as his father.

Yet in spite of all these excesses his health was remarkably good. A court physician stated at his death that during his whole life he had been sick for only 13 days. He was not without a sense of humour, too. A certain Abú Bakr al-Shiblí, a retired government official and a poet, turned Ṣúfí in his old age and renounced the world. To escape martyrdom for his heretical views he feigned madness. For a while he was interned in a mad-house from where he used to throw stones at all visitors. 'Alí the *wazír*, who was a friend of his in former times, persuaded al-Muqtadir to send a physician to the asylum to see what he could do. Al-Muqtadir complied and sent a Christian doctor. To the amazement of all, al-Shiblí remained in the asylum and the doctor turned Musulman. When al-Muqtadir heard of it, he exclaimed: 'We thought we had sent a doctor to a patient, but it seems we sent a patient to a doctor.'

In A.D. 929, on account of the flagrant misuse of public money and the part that al-Muqtadir gave to eunuchs and women in the administration of the kingdom, a revolt broke out headed by Mú'nis the Eunuch, a general named Názúk and others. Mú'nis entered Baghdad with his army and the caliph together with his mother, his sister and favourite slave girls was made a prisoner and sent to Mú'nis' house up the river. Muḥammad, a son of al-Mu'taẓid, was saluted as caliph by Mú'nis and the successful rebels and began to reign under the title of *al-Qáhir b'Illah* or 'The Conqueror by God'. Two days later he held his first public court. The army attended to demand the accession present and a year's pay. But the treasury was empty and unable to meet their demands. Mú'nis in expectation of this awkward situation had remained at home and refused to meet the soldiers face to face. Názúk was within the palace, but was too timid to attempt to control either his own men or the mob. Very soon the situation got out of control and the soldiery began to force their way into the palace. Názúk then attempted to reason with them, but still half-drunk from his orgy of the previous night he lost his head, turned and fled. He was soon overtaken and killed by the mob. The rest of the courtiers abandoned the throne room and al-Qáhir was left alone.

The mob seem to have been satisfied with the blood of Názúk, for they now made off to the house of Mú'nis, shouting for the restoration of al-Muqtadir. No one was more surprised at this turn of affairs than al-Muqtadir himself. Fearful of treachery he declined to meet the mob. At last he was carried by force from the house of Mú'nis to the royal barge and from the barge to his own palace. Here he was saluted for the second time as caliph. Among the first to do him homage was al-Qáhir who had managed to lie concealed all that day. 'Brother, you are not to blame,' said al-Muqtadir with a ready wit as he kissed him on the forehead, 'for I know that you were forced.' For al-Qáhir not only means 'The Conqueror' but also 'He who is Forced'.

On his restoration to the throne al-Muqtadir confirmed Ibn Muqla in the wazirate and determined to make the customary presents to the troops. All the ready cash he gave away first. Then he brought out clothes from his stores and sold these. When this did not suffice, he disposed of the royal lands at a very low rate. Among the properties thus sold was the estate of Jibrá'íl bin Bukht Yishú'. Sinán bin Ṣábit, who was present in the office when the *wazír* was signing the deeds of sale, records that 'Alí bin 'Ísá, when he saw the price it fetched, could not restrain an exclamation of surprise. Ibn Muqla put down the deed which was in his hand, saying:

> I was told by my Chief that when al-Mutawakkil became displeased with the physician Bukht Yishú', he sent to his house to make an inventory of the contents of his stores. There was found in his clothes store a statement of the estates which he had purchased. The price was more than ten million dirhams. They have come now to be sold for this small figure.

In A.D. 931 Mú'nis again began to be impatient and to show signs of disloyalty to al-Muqtadir. Having defeated his Ḥamdánid rivals he once more marched on Baghdad. To secure the troops the caliph again distributed as much cash as he could lay hands on. He then prepared to resist or fly as circumstances might demand. The soldiery rallied to him and a pitched battle was fought. His generals begged him to show himself to the troops to encourage them, but al-Muqtadir refused to leave the palace. Too late he consented. By the time he reached the battlefield his followers had been routed and were in flight. Some African hirelings of Mú'nis discovered him and one of them struck him from behind a blow which brought him to the ground. His head was raised on a sword, he was stripped of his royal robes, and his naked body was left where it fell until a labouring man, who passed by, covered him with grass and dug a grave for him just where he lay.

Mú'nis thereupon entered Baghdad in triumph and took possession of the capital. He restored al-Qáhir to the caliphate, ibn Muqla to the wazirate. Al-Qáhir's first act was to seize al-Muqtadir's mother, who was ill at the time with dropsy, and torture her in order to make her reveal where her son had kept his wealth. Though he tied her up by one foot and beat her all over, she would not or could not tell him anything. He then turned upon Ibn Qarábah, one of the wealthiest of Baghdad's citizens. This man had already consulted Sinán bin Ṣ̈ábit about the advisability of continuing his political career. Sinán strongly advised him to retire from public life and enjoy his health and wealth. Ibn Qarábah rejected the advice. Sinán, with his usual perspicacity, remarked to his son: 'I have never seen a greater fool than that man. Men of that kind either get themselves killed or die in the most abject poverty.' And he was right, for al-Qáhir now seized his goods and pulled down his house and would indeed have taken away his life had he not been deposed before he could sign the order.

In practical politics Sinán was a wise counsellor: in medicine his skill lay in organization rather than treatment. He found in the *wazír* 'Alí bin 'Ísá al-Jarráḥ a sympathetic and helpful chief.

These two raised the public health services to a degree of perfection never before reached. Baghdad was at that time very short of hospital accommodation. There existed only four hospitals to supply the needs of the whole city. A recent epidemic of plague had brought this question of shortage of beds to the front. 'Alí therefore built another hospital at his own expense at the western limit of the city close by the Muhawwal Gate in the Ḥarbiyyah quarter, a point at which the plague had raged with special vehemence. By the advice of Sinán this hospital was placed under the direction of Abú 'Uṣmán Sa'íd ibn Ya'qúb al-Damashqí, who was the *wazír's* personal physician and at that time physician-in-chief to all the hospitals in Baghdad. 'Alí also improved the accommodation and status of the attendants in the hospitals that already existed.

Sinán was now promoted to the rank of one of the two chief court physicians, the other being the Christian Bukht Yishú' IV, the son of Yaḥyá or Yúḥanná, the grandson of Bukht Yishú' III. Sinán also took over the post and duties of Sa'íd bin Ya'qúb, thus assuming charge of all the metropolitan hospitals. He was also given authority over the hospitals at Mecca, Medina and Tarsus. In June 918 there was inaugurated in Baghdad yet another hospital, this one being founded by a woman, and was named in consequence the Bímáristán-ul-Sayyida. Six hundred dinars a month were allocated for its support. The administration of the establishment was confided to the celebrated astronomer Yúsuf ibn Yaḥyá.[1] This foundation was to the east of the city and was built upon the banks of the river. Its main gate opened upon the Yaḥyá Bazaar, so called because the market had been given by al-Rashíd to Yaḥyá ibn Khálid the Barmecide. After the fall of the Barmecides it passed into other hands and was finally destroyed with the hospital when the Seljúqs entered Baghdad.

In the same year, by the advice of Sinán, the caliph founded another hospital by the Syrian Gate, that is, in the western quarter of the city. This was the famous Muqtadirí hospital which the

1 Ibn Khallikán, vol. II, p. 45, n. 2.

caliph supported at a cost of 200 dinars a month from his privy purse. Many were the great physicians who served this hospital. It is claimed that Rhazes is to be numbered among them, but the evidence for this is very conflicting. Yúsuf al-Wásiṭí, a personal physician to the Caliph al-Muqtadir, was one of the staff and here he had among his pupils Jibrá'íl bin 'Ubayd-Ulláh, a great-grandson of Bukht Yishú' II. In due course Jibrá'íl succeeded to the staff of the hospital. He did not stay there long, for his astonishing clinical acumen caused him to be in great demand outside Baghdad.[1] His first success was with a woman afflicted with a haemorrhage whom the physicians of Kerman, Fars and 'Iraq had failed to cure. Next he was honoured by a summons to the court of 'Aẓud-ul-Doula at Shiraz and there he composed for him a book on the nerves and muscles of the eye. When 'Aẓud-ul-Doula founded the 'Aẓudí Hospital at Baghdad, Jibrá'íl returned to practise in Baghdad and became a physician to the new hospital. His fame was now at its height and he was in greater demand than ever. He was sent to Ray to treat al-Ṣáḥib bin 'Albád for whom he wrote his *Káfí* or 'Sufficiency'. Next he went to Daylam, then to Jerusalem, probably as a pilgrim, then to Ray again and Mosul, and finally to Mayáfáriqín, where he retired and died in the year 1005 at the great age of eighty-five.

When Sinán died, he left two sons behind who both became physicians. The elder, named Ṣábit after his grandfather and hence usually called Ṣábit II, was born in A.D. 907/8. He served the 'Abbásid family during the reign of four successive caliphs. He showed the same interest as his father in the work of the public hospitals of Baghdad, so that at the early age of eighteen he was put in charge by the *wazír* al-Kháqání of a new hospital which had recently been founded by Ibn ul-Firát, who was three times *wazír* to the caliph and who came to a violent end in A.D. 924. This hospital served the centre of the city.[2]

Ṣábit II died in the year A.D. 973 or 976. His most famous written work is not medical, but historical, and deals with the

1 *I.A.U.* vol. I, p. 144. 2 Ibid. p. 224.

history of Baghdad during the century in which he lived. After his death the poet Sarí al-Raffá composed the following epitaph over him, which according to Ibn Khallikán are the finest lines ever written on medicine.[1]

Has the sick man any help but Ṣábit,
Next after God? Is anyone sufficient but him?
It is as though Jesus, the Son of Mary, were talking;
For he gives life by his simplest prescription.
He has revived for us the Science of Philosophy, which
Had perished, and reformed the Science of Medicine, which had pined away.
I presented to him a phial of my urine:
He saw therein that which was concealed between my ribs and my heart.
Hidden sickness is as clear to him
As a pebble in translucent water.

Among his many pupils was Aḥmad bin Yúnis, who journeyed from Spain to work under him. This pupil after studying medicine under Ṣábit and ophthalmology under Ibn Waṣíf[2] returned to Spain and became a personal physician to the Amavi caliph. Another pupil was Isḥáq bin Shalíṭa.[3] Through the marriage of his daughter Ṣábit became the father-in-law to the famous Abú ul-Ḥasan Hilál bin al-Muḥassin the Sabean, man of letters, historian and secretary in the service of more than one caliph, who continued the history which Ṣábit had left unfinished.

Sinán's other son was named Ibráhím and is usually known by his *kunya*—Abú Isḥáq. He was born in A.D. 908/9 and died in 947 of a swelling of the liver. He is said to have been a physician and to have occupied the post of president of the board of examiners[4] after the retirement of his father. The story that the Muqtadir hospital was planned by him, as some oriental writers relate, is manifestly untrue, because he was only 10 years old when the hospital was built. There is no evidence to show that his son Isḥáq was a doctor. With Ibráhím the medical genius of the Qurra family seems to have died out.

1 Ibn Khallikán, vol. 1, p. 289.
2 *Maṭraḥ-ul-Anẓár*, pp. 177, 196.
3 *I.A.U.* vol. 1, p. 237.
4 *Maṭraḥ-ul-Anẓár*, pp. 32, 119.

CHAPTER V

THE PLACE OF OPHTHALMOLOGY IN ARABIAN MEDICINE

Of all the branches of Arabian medicine which most deserve study and which indeed have been most studied, ophthalmology is certainly the foremost. Pharmacy follows a bad second: of that later.

The science and art of optics and ophthalmology was not very highly developed among the Greeks and Romans. The Arabs borrowed all that they knew and, though borrowing many errors, built up a very successful, though limited, superstructure. The oculist, a somewhat despised figure in Galen's time, in the days of the caliphs was an honoured member of the medical profession and occupied a unique place in the royal household. From a purely scientific point of view it has to be recorded that pannus was first described not by the Greeks but by the Arabs. The operation for the relief of the chronic form was borrowed by later generations from the Arabs. Glaucoma under the name of 'headache of the pupil' was first described by an Arab. Phlyctenulae and the 'string of pearls' vesicles on a blanched eye-ball appear for the first time in Arab literature. The 'white ulcer' of the cornea was better described by the Arabs than by the Greeks and was separated by them from corneal ulcers. The operation of circumcision of the conjunctiva, which Furnari reintroduced in 1862 as a new method of treatment, was in fact the revival of a technique which the Arabs had introduced many centuries before. Many remedies, known to the Greeks it is true, but not so used by them, were introduced into ophthalmological circles by the Arabs. Camphor, musk and amber were entirely original. On the other hand midriatics were unknown to them. Finally, even the terminology of the Arabs has survived and passed into modern use. Words such as retina and cataract we owe to Arab descriptive anatomy.

It was the Arabs who first upset the traditional theory of vision. The natural philosophers of the pre-Hippocratic days had taught that vision was the result of information gathered by antennae-like rays emitted by the eye. These rays, striking any object, were reflected back to the eye and thus conveyed to the individual information about the outer world. This information was carried to the brain by a hollow tube which connected it to the eye. This hollow tube is what is now known as the optic nerve, which the Arabs, following the Greek anatomists, called the hollow nerve.

This bald theory did not, of course, remain unchallenged or unmodified until the days of the Arabs. Plato suggested that there was also another set of rays which emanated from the object seen. Alexandrian naturalists fixed the seat of vision in the lens. The Atomists put forward an atomical theory; and Aristotle in his own theories was very near to the modern conception. In his 'Questions on the Eye' Ḥunayn developed a theory of vision which approximated to that of Plato. He regarded the lens as the central organ of vision. Here were received the visual force, which came from the brain, and the image of the object which came from without. Rhazes, too, wrote on the subject a monograph which he called 'On the Nature of Vision: wherein it is shown that the Eyes are not radiators of Light'.

It is in the realm of optics rather than in the physiology of the eye that the Arabs have contributed most to the world's knowledge. For this the greatest credit must be given to Abu 'Alí Muḥammad bin al-Ḥasan bin al-Hayṣ̱am of Basra. Early in life Ibn al-Hayṣ̱am moved to Cairo, so that the two caliphates must share the honour which his researches gave to all Islam. His main book on optics is lost in its Arabic form, but the book survives as the *Opticae Thesaurus* of Alhazen in its Latin translation by Witelo the Pole. Basing himself on the geometry and physics of the day Alhazen solved a number of optical problems and conclusively proved that objects are seen by rays passing from them towards the eye and not by the opposite process. Most of his successors did not adopt his views. But al-Bírúní and Avicenna both agree independently and fully in his unorthodox opinions. So far did he carry his theory of vision that he was within an ace of the discovery of the use of spectacles. In his days the only method of aiding weak sight was that recommended by 'Alí bin 'Ísá. Those who do not see in the near, he says, should use styptic medicines; those who see well in the near but not in the distance require medicines which give moist nutrition and bring the moist principle to the eye. With Alhazen began not only modern physiological optics, but also the whole science of modern optics.

The work of Alhazen was repeated and extended by a Persian named Kamál-ul-Dín, who died about 1320. This scientist also observed the path of the rays in the interior of a glass sphere in order to examine the refraction of sunlight in rain-drops. This led him to an explanation of the genesis of the primary and secondary rainbows.

The greatest contribution of the Arabs in practical ophthalmology was in the matter of cataract. The old Greek name for this condition was ὑπόχυμα, the Latin *suffusio*. Both suggest the supposed pathology. The Arabs adopted their view that it was due to a pouring out of humour into the eye. Hence the Persians called the condition *Nazúl-i-Áb* or 'Descent of Water'. According to Celsus suffusion is characterized by corrupt, inspissated humour, collected in the locus vacuus between the pupil and the lens, thus obstructing the visual spirit. By clearing this empty space vision could be restored. Galen, though he did not admit the existence of a locus vacuus, admitted this pathology. The Arab ophthalmologists adopted as their own the views of Celsus.

The operation of couching for cataract, that is, a violent displacement of the lens, dates back to Babylonian and even prehistoric days. The method of extraction is essentially the method introduced in the eighteenth century. Yet there are reasons for believing that surgeons were groping vaguely towards this technique many centuries before. There is the significant passage in Galen where he speaks of someone who instead of displacing the cataract 'attempted to extract it, as I shall show in the book dealing with operations'. This book is lost and unfortunately not even an Arabic translation is now known. Rhazes is reported by Ṣaláḥ-ul-Dín to have said that according to Antyllus some divide the inner part of the pupil and extract the cataract. But neither the original work of Antyllus is extant nor does this passage occur in any of Rhazes' works known to-day.

There must have been, therefore, in the days of Galen and Antyllus some method of radical cure similar to that practised to-day. Apparently it lost favour, for the Arabs were forced to develop a technique of their own. The most significant development was that of 'Ammár bin 'Alí of Mosul, who elaborated the operation of suction. His operation consisted of introducing a hollow needle through the sclerotic and extracting the lens by suction. This avoided an incision into the anterior chamber and the consequent loss of aqueous humour. His operation was accepted in the East, but gained no adherents in the West. Europe rediscovered the principle in the nineteenth century.

The foundation of all Arab ophthalmology was, as is equally true of all their medicine, Greek, and of the Greek works, as usual, those of Galen. Galen's book on 'Diseases originating in the Eye' is lost, but there is an early Arabic translation entitled *Jawámi' Kitáb Jálínús* or 'Collection of Galen's Works' which enumerates 91 eye diseases and their symptoms and which may possibly be an extract from the lost book.

Of surviving Arab original works the earliest is that of Mesue Senior, that is Yúḥanná bin Másawayh. This was written about A.D. 850 and is composed in bad Arabic with many Greek, Syriac and Persian technical terms, according to Meyerhof, who has published a short analysis and extract from the work.[1]

1 'Die Augenheilkunde des Juhanna ibn Masawaih', in *Der Islam*, vol. VI, pp. 217–56. Mesue's book is called *Daghal-ul-'Ayn* or 'The Alteration of the Eye'.

Contemporary with this was the far more important 'Ten Treatises on the Eye' by Ḥunayn, to whom I have already referred. This is the earliest known systematic text-book on ophthalmology and from this all later works borrow more or less. It is available for study in the original Arabic and in a translation into English, for it was published in Cairo in 1928 with a glossary and notes by Dr Meyerhof.

As a text-book the work has its faults. There is a want of balance between the theoretical and the practical parts; the theoretical is relatively too long. Ibn abí Uṣaybi'a sums up this criticism when he wrote:

There exist of this book very different copies, and the arrangement of the treatises is not uniform. In some of them the contents are found to be abridged; in others Ḥunayn enlarged and increased them more than is required by the composition of the book. The reason for this is that each of its treatises is a separate book without connection with the others. He himself says in the final treatise: 'For more than thirty years I have been composing various treatises concerning the eye, in which I pursued divergent aims about which I was questioned by several people one after another.' Then Ḥubaysh asked me to collect these treatises—there were nine of them—and to make one book of them and to add for him to the nine preceding treatises a tenth in which I discussed a commentary on the compound remedies composed by the Ancients and laid down in their books for the treatment of eye diseases.[1]

Ibn abí Uṣaybi'a also states that he knew of an eleventh treatise by Ḥunayn which dealt with operative treatment. That such a treatise once existed is confirmed by the fact that Rhazes quotes from it in his *Continens*.

Ḥunayn also wrote a second ophthalmological treatise for the use of his sons Dá'úd and Isḥáq, which he called the *Kitáb-ul-Masá'il fi il-'Ayn* or 'Book of Questions on the Eye'. This is a treatise on the physiology and pathology of the eye, couched in the form of question and answer. Meyerhof doubts its authenticity and is inclined in spite of the testimony of the Ancients to

1 *I.A.U.* vol. 1, pp. 184–200.

attribute it to one of his pupils. The text and a French translation have recently been published in Cairo.

With the publication of Ḥunayn's works the interest in ophthalmology seems to have become more pronounced, for all text-books of medicine now contain a long section devoted to diseases of the eye. Notable among these are the *Firdaus-ul-Ḥikmat* of 'Alí bin Rabbán al-Ṭabarí, the *Continens* of Rhazes, the *Canon* of Avicenna (of which the ophthalmological section has been translated into German by Hirschberg and Lippert) and the *Liber Regius* of Haly Abbas. It is unnecessary to continue the list, for all writers of importance deal at length with this subject.

Following Ḥunayn the next important monograph is that of 'Alí bin 'Ísá, a Christian oculist of Baghdad and a pupil of Abú ul-Faraj bin al-Ṭayyib. He died early in the eleventh century. His is the most complete text-book on eye diseases which the Arab school produced, besides being the most original of all the early written treatises on the subject. Exactly how much is original and how much is borrowed it is difficult to say. 'Alí himself says in his preface: 'I have searched the works of the Ancients throughout and merely added a little of my own thereto, which I have learned publicly from the teachers of my own time and which I have acquired in the practice of this science.'

It is a work which can be easily studied, even by those who do not know Arabic, for a translation of it into German by Hirschberg appeared in 1904 and another into English by Casey Wood in 1936. The book is called the *Tazkirat-ul-Kaḥḥálín* or 'Note-book of the Oculists'. There is, or was, some dispute about the identity of the 'Alí who wrote it. Al-Qifṭí and Ḥájjí Khalífa both state that he was a pupil of Ḥunayn. This is quite incompatible with the statement of Ibn abí Uṣaybi'a that he died after A.H. 400, that is A.D. 1010, which is at least 125 years after the death of Ḥunayn. Nor is it likely that a pupil of Ḥunayn's would attempt to write a work dealing precisely with the subject upon which his master and a favourite pupil had so notably excelled.

The author of the *Tazkirat* moreover attacks Ḥunayn. From a negative point of view, too, the fact that Rhazes fails to quote from the *Tazkirat* suggests that the later date is the more correct. In all probability, 'Alí bin 'Ísá being an extremely common name, there were two physicians of this name, one the pupil of Ḥunayn and not particularly interested in ophthalmology, and a second who composed the *Tazkirat* a century and a half later.

Of the work itself there is no need to say very much. The first part is devoted to anatomy, the second to the external diseases of the eye, and the third part to internal diseases of the eye which are not visible upon inspection. This last section is perhaps the most interesting from a modern point of view, for it shows the very definite limitations of Greek and Arab ophthalmology. The ophthalmoscope and the power of seeing the retina have revolutionized ophthalmological practice. When 'Alí speaks of internal diseases of the eye, he literally means diseases confined to the eye. The possibility of first diagnosing diabetes, kidney disease and cerebral tumour in the ophthalmic consulting room is not conceived of by the oculists of those times. The nearest approach that 'Alí makes to the modern conception of eye disease as a manifestation of general disease is when he urges the practitioner to realize that defective vision may be due to a disease of the stomach or brain just as much as to an incipient cataract. And with that he leaves the question.

This limitation was, of course, common to all oculists of his day and continued for many centuries after. Al-Qifṭí and Ibn abí Uṣaybi'a say that his *Tazkirat* became the text-book upon which most ophthalmologists worked. It then passed over to Europe to become the foundation of western practice. It was translated into Latin under the title of *Tractatus de Oculis Iesu Halis* and was printed in Venice in 1497 and again in 1499 and 1500. And indeed, as Casey Wood remarks, it was not until the beginning of the fifteenth century, when Kepler published his complete work on dioptrics, when the prescription of glasses became common, and such important matters as the true character of cataract was settled, that any really better treatises on ophthalmology than the *Tazkirat* began to appear.

Contemporary with 'Alí bin 'Ísá were three other ophthalmologists who published works of note. One was Jibrá'íl bin 'Ubayd-Ulláh of the great Bukht Yishú' family, who was oculist to 'Azud-ul-Doula. He wrote a book called *Ṭibb-ul-'Ayn* or 'Medicine of the Eye'.

The second is 'Ammár bin 'Alí of Mosul, who is most unjustly overshadowed by his contemporary, the more famous but less original, 'Alí bin 'Ísá. 'Ammár first lived in 'Iraq and later in Egypt. He travelled widely, visiting Khorasan and Palestine; throughout his travels he practised and performed operations. It was in Egypt that he wrote his great treatise which he called the *Kitáb-ul-Muntakhab fi 'Iláj-il-'Ayn* or 'Book of Selections in the Treatment of the Eye'. He commences the work with a preface on the story of the composition of the book. Then he deals with the anatomy and pathology of the eye. In the course of the book he describes six cases of operation for cataract. A German edition of the text has recently been published. Previous to that, apart from manuscripts, the work was only available in a Hebrew translation made in Rome by Nathan the Jew in the thirteenth century. The Latin *Tractatus de Oculis Canamusali* of David Hermenus or David Armenicus, which was printed in Venice in 1497, is generally considered to be a forgery and to be unconnected with the original work of 'Ammár.

Thirdly there was the Persian Abú ul-Ḥasan Aḥmad bin Muḥammad al-Ṭabarí, who in his *Kitáb-ul-Mu'álaja-ul-Buqráṭiyya* or 'Book of Hippocratic Treatment' says that he wrote a long special treatise on diseases of the eye. This treatise is unknown to-day.

The first ophthalmological treatise to be written in the Persian language was, as far as I know, that of Abú Rúḥ Muḥammad bin Manṣúr of Jurjan, who was known by the very suggestive title of *Zarríndast* or 'Golden Hand'. His work was called *Núr-ul-'Ayún* or 'Light of the Eyes' and was composed in A.D. 1088.

Only two manuscripts of this work are known to exist, preserved, one in Oxford and one in Calcutta. The contents follow the example set by the *Tazkirat*, but the work is distinguished by a chapter, the seventh out of the ten discourses, which deals with operative technique. This has been translated by Hirschberg. As a whole the work is said to be disappointing, for it is a slavish imitation of the earlier Arab models and gives no indication of pre-Moslem Iranian methods or of anything peculiarly Persian, which would be so much more interesting to a later age. Its importance is its language, not the contents.

Later Ophthalmology in Persia seems to have produced but few outstanding names. After these great men whom I have just described, I can find no one who has composed any monograph on the eye, far less who has made any original contribution to the speciality. Bar Hebraeus, indeed, speaks of a certain Najm-ul-Dín Qazvíní, who was a famous logician and the author of a work[1] called *Al-'Ayn* or 'The Eye'. He flourished at the end of the thirteenth century. There is, too, in existence a Persian manuscript entitled *'Ilm-i-Ḥikmat-i-'Ayn* or 'The Science of the Wisdom of the Eye', composed by one Muḥammad bin Muḥammad 'Arab. This being dedicated to Abu Sa'íd the Il-Khan dates itself to within a few years of A.D. 1336, for in that year Abu Sa'íd died. All original work on diseases of the eyes seems to have shifted with 'Ammár bin 'Alí to Cairo and it is in the history of Egyptian medicine rather than in that of Persia that the later developments of Islamic ophthalmology should be sought.

1 *Hist. Dynst.* vol. x, p. 358.

CHAPTER VI

THE RISE OF THE BUWAYHID FAMILY

TO the south-west of the Caspian Sea between the modern provinces of Gilan and Azerbaijan once lay the small state of Daylam. The Daylamites were late in accepting the authority of Islam. Al-Ḥasan ibn 'Alí, known as Al-Uṭrush or 'The Deaf One', having failed to secure a temporal kingdom in Tabaristan, was more successful in his spiritual warfare in Daylam. Himself a Shí'ah his converts too became Shí'ahs. Having saved their souls he then returned to his former ambition of carving out for himself a throne in northern Persia. The Daylamites being good and willing fighters he was now successful. He captured Amul in A.D. 913 and ruled from there as an independent chieftain for the remainder of his life.

By his will he set aside the claims of his children to succeed to his throne and, as so often follows, the consequence was civil war. Two leaders emerged as a result of the fighting; one was Mákán ibn Kákúy and the other Asfar ibn Shiravayh. Mákán occupied Ray, but was soon driven out by Asfar, who followed up his success by defeating an army from Baghdad which had been sent north to assert the authority of the caliph in those parts.

Asfar, though an excellent fighter, was no ruler and before long his subjects were in revolt. Led by Mardávíj ibn Ziyár, who for the moment was united with Mákán, they drove Asfar out of Ray and killed him on the road. Mardávíj now became supreme, extended the boundaries of his principality by a successful attack on Hamadan, and defeated another army sent up from Baghdad. He even dreamed of leaving the highlands of Persia, of capturing the caliph himself, and of founding a new empire on the Sassanian model with his headquarters at Ctesiphon. But his plans were cut short. For some of his Turkish soldiery, jealous of the favours that he showed to his Daylamite followers, murdered him one winter morning and placed his brother Vashmgír upon the throne in his stead.

Although the plans of Mardávíj were thus misplaced, there was in his retinue a young officer who was destined to see them accomplished by his own family. This was 'Alí ibn Buwayh. Buwayh himself was a simple Caspian fisherman. His eldest son attached himself to Mákán and, when Mákán's fortunes began to wane, transferred his services to Mardávíj. A younger son Aḥmad was a simple cutter of wood in his early days and now threw in his lot with his brother. 'Alí, living at Ray, ingratiated himself with the *wazír* and was rewarded with the post of a tax-collector in some obscure village on the fringe of the Great Salt Desert. But his dealings with the villagers, with the landed gentry around, and with some soldiers who were quartered in the village so endeared him to all that he was able to lay the foundations of a following with which he could ultimately defy even the caliph.

As soon as he felt himself strong enough to take independent action, he moved towards Ispahan. But considering himself still too weak to defy Mardávíj alone, he offered his services to the caliph; for al-Qáhir still controlled Ispahan. His offer was rejected and against his wishes he found himself obliged to attack the city. A large desertion of the hired Daylamite soldiery to his side gave him an unexpected advantage and he routed the caliph's forces with ease. Strengthened by this success he went south and again put to flight the orthodox governor in a battle near Shiraz. Thus all Fars came into his possession.

The murder of Mardávíj left 'Alí ibn Buwayh in almost undisputed possession of Persia. He therefore determined to go down to the plains and attack the cities of the caliph in the Euphrates valley. He dispatched his brother Aḥmad against Basra. He, although failing to capture the city, was strong enough to remain encamped in the neighbourhood, awaiting a favourable opportunity either to attack again or to march north upon Wasit and Baghdad.

During these years Baghdad itself was the scene of intrigue and plots beyond number. The Caliph al-Qáhir was only a puppet of his generals. The mere breath of suspicion that he was plotting to assert his authority caused Mú'nis, now the generalissimo of the army, to keep him in even closer confinement and to banish his favourite physician 'Ísá bin Yúsuf ibn ul-'Aṭṭár to Mosul.

A change in the situation gave the caliph the upper hand. Mú'nis and his lieutenants were promptly thrown into gaol. 'Ísá was recalled to Baghdad, and another favourite, Muḥammad ibn ul-Qásim, was installed as *wazír*. These three now ruled the State. The *wazír* and the physician shared the privilege of the use of the royal barge. Upon their advice al-Qáhir assumed a pose of sanctity and began by decreeing the banishment of wine and singing girls from the city. The pious union did not last long. First 'Ísá began to plot against Ibn ul-Qásim and in October 933 persuaded al-Qáhir to replace him by a favourite of his own. Next it became known in the city that al-Qáhir, so far from following the laws of Islam and his own regulations, was in fact rarely sober and was a lewd fellow who coveted other men's singing girls. His overthrow was determined upon. Ibn Muqla, now in hiding, stirred up the troops against him. They were told that the caliph was building new dungeons in which to imprison their officers. A popular astrologer was bribed to add to their fears by his terrifying predictions. 'Ísá the physician did his utmost to warn al-Qáhir of his danger. For a short time his advice was heeded. Then al-Qáhir returned to his cups and nothing more could be done.

In the morning of 22 April 934 the attack on the palace was made. 'Ísá tried to rouse al-Qáhir, but found him comatose with wine. He had been drinking till sunrise and even when awakened was too drunk to understand what was told him. When at last the troops entered his private quarters, he sobered up and fled to the ceiling of the bath-room for concealment. He was found, arrested and deposed. That same night orders were given to Bukht Yishú' bin Yaḥyá, that is Bukht Yishú' IV, his personal physician, for the depriving him of his eyes. Bukht Yishú' summoned a surgeon who blinded the deposed caliph then and there.

Al-Qáhir was succeeded by al-Rá̤zí, who at once chose Ibn Muqla for his *wazír*. A few months later al-Rá̤zí yielded to the wishes of his courtiers and deposed him and offered the post to the aged 'Alí bin 'Ísá in his stead. This 'Alí refused, but suggested the name of his brother. Ibn Muqla, thus deprived of office, left no stone unturned to secure his return to power. He even persuaded al-Rá̤zí to join him in plotting against the new *wazír*. Al-Rá̤zí, however, failed at the last moment to play his part and revealed the plot. Ibn Muqla was punished by the amputation of his right hand.

No sooner was the punishment carried out than al-Rá̤zí repented of his weakness and sent his own physician Sinán bin Ṣábit to attend him. Being a fine calligraphist the amputation of his right hand was the greatest punishment that could be inflicted upon Ibn Muqla, short of depriving him of his life. Sinán found him weeping. 'I have laboured', he said, 'in the service of the caliphs, three times have I been minister to three caliphs, and twice have I transcribed the Qur'án. Yet they cut off my hand as though it had been the hand of a thief.'[1]

Sinán has left among his clinical notes a description of the scene:

'I found him in a terrible plight [he writes]. The fore-arm was dreadfully swollen with a coarse blue kardawání rag tied round it with a hempen cord. Undoing the cord and removing the rag, I found beneath it, where the hand had been severed, a layer of horse dung. This I shook off. The top of the fore-arm proximal to the amputation was ligated with a cord of hemp which owing to the swelling had sunk into the tissues of the arm which was beginning to turn black. I told him that the cord must be undone and that in place of the dung camphor must be applied and the arm anointed with sandal, rose-water, and camphor. He told me to proceed. So I undid the cord, emptied the box on the wound, and anointed his arm. He revived, was eased, and the palpitation calmed down.[2]

1 Ibn Khallikán, vol. III, p. 266. Quoted in *Eclipse of 'Abbasid Caliphate*, vol. IV, p. 438.
2 Ibid. p. 437.

His arm healed and he was even able to write again by fastening a pen to the stump. But his troubles were not yet over. He was removed to a darker prison and even the visits of Sinán were forbidden. His rival, who continued in office, next ordered the amputation of his tongue. Through this too he lived. In his prolonged confinement he was attacked with a diarrhoea and having no person to attend him was forced himself to draw the water from the well for his use. This he did by seizing the rope alternately with his left hand and his teeth. He continued in this miserable state until his death. He was even buried within the prison walls.

The caliph had now become the objective of three rival parties, each of whom strove to possess themselves of his physical person in order to preserve a semblance of constitutional rule. At one moment the powerful Arab tribe, the Ḥamdánids, would be successful and the caliph would be tossed between Mosul and Baghdad. At another moment the Turks under Bachkam would gain the upper hand and the caliph would be a prisoner in his own palace on the Tigris. The third party was that of al-Barídí, a Persian chieftain who had once held the office of *wazír*.

Bachkam had had a hand in the murder of Mardávíj. He himself in turn was slain by a Kurdish lad when engaged in an attempt to seize some wealthy Kurdish tribesmen. He died possessed of considerable riches the greater part of which he had buried for safety. The diggers who were sent to search for it, after they had discovered and unearthed a vast number of jars filled with silver and gold, were offered as their hire either a sum of 2000 dirhams down or the mould which had covered the jars. They chose the former. The caliph then ordered the mould to be sieved and from it is said to have recovered 36,000 dirhams.

It was commonly said that Bachkam slew his servants who were privy to the palaces where the treasure was buried, but Sinán bin Ṣábit denies that this was true. He writes that 'Bachkam himself told him that he had never found it necessary to kill any of his slaves; for he used to convey the diggers to the secret spot shut up in chests so that they were always quite ignorant of where they were and he himself used to drive the mules'.

In his old age Bachkam became a model of philanthropy, for he founded a soup kitchen at Wasit during a time of famine and a hospital at Baghdad. His appeal to Sinán to come and help him reform his life is well known. As long as al-Rází was alive, Sinán refused to leave Baghdad. On the death of the caliph Sinán joined Bachkam at Wasit. The words of his welcome are quoted in many histories and biographies:

> I wish to rely on you. You are to look after my body and give me what is useful for it. And there is another matter which is even more important than the affairs of my body and that is the matter of my character. For I have confidence in your intelligence, your good qualities, your religion, and your affection. Verily the supremacy over me of my anger and my passions and their excesses have brought me to repentance. For often do I act in a manner of which I repent me when my passions subside. So now watch what I do. If you note anything which deserves reproach, do not refrain from telling me. Hide it not, but make it clear to me. Thus direct me on the right path and cure me a perfect cure.[1]

The successor to Bachkam as commander of the Turkish troops was Túzún, who having defeated al-Barídí entered Baghdad in triumph and was saluted with the title of Amír-ul-Umara' or 'Lord of Lords'. During Túzún's temporary absence a conspiracy broke out which threatened the caliph's life. Al-Muttaqí, who had succeeded al-Rází in 940, was obliged to appeal to the Ḥamdánids for help. With their aid he left Baghdad and took up his residence at al-Raqqa, now a suppliant and a refugee and shorn of all his glory. Túzún was furious when he heard that his puppet master had fled. The fact that he was in the hands of his rivals added to his fury. Accordingly, as soon as he heard that al-Muttaqí was dissatisfied with his position, he offered to restore him to his palace in Baghdad and guaranteed him his safety. On these conditions al-Muttaqí left al-Raqqa. He met the *amír* in

1 *I.A.U.* vol. 1, p. 222.

the winter of 944, and even before he had set foot within his palace, Túzún broke his word and had the unfortunate caliph blinded. On the same day he installed his brother as caliph with the title of al-Mustakfí.

The personal physician of Túzún was a certain Hilál bin Ibráhím bin Zahrún, a Sabean of Harran. Túzún, though generous in his dealings with his physician, was not an intelligent patient. Hilál one day, having reason to administer a purge, gave him in error such a large dose that the bowels were excoriated and Túzún began to pass blood. Hilál rapidly gave him another drug to undo these bad effects. Túzún, believing that the voiding of blood was the passing out of diseased matter, rewarded his physician with a robe of honour and much money. Instead of being pleased Hilál was considerably upset; for he considered that if his master thus mistook the bad for the good, one day perhaps his loyal services would be similarly misinterpreted and an undeserved punishment be meted out upon him.[1]

Hilál's son Ibráhím was brought up among the schoolmen of Baghdad and preferred astronomy and mathematics to medicine. He is said to have written excellent prose and verse, to have published a collection of his letters, and to have written several books on astronomical subjects in one of which he described his observation of the entry of the sun into the Signs of the Crab and the Scales. This was considered an observation of the utmost importance.[2]

Both the father of Hilál and his brother Abú ul-Ḥasan Ṣábit were also physicians. Abú ul-Ḥasan later became a personal physician to 'Aẓud-ul-Doula Daylamí and appears to have been a skilful practitioner and one who glories in the trial of new remedies. Many are the stories told about Abú ul-Ḥasan. Ibn Buṭlán says that in those days the practice of bleeding for cerebral haemorrhage was just coming into fashion. Up till then it had been the custom only to administer stimulants. One day a certain nobleman had an apoplectic fit and was accounted for

1 *Hist. Dynst.* vol. IX, p. 204. 2 Ibid. p. 217.

dead by all the attendants. Abú ul-Ḥasan seized the opportunity to try out the new method of treatment. 'For if he is already dead', he said, 'it can do no harm. And if there is still life and if the method is good, it may save his life.' Accordingly he opened a vein and the supposedly dead man was saved.

It is also said that when a certain nobleman of Baghdad wished to purchase a slave girl for a very high figure, he first sent her to Abú ul-Ḥasan to ascertain whether she suffered from any hidden disease. Abú ul-Ḥasan sent back the extraordinary report that the clinical signs were unfavourable for purchasing unless the girl had eaten a dish of sumach and unripe grapes on the night previous.

His deductions from the pulse were equally marvellous. To a poet who had allowed him to feel his radial artery, he replied that he had overloaded his stomach and that he had had the temerity to eat soured milk with veal. To an astrologer in the same company he stated that he had exceeded the amount of cold food proper to his temperament by eating eleven pomegranites. Upon which the astrologer exclaimed: 'This is clairvoyance, not medicine.' These powers of accurate diagnosis Abú ul-Ḥasan ascribed to the fortune of his birth as revealed by his horoscope.[1]

Two works from his pen were well known among his contemporaries. One was a 'Rectification of the Discourses of Yúḥanná ibn Sarábiyún'; the other was a collection of his replies to various medical questions put to him. He died in Baghdad in the year A.D. 975 or 979.

Less than a year after the installation of al-Mustakfí as caliph Túzún himself died, and the lawless state of Baghdad became worse than ever. The solution of the troubles came from Wasit. The governor of that town, doubting the capacity of any of the officers of Baghdad to maintain order, invited Aḥmad ibn Buwayh, who was still hovering round, to advance to the capital. Aḥmad required no second invitation. On this news the Turkish soldiery, who had now neither a Bachkam nor a Túzún to lead

1 Ibid. p. 213.

them, fled. The caliph and his *wazír* went into hiding. The populace willingly opened the gates of the city to the Buwayhid troops.

It was on Saturday, 18 January 946, that Aḥmad ibn Buwayh entered Baghdad. On the next day he had an interview with the caliph and swore to uphold his rights. In return he was invested with the office and title of Amír-ul-Umara' and the further title of Mu'izz-ul-Doula. His absent elder brothers were at the same time given the titles of 'Imád-ul-Doula (this was for 'Alí, the eldest) and of Rukn-ul-Doula (this for al-Ḥasan, the second). But all these honours were in vain. The new *amír* was suspicious of al-Mustakfí's pro-Turkish tendencies. Was not the *amír* a Shí'ah and the caliph a Sunni? The story goes that he took offence at an entertainment provided by the chief lady in the caliph's harem. Whatever the reason, political, religious or petty, a few days later the wretched caliph was dragged to the *amír's* house and there deprived of his eyes. In this state he went to join his predecessors. Al-Muttaqí had been blinded and was still alive; al-Qáhir was not only blinded and still alive, but was now destitute and begging his daily bread in the street.

The accession of Mu'izz-ul-Doula to the throne—for a sovereign he was in fact—marks the beginning of a new period. Politically it meant that the supreme ruler of Baghdad was for the first time a Shí'ah, a heretic in the eyes of the people; and this became the cause of much trouble and ultimately of the fall of the house before the Seljuq invaders. It also meant the dominance of Persia over the whole of eastern Islam. Mu'izz-ul-Doula was by birth, by training, and by preferences frankly Persian. He could not even speak Arabic. In his first interview with 'Alí bin 'Isá, the aged *wazír*, he was obliged to use an interpreter, for 'Alí would not, and possibly could not, speak Persian. The position of the ruling caliph of the day now reached its lowest ebb. Up till now the caliph had had a *wazír* as his right-hand man; the *amír* had contented himself with a secretary. Now the custom was reversed. The caliph became a mere dependent upon the *amír* and was often even carried in the *amír's* train when fighting at a distance from the capital.

On the other hand the presence of a strong ruler, uninfluenced by Turkish or Arab sympathies, as was Mu'izz-ul-Doula, gave to the city the peace which it so much demanded. Though the period that was about to begin can by no means be said to rival the days of al-Ma'mún, yet in his encouragement of hospitals and medicine in general, the entry of Mu'izz-ul-Doula into Baghdad must be considered as the inauguration of the Silver Age of Arab medicine. Under the patronage of the Buwayhids flourished Rhazes, Haly Abbas and Avicenna.

Mu'izz-ul-Doula had only ruled as *amír* for a few years when he began to suffer from distressing attacks of priapism. Fearing that this impended his early death, in the year 955 he nominated his son Abú Manṣúr Bakhtiyár as his successor. His disease was evidently a calculus of the urinary bladder, for a few years later he was again taken ill in the night with difficulty in passing water and with a discharge of blood and gravel. He summoned his *wazír* Muḥallabí and his chamberlain Sabuktagín and bequeathing his empire to his son formally abandoned the government of the country. But this was not the moment for his death, and it was not until March 967 that Bakhtiyár, now glorified with the title of 'Izz-ul-Doula, was able to assume the amirate. The night that Mu'izz-ul-Doula died, it began to rain. For three days and for three nights it rained in Baghdad so hard that the soldiery and the mob were unable to venture out-of-doors. By the time the sun shone again the position of Bakhtiyár on the throne was established.

His father's advice to obey his uncle Rukn-ul-Doula and to consult him on all matters of importance and to obey his cousin 'Aẓud-ul-Doula, the son of Rukn-ul-Doula, his senior and a more skilled administrator, Bakhtiyár rejected from the first. He spent his time in sport and the society of buffoons, singers and women. He exasperated his courtiers, especially Sabuktagín now his commander-in-chief. His neglect of his duties very soon brought difficulties which threatened his position. Sabuktagín openly mutinied and demanded that he should give up Wasit and Baghdad. The Turkish troops followed his lead. Before Bakhtiyár had made up his mind what course to follow, Sabuktagín died and Bakhtiyár thought the moment opportune to swallow his pride and to appeal to 'Aẓud-ul-Doula for help. This help 'Aẓud-ul-Doula very readily gave and in January 975 he put the Turkish troops to flight and entered Baghdad at the head of his army.

It was not long before 'Aẓud-ul-Doula's real motives became apparent. He fomented a mutiny among the followers of Bakhtiyár and then refused to act as a mediator unless Bakhtiyár abdicated and left him as sole *amír* of the caliph. Though opposed by Marzubán, a son of Bakhtiyár, and even by his own father who thought that he was carrying matters a little too far, 'Aẓud-ul-Doula persisted in his demands and ultimately received all that he demanded.

He now found time to devote himself to those social works which are the glory of the Buwayhid house. In the midst of his triumphs when still a man of only forty-seven, he died of what is usually held to have been epilepsy, though it may well have been uraemia.[1] His biographer says that he was attacked when a young man 'by an ailment which became recurrent, resembling epilepsy, which was followed by a brain disease called Lethargos'. He was a sovereign greatly respected,[2] supremely munificent where bounty was proper, yet as close-fisted as a miser when it was more fitting to withhold. He used to rise early in the morning, take his bath and then say his prayers. The morning he devoted to affairs of State. A large mid-day meal followed with his physician-in-attendance standing before him and discussing the value of his various dishes and similar subjects. The afternoon siesta came next. The evening was again given over to affairs of State, but the task was then lightened by interludes of songs and stories.

The highest of his honours were bestowed upon men of

1 *Hist. Dynst.* vol. IX, p. 211; Ibn Khallikán, vol. II, p. 484.
2 Ibid. vol. V, p. 456 and vol. VI, p. 36.

learning. He encouraged ascetics, jurists, theologians, poets, grammarians, physicians, astrologers and mathematicians. In his palace he set apart a special room for men of attainments and distinction. It was near his own room and was so far removed from the halls of public audience that there was no danger that these sages would be interrupted in their researches or their discussions. 'So these studies', says Ibn Miskawayhí, 'were brought to life after they had been defunct. Their devotees reassembled after they had been dispersed, the young were encouraged to study and the old to instruct, talent had free scope, and there was a brisk market for ability which had previously had none.'[1]

The period of translating Greek texts into Arabic, which had never completely ceased, now revived. As his chief translator 'Aẓud-ul-Doula employed a Greek physician named Naẓíf the Priest,[2] who is said to have been as skilful in his translations as he was inept in his clinical work. His mistakes became so well known that patients dreaded his approach. A sick general to whom Naẓíf[3] announced that 'Aẓud-ul-Doula had sent him to give treatment, made sure that this was a sign that he had in some way offended him and sent at once to know what his offence might be. The books which 'Aẓud-ul-Doula thus had composed, he guarded carefully in his own library and in some cases refused to allow others even to see them. When someone once succeeded in making by stealth a copy of *The Elucidation*, a book on grammar by Ḥasan bin Aḥmad Farisi, he ordered the hand of the culprit to be amputated. It was now that Haly Abbas composed in his honour the *Liber Regius*, a work which a contemporary described as 'clearer, better arranged, and more complete than any other encyclopaedia of medicine'.[4]

'Alí ibn ul-'Abbás al-Majúsí, known to the West as Haly Abbas, studied medicine under Abu Máhir Músá ibn Yúsuf ibn Sayyár of Shiraz[5] and refers to him in grateful terms more than

1 Ibid. vol. v, p. 447.
2 *I.A.U.* vol. I, p. 238.
3 *Hist. Dynst.* vol. IX, p. 215.
4 Niẓámí, *Chahár Maqála*.
5 *I.A.U.* vol. I, p. 236.

once. Of the master very little is known. He is said to have written works on surgery, phlebotomy, and on more general topics. Nafís bin 'Iwaz̲ of Kerman states that he offered to cure Ī'sá̲ bin Másawayh of a melancholia brought on by excess of study. But on chronological grounds alone this story must be doubted.

Of his greatest pupil also very little is known. The title al-Majúsí or 'The Magian' seems to show that he was of Zoroastrian origin. It has been suggested that he was himself a Zoroastrian and that the orthodox names of his father and grandfather are not proofs of their conversion to Islam. His biographical note by al-Qifṭí is so short that it may be quoted in full. I use Professor Browne's translation:

> 'Alí ibn ul-'Abbás al-Majúsí was an accomplished and perfect physician of Persian origin and was known as 'the Son of the Magian'. He studied with a Persian professor known as Abu Máhir and also studied and worked by himself with the writings of the Ancients. He composed for the king 'Aẓud-ul-Doula Fanák̲h̲usrú the Buwayhid his system of medicine entitled *al-Malikí*, which is a splendid work and a noble thesaurus comprehending the science and practice of medicine, admirably arranged. It enjoyed great popularity in its day and was diligently studied, until the appearance of Avicenna's *Qánún*, which usurped its popularity and caused *al-Malikí* to be somewhat neglected. The latter excels on the practical and the former on the scientific side.[1]

Of his great book, called in Arabic the *Kámil-ul-Ṣaná'at* or *Kitáb-ul-Malikí*, that is, 'The Perfect Practitioner' or 'The Royal Book', and in Latin *Liber Regius*, copies abound in manuscript form in public and private libraries. It was translated into Latin and printed in Venice in A.D. 1492 and again at Lyons in 1523. During the last century it was published in lithograph form in Lahore and printed in Cairo. It has been so admirably analysed and discussed by Professor Browne in his *Arabian Medicine* that there is no need to recapitulate what he says there. It is notable that Professor Browne disagrees with the judgement of al-Qifṭí, Bar Hebraeus and other medieval writers in holding that this

1 Al-Qifṭí, *Ta'rík̲h̲-ul-Ḥukamá*, quoted in Browne's *Arabian Medicine*, p. 53.

work of Haly Abbas is far superior in style, arrangement and interest to Avicenna's *Canon*.

Arabic and Persian biographers ascribe to him only this work. Brockelmann[1] mentions a manuscript at Gotha which contains another medical treatise attributed to him. The Royal College of Physicians in London, although it possesses no copy of the *Liber Regius* either in Arabic or in a translation, holds among its treasures a small Latin work, printed in Venice in 1485, entitled *De Fatis Stellarum*, which is said on the title-page to be a translation of an Arabic work by Albohazen Hali filius Abenragel. Is Haly Abbas to be recognized in this name, as the catalogue of the college says? I think not. The names put into modern transliteration run Abú ul-Ḥasan 'Alí ibn abí il-Rajal, which are a long way removed from the names of Haly Abbas. The book is mainly concerned with the stars, although it contains also a lot of medical lore. Part I, pp. 15–17, for instance, deals with pregnancy and the influence which the stars can have upon it; as also does p. 28 in Part II. The fifth part of the book is confined to pregnancy and generation: the seventh part, pp. 116 and 117, deals with the administration of medicine and drugs.[2]

Haly Abbas was court physician to 'Aẓud-ul-Doula while the latter was still in residence in Shiraz. Apparently he did not follow him to Baghdad and outlived his royal patron, for he died in A.D. 994/5. Among the physicians in his suite 'Aẓud-ul-Doulá had as his treasurer a Persian named Abú 'Alí Aḥmad bin Muḥammad bin Miskawayhí. As a physician Ibn Miskawayhí is of no importance. But his great historical work, the *Kitáb Tajárib-ul-Umám wa Ta'aqíb-ul-Ḥimám* or 'The Book of the Vicissitudes of Nations and the Results of Efforts', assures him of a place among the writers of his day.[3] He is one of the earliest

1 Brockelmann, *Gesch. d. Arab. Litt.* vol. I, p. 237.

2 See Mourad, *La Physiognomie Arabe* (Paris, 1939), p. 38, who there discusses this book.

3 Vols. I, V and VI have been published in facsimile in the Gibb Memorial series.

historical writers in the Arabic language, for though a Persian he wrote in Arabic. He presents this work not as a collection of facts but with a central idea running through it so that the whole forms an organic structure.

Very little is known about the life of Ibn Miskawayhí. His name is associated with Avicenna in the court of the Khwárazmsháh. He was one of the few who preferred liberty to service under Maḥmúd Ghaznaví. He died a cripple in the year A.D. 1029, leaving behind him many works which Avicenna stigmatized as 'prolix and unintelligible'.

The concluding portion of his big history has been published. Among his many works al-Qifṭí mentions three on medical subjects, which he describes as sound and exhaustive. He says that Avicenna once put a question to him, but after repeated attempts Ibn Miskawayhí failed to grasp it. It is also said that Avicenna, wishing to show off his own superiority once produced a nut before a class of students and asked Ibn Miskawayhí to measure it in barley corns. Ibn Miskawayhí replied by handing Avicenna some sheets of paper and bidding him write an essay on good manners. One of his books, which he called the *Kitáb-ul-Ṭaharat* or 'The Volume of Purity', forms the basis of that popular Persian book on ethics called the *Akhláq-i-Náṣirí*, which Naṣr ul-Dín Ṭúsí Muḥaqqiq wrote 200 years later. Another, entitled *Kitáb-i-Adab-ul-'Arab wa ul-Fárs* or 'The Manners of the Arabs and the Persians', embodies a much earlier work called *Jáwídán-i-Khird* or 'The Everlasting Wisdom', a book of practical maxims ascribed to Hóshang Sháh.[1]

Another member of the staff of personal physicians attached to 'Aẓud-ul-Doula was a great-grandson of Bukht Yishú' II, named Jibrá'íl, being the son of 'Ubayd-Ulláh who had been physician to the Caliph al-Muttaqí. Jibrá'íl II, whom I must so call to distinguish him from his grandfather, also outlived his master, dying in the year A.D. 1006. The names of two of his written works are known—the *Káfí* or 'Sufficiency', a work in five parts,

1 See *I.A.U.* vol. I, p. 245.

and the *Muṭabiqat bayn Qol-il-Inbiya' wa il-Falásifat* or 'The Common Ground between the Prophets and the Philosophers'.

This same 'Ubayd-Ulláh tells the story of 'Aẓud-ul-Doula's first coming to Baghdad and his rude treatment of the two leading physicians of the city. In those days Abú ul-Ḥasan Ṣ̤ábit bin Ibráhím was at the height of his fame. Accompanied by Sinán he went to pay his respects to the ruler of Fars and the virtual lord of Baghdad. 'Aẓud-ul-Doula inquired who the two newcomers were and learning that they were physicians rudely called out that he was in good health and had no need of them. The two left his presence unpresented, put to a public shame. Sinán, who was the younger of the two, was considerably angered by this behaviour and suggested to Ṣ̤ábit that they should return and offer some suitable reply in order to uphold the dignity of the profession. Ṣ̤ábit agreed. The two physicians returned and being readmitted to the presence cried out to the king: 'May God prolong your life, all the more because it is the function of our knowledge to preserve that life and a king has a greater need of that function than has any other man.' 'Aẓud-ul-Doula was pleased with this remark and appointed the two physicians to his personal staff.

The memorials to 'Aẓud-ul-Doula are not confined to literature. All over Fars and Khuzistan, not to mention Baghdad, he raised new buildings. He constructed caravanserais, mosques, palaces and hospitals. His hospital at Shiraz is famous. All these are overshadowed by the hospital that he founded in Baghdad, complete with equipment, numerous trust funds and a pharmacy stocked with drugs brought from the ends of the earth. It was almost at the end of his life that he determined upon the foundation of this great hospital. It has often been stated that Rhazes was consulted upon the choice of the site and that he gave his decision after hanging up pieces of meat in various quarters of the city and selected as the site that area where the meat showed least decomposition. But this is manifestly incorrect, for whatever date is assigned to the death of Rhazes, he must in any case have been dead some 50 years before 'Aẓud-ul-Doula determined upon the foundation of his hospital.

The original city of al-Manṣúr, as I have already said, was round and lay altogether on the western side of the Tigris. Al-Manṣúr even in his own lifetime abandoned his plan of confining the city to within the wall; for, in the angle which a bend of the river makes between its right bank and the circumference of the walls, he began to build a great palace, which he called the Qaṣr-ul-Khuld or 'Palace of Eternity'. This space of ground was nearly a mile in length, though much less in breadth. Probably this site was chosen for a palace because here the ground was higher than the rest of the river bank and hence the risk of flooding and the plague of mosquitoes were both less. In this palace Hárún-ul-Rashíd kept state. Here al-Amín, his son, made his last defence when attacked by the arms of his brother, al-Ma'mún. And from the palace wharf he embarked to meet his death.

Al-Ma'mún at first held his court in the Khuld Palace, but later moved to another. During the sixty odd years when the seat of government was transferred from Baghdad to Sámarra, the palace was entirely neglected and must have fallen into complete ruins. Hence in the year A.D. 979 the prince 'Aẓud-ul-Doula had available an excellent and unoccupied site for his new hospital. Yáqút, indeed, states that the new hospital stood on the bank of the river somewhat higher up than the Khuld Palace. But as Muqaddasí says that it lay close beside the main bridge of boats, there is no difficulty in reconciling Yáqút's statement with the claim that the hospital occupied the site of the ancient palace, for the Khuld Palace was separated from the bridge by stables and servants' quarters. These, too, having collapsed while the palace lay unoccupied, the new buildings were erected on the site of the stables, extending along the river bank until they reached the site of the old palace.

The new hospital took three years to build. Like the old hospital, it served what had now become the most important and populated portion of Baghdad. Behind it lay the old round city.

Before was the river with the teeming, busy eastern suburbs beyond. To the left was the Khorasan Gate with the great main road to Persia running through the review ground, over the main bridge, through the market of Yaḥyá and on to the desert. On the other side was the Palace of Zubayda and the Maqbarah Báb-ul-Dayr or 'Cemetery of the Convent Gate', the most famous tomb of which, that of Ma'rúf Karkhí, still exists, and therefore marks the extreme lower limit of where the hospital must once have stood.

The hospital was completed in the year A.D. 982.[1] To staff it 'Aẓud-ul-Doula called upon the best physicians which the two 'Iraqs could provide. Jibrá'íl, who had been his physician in Shiraz, was summoned. Abú Sa'íd 'Ubayd-Ulláh wrote:

> My father was called from Shiraz by 'Aẓud-ul-Doula and was engaged among the physicians of the hospital. He was attached at the same time to the private suite of the caliph. There were also in the hospital skilful ophthalmologists, such as Abú Naṣr ibn ul-Duḥalí, surgeons such as Abú ul-Khayr and Abú ul-Ḥusayn ibn ul-Naqáḥ, and orthopaedic surgeons of high repute, such as Abú ul-Ṣalt.[2]

Al-Qifṭí says that the medical staff numbered eighty in all and that Ibn Mandúyah of Ispahan was also among those summoned from central Persia. 'Abd-Ulláh ibn Jibrá'íl gives the names of several more of the original staff. Among them were Abú ul-Ḥasan 'Alí Ibráhím bin Baks, who was engaged for the most part in the teaching of medicine to the unqualified. There were also to be found in the hospital Abú ul-Ḥusayn 'Alí ibn Kashkaráyá, who was a pupil of Sinán's, Abú Ya'qúb of Ahwaz, Abú 'Ísá Baqia, Naẓíf al-Rúmí the priest and the sons of Ḥasan.

The physician Ibráhím bin Baks was famous as a teacher, as a translator and as an original author. Among his works are a large and a small compendium of medicine and monographs on diseases of the skin, of the eyes, on anatomy and on antidotes. Towards the end of his life he became blind and was compelled

1 Or in A.D. 978 according to Ibn Khallikán, vol. II, p. 484.
2 *I.A.U.* vol. I, pp. 144, 310.

to ask his pupil to describe to him the colour of the urine of his patients and their physical appearances. His excellence as a teacher made him a valuable member of the staff of the hospital even with these disadvantages and his services were retained at a salary sufficient to remove all fear of want in his old age. He is said to have died in the year A.D. 1003.[1]

It is also said that he had among his pupils in the hospital a namesake, who was a lover of wine and a drunkard. Ibn ul-Khammár, the associate of Avicenna, who later resided in the court of Maḥmúd Ghaznaví, refers to these two when he wrote in his treatise 'On the Examination of Physicians': 'Medicine in Baghdad has come down to such a level that someone who was the guide of a blind man for two months opened an office and announced that he gave medical treatment.' This pupil according to Ibn Buṭlán was dismissed from the hospital on account of his intemperate habits, which prevented him from giving a clear mind to his work and from being capable of inspecting the urine or taking the pulse of his patients. In spite of this disadvantage he apparently opened a consulting room in Baghdad on his own account and wrote a book in which he showed how much practical anatomy he knew by asserting that man has one rib less than a woman.

Of Abú ul-Khayr it is known that he was the first senior surgeon to the hospital. He was an old man even when he took office. The date of his death is uncertain. He is said to have invented two ointments which continued to be incorporated in all Persian pharmacopoeias long after his death, although one was ascribed (falsely, so the author of the *Maṭraḥ-ul-Anẓár* says[2]) at a later date to Ibn ul-Tilmíẕ.

The other surgeon mentioned by 'Ubayd Ulláh, Abú ul-Ḥusayn ibn ul-Naqáḥ, or Abú ul-Ḥasan bin ul-Tafáḥ according to Ibn abí Uṣaybi'a, was a well-known surgeon of Baghdad of those days. His brother was also a surgeon. Later he became an official in the court of 'Aẓud-ul-Doula on account of his skill in re-

1 *I.A.U.* vol. 1, p. 244. 2 *Maṭraḥ-ul-Anẓár*, p. 115.

moving a fragment of steel in the thigh of a courtier, which other surgeons had failed to extract. The date of his death is unknown.[1]

Of the orthopaedic surgeon Abú ul-Ṣalt nothing is known.

Abú ul-Ḥusayn 'Alí ibn Kashkaráyá was another physician whom 'Aẓud-ul-Doula summoned from Persia. He was originally physician to the Prince Sayf-ul-Doula bin Ḥamdán. He is said to have made his studies under Sinán bin Ṣábit bin Qurra and to have delighted in the unsocial pleasure of excessive talking and confuting of his colleagues. Because he invented a successful clyster for the treatment of troubles of the liver, they got their own back by giving him the nickname throughout the hospital of 'Master of Enemata'. The names of a few of his works have been preserved. He is said to have died in 980/1.[2]

Another interesting name on the hospital list is that of Abú Aḥmad 'Abd-ul-Raḥmán ibn 'Alí ibn ul-Marzubání of Ispahan. It would seem that he was a lecturer in forensic medicine, for his biographers state that he distinguished himself both in Islamic law and in medicine. At the beginning of his career he acted as a judge in Shustar and in other parts of Khuzistan, but later he was invited to become director of the 'Aẓudí Hospital. He died in February 1005.

Also from Ispahan came Ibn Mandúyah, whose full name is Aḥmad bin 'Abd-ul-Raḥmán bin Mandúyah. He was a pupil of Abú Máhir and thus probably a colleague of Haly Abbas. He was one of the original staff of the hospital. The dates of both his birth and death are unknown. He left behind him an enormous number of works dedicated to his various pupils. His 'Sufficiency' was so popular that it was commonly called 'The Lesser Canon'.[3]

Of Abú Ya'qúb of Ahwaz nothing of importance is known, though the name of some of his pharmacological works have survived. With regard to the physicians known collectively as the

1 *Maṭraḥ-ul-Anẓár*, p. 109. 2 Ibid. p. 108; *I.A.U.* vol. I, p. 238.
3 *I.A.U.* vol. II, p. 21.

Banú Ḥasnún or 'Sons of Ḥasan', no writer except Ibn abí Uṣaybi'a mentions them and it must remain a matter of conjecture who they were.[1]

After the death of 'Aẓud-ul-Doula the first glory of the hospital passed away. But the fame of its staff did not cease; it still attracted the best physicians of both Iraq and Persia. Among the later court physicians who were also on the staff of the hospital was Abú ul-Ḥasan Sa'íd bin Hibat Ulláh, who was born on 16 January 1044 and died on 30 December 1101. He was physician-in-chief to the Caliphs al-Muqtadí and his son al-Mustaẓhir. In spite of his high rank his extraordinary humility is illustrated by a story told by a contemporary physician, a certain Rashíd-ul-Dín abú Sa'íd bin Ya'qúb the Christian. Hibat Ulláh was one day engaged in his professional work in the 'Aẓudí Hospital when a woman came up to him and begged him to help her by examining her son and seeing that he had the right treatment. After examining the case he ordered her to give him a special regime and to provide only food which produces a cold and damp effect on the body. One of the physicians who happened to be present criticized this advice and asked, very pertinently it would seem, how an ordinary person was to know what foods produce cold and what produce damp, and said that it would be much better to tell the woman exactly what to give and what to withhold. Sa'íd bin Hibat Ulláh acknowledged that he was right. The first physician then said:

> Then I will not blame you in this matter for you have done an even stranger thing. It is this. You have composed a very short book on Medicine and given it the title of *al-Mughní* or 'The Sufficiency' and a very prolix work on the same subject which discusses medical problems at great length. And this you have called *al-Iqná'* or 'The Satisfaction'. It would have been better to have changed the names round.

Sa'íd bin Hibat Ulláh acknowledged that he was right again and exclaimed that if it were possible to change the names now he would do so, but that it was too late for several copies of each

1 *I.A.U.* vol. I, p. 310.

were in circulation. According to some versions of the story it was not a physician who administered this rebuke but a lunatic among the patients whom he was examining.[1]

The next famous name on the list of the hospital staff is that of Abú ul-Ḥasan Hibat Ulláh bin abí il-'Ala' Sa'íd bin Ibráhím, whose title was Amín-ul-Doula. He succeeded his uncle Abú ul-Faraj Yaḥyá ibn ul-Tilmíz, a Christian physician of Baghdad, and was called Ibn ul-Tilmíz after him. He was born in 1073. His father also was a doctor and a Christian; the son followed both these professions. He made his medical studies under Sa'íd bin Hibat Ulláh. He had leanings to pure medicine and can never have practised any surgery, for he once said that he would never willingly pull a thorn out of the skin for fear lest it break off.[2]

Before settling down to practise, he travelled through Persia. Here he perfected his knowledge of the Persian language, so that when he returned to Baghdad, he was proficient in Arabic, Persian and Syriac. In his native city honours awaited him. He was attached to the 'Aẓudí Hospital and became a court physician to the Caliph al-Muqtafí and to his successor al-Mustanjid. The former is said to have received him regularly once a week and to have allowed him the privilege of sitting in the royal presence.

All writers agree in praising him from every point of view. The Kátib 'Imád-ul-Dín al-Ispahání writes:

> In the science of Medicine he was for the whole world the point to which they had recourse. He was the Hippocrates of the Age, the Galen of the Epoch. His talents carried medical science to the acme of perfection; none of the ancient doctors reached the height to which he attained. His life was long and his days prosperous. When I saw him, he was an old man of a pleasing aspect. His sweetness of character, indicated by his looks, was found on trial to be real. His mind was quick, his body graceful, his sentiments exalted, his thoughts aspiring, his sagacity felicitous, and his judgement solid. He was the Elder of the Christians, their priest, their head, and their chief.

1 Ibid. p. 254.

2 *Hist. Dynst.* vol. IX, p. 258; Ibn Khallikán, vol. III, p. 596; *I.A.U.* vol. I, p. 259; Yáqút, *Dict.* p. 243.

His conduct was so regular and his gravity so remarkable that it is said that during the frequent visits that he made to the palace of the caliph, he was only heard once to speak in jest. That was in the presence of al-Muqtafí. A pension, which had been assigned to him on the glass bottle manufactory at Baghdad, was stopped without the caliph's knowledge. One day that he was in the caliph's presence, when the time came to withdraw, he had great difficulty in rising owing to his advanced age. The caliph remarked: 'Doctor, you are growing old.' To which he replied: 'It is true, my Lord; my bottles are broken.' This is an expression used by the people of Baghdad to indicate that a man is old. The caliph, surprised at the unaccustomed joke, guessed that there was some further meaning, and inquiring into the matter had the pension restored to him.

Remarkable cures are, of course, ascribed to him. In one case he cured a girl in coma by subjecting her to a cold bath followed by sudorifics. Another time a patient was brought to him who sweated blood in the summer. This was cured by a diet of bread and apples.

He died on Christmas Day in the year A.D. 1164. In so great affection was he held by the people of Baghdad that the inhabitants of both sides of the river accompanied his corpse to the church and attended the funeral service. Not one of them, it is said, stayed away.

Late in life he became chief of the physicians of Baghdad and president of the board of examiners. At the height of his fame, when he was physician-in-chief in the 'Aẓudí Hospital, he refused to see any patient below the rank of a prince, excepting the very poor. An enormous fee he once refused to accept from a merchant for this reason. Yet when pressed to enter the political service of the Khwárazmsháh, he remarked that he was only a simple physician, who knew nothing about anything except barley water and syrup of violets, and begged to be allowed to continue his medical profession. His house is said to have backed on to the Niẓámiyya college. When any of the law students there fell ill, he used to have them brought to his house and would take care of them himself until cured and able to return to work.

Like so many other men of his age, Ibn ul-Tilmíz̲ was also something of a poet. Bar Hebraeus quotes a couplet of his, which may be translated:

Sweet was the state of youth and youth's wild state.
Now that is left behind: the narrow path I tread.
I sit awaiting Death, like the benighted traveller who
Knows where his journey ends, and still lacks house and bed.

Among his medical works are many commentaries on the writings of the Greeks and his own countrymen. He also wrote a 'Commentary on the Traditions of the Prophet' which have reference to medicine, being probably the earliest of the many *Ṭibb-ul-Nabbí* which were to follow, and a pharmacopoeia which replaced that of Jundí S̲h̲ápúr, which Sahl bin Sápúr had composed and which had been in general use until that time. On his death his library is said to have filled twelve waggons. He left a son behind him who followed in no way his father's footsteps, for he embraced Islam and did not practise medicine.

A curious fact, which did not escape the notice of the ancients, was that at that period the three leading physicians all were named Hibat Ulláh and that these three represented the three leading faiths of the city—the Christian, the Mohammedan and the Jewish. With the Christian Hibat Ulláh I have just dealt. The second of the three was his bitter enemy Ibn Malka the Jew. This Hibat Ulláh, better known by his *kunya* Abú ul-Barkát, was born in a village named Balad and hence is sometimes known as al-Baladí. He came to Baghdad as a young man, and full of enthusiasm tried to join the medical classes of Sa'íd bin Hibat Ulláh, the Christian. Being a Jew he was refused admission. Not to be thwarted he bribed the door-keeper to let him in and hiding in the corridor attended secretly all the lectures. At the end of a year, so the story goes, the professor propounded a question which none of the students could answer. Abú ul-Barkát could contain himself no longer and bursting forth begged for permission to reply. So good was his answer that he was admitted to the classes and finished his training with the Christians.[1]

His success in practice was enormous and reached its highest point when he was summoned to Persia to attend one of the Seljuq princes. On his return his haughtiness so annoyed the Baghdadis that he became the subject of frequent scurrilous poems. Above all he was taunted with his faith which gave him a rank below the dogs of the street. He therefore embraced Islam, but not before he had obtained from the caliph a ruling that his daughters, if they remained in the Jewish faith, should not be deprived of their inheritance. At the height of his glory he received the title of Wáḥid-ul-Zamán or the 'Unique One of the Age'. Then a terrible tragedy befell him. He contracted elephantiasis. To cure himself he allowed himself to be bitten by vipers which he had kept for some time without food. He was cured of the elephantiasis, but lost his sight. It is said that later still he became deaf and afflicted with leprosy. His scheming ambitions, which culminated in an attempt to overthrow his old master on a charge of high treason by means of a forged letter left lying in the caliph's room, deprive him of any sympathy which his pathetic end might call forth. Deserted by all, in poverty and misery he died at the age of eighty-four. Al-Asṭralábí, contrasting the two, wrote: 'Hibat Ulláh ibn ul-Tilmíz̲ and Hibat Ulláh abú ul-Barkát: the two rivals: how different their ends. Humility lifted the one to the Pleiades: pride chained the other to the Earth.'[2]

Abú ul-Barkát wrote several books. He himself considered that his best was the one entitled *al-Mu'tabar*, or 'The Worthy of Honour', a book which deals with metaphysics, and he requested that there might be inscribed on his tombstone: 'Here lies Abú ul-Barkát, who knew both good and bad fortune, and who wrote *al-Mu'tabar*.' A modern student of this work reports that the intelligence and style of the author is excellent and that he is a

1 *I.A.U.* vol. I, p. 278; *Hist. Dynst.* vol. IX, p. 259.
2 Ibn K̲h̲allikán, vol. III, p. 600; al-Qifṭí, p. 343.

worthy successor to Rhazes in his Platonic conceptions of philosophical thought.[1]

The third of the Hibat Ulláhs was the Moslem Hibat Ulláh ibn ul-Ḥusayn ibn 'Alí of Ispahan, who died of apoplexy and was buried in a cellar in his own house. Presumably he was still alive, for several months later, when the door was opened to carry the body to its permanent tomb, he was found sitting upright, but dead.

A contemporary of Hibat Ulláh, which seems to have been a very popular name about this time, was Badí'-ul-Zamán, a physician of Baghdad, who on account of his skill in making astronomical instruments was known as al-Badí' al-Asṭralábí.[2] He was a man of very wide learning, and was equally distinguished as a physician, as a poet, and as an astronomer. For a while he lived in Ispahan and while there dedicated his book of Astronomical Tables to Maḥmúd, the grandson of Maliksh____áh the Seljúq, who had his seat of government there. Al-Badí' died of a stroke in A.D. 1139 and was buried in the cemetery called al-Wardiyya or the Rose Garden in the eastern quarters of Baghdad. Whether any of his scientific work survives, I am unable to say. Fragments of his poetry are quoted by various writers, though he is said to have been extremely licentious and to have admitted into his poetry such indelicate ideas that he was forced to use very obscene language. Among the less obnoxious of his poems is a scurrilous ode against some surgeon of his day, which begins:

He is a bleeder who wields his lancet as though going to a war.
Worthless are his operations: nothing comes of them except blood.
Even though he walk upon the pavement, those in the road perish.
Summon him when your foes press upon you: for then you will have no need to fight.

To return to the 'Aẓudí Hospital from which I have strayed a long way. In A.D. 1068 the hospital benefited from the legacies

1 Dr Paul Kraus, quoted in Meyerhof, 'Mediaeval Jewish Physicians in Near East', *Isis*, (May 1938), p. 444.

2 Ibn Khallikán, vol. III, p. 580.

of a certain 'Abd-ul-Malik who repaired the buildings and re-endowed it. At the same time the staff was increased to 28 physicians. In the year of the flood of A.D. 1074 it must have suffered great damage, for the waters are reported to have entered the windows, and the whole building was flooded. A similar disaster occurred in 1159. A third and even greater flood occurred in 1173. Ibn ul-Aṣír thus described it in his diary:

In the month of Ramazan, although it was spring, there was a very heavy rainfall at Gezireh, at Diarbekir, and at Mosul. It continued for forty days during which time we saw the sun only twice and then only for a short time. Several buildings collapsed and some houses fell, burying their inhabitants, who were suffocated in the ruins. The Tigris overflowed its banks, causing floods on both sides, especially at Baghdad where the flood level rose three feet above the maximum level ever reached since the founding of the city. Fearing wreckage the inhabitants abandoned the city and took up their residence on either side. In an attempt to escape the floods caused by the bursting of the banks, every time that a crack appeared in an embankment, it was filled up with earth. But the water entered the drains and destroyed the houses. It even forced its way into the 'Aẓudí Hospital and boats rowed past the windows whose shutters had been carried away by the water. But then God had pity upon His creatures and the flood subsided just when destruction seemed imminent.

When in 1184, that is 11 years later, Ibn Jabír reached Baghdad, he found that the hospital had been completely restored and was carrying out faithfully the intentions of its founder. He wrote:

Between the main street and the quarter of the Basra Gate lies the hospital bazaar. In this district there has been built on the bank of the river the well-known hospital of Baghdad. It is visited by physicians every Monday and Thursday, who examine the patients, prescribe for them the proper treatment, and order them the food that they require. These physicians have under them nurses whose duties it is to prepare the medicines and the food. This hospital was once a large palace and consists of a number of halls and rooms. It is provided with every comfort, such as is found in the royal establishments. The water supply is from the Tigris.

It must have been about the time of the flood that Abú Bakr 'Ubayd Ulláh bin abí il-Faraj 'Alí bin Naṣr bin Ḥamza, usually known as Ibn ul-Máristání, became director of the hospital. In spite of his good reputation and high position his rivals succeeded in poisoning the ear of the caliph, at that time al-Náṣir, and he was thrown into prison. He was released two years later and left Baghdad on an embassy to Tiflis. After successfully carrying out his commission he was returning to Baghdad, but died in the year 1202/3 before he reached home. He wrote a history of Baghdad which was incomplete at the time of his death and which he called the *Díwán-i-Islám*.

After the flood the restoration of the hospital must have been complete, for in later years a small suburb sprang up to the south, lying between the hospital buildings and the Basra Gate of the old round city. This was known as the Súq-ul-Máristán or 'Hospital Bazaar' and occupied the site of the gardens of the old Khuld Palace. The lower end of this bazaar was occupied by the shops of papersellers and booksellers. The paper itself was manufactured in the Súq-ul-Hayṣam, which lay between the Syrian and Kufah Gates, not very far from the old hospital. The market was rebuilt by 'Aẓud-ul-Doula, although by his days the surrounding buildings were for the most part in ruins. In the hospital bazaar there are said to have been over 100 sellers of books.

When in 1258 Húlágú besieged Baghdad, he made the hospital the centre of his attack from the west. The hospital must have suffered very severely, for when Ibn Baṭúṭah visited Baghdad in 1330, he found the place a complete ruin,[1] only traces of the walls being left. Yet it is quite possible that the destruction of the hospital had already been accomplished before the inroads of the Mongols. For there is every reason to believe that it was dismantled some time prior to 1233, when the Caliph al-Mustanṣir decided to found another hospital in the grounds of the Mustansiriyya college in east Baghdad.

It must not be thought that all the wealth and energy of

1 Ibn Baṭúṭah, *Travels*, vol. II, p. 107.

Baghdad were concentrated upon the 'Aẓudí Hospital alone. In addition to the other hospitals already mentioned a new one was founded as late as A.D. 1113 by a certain Kumashtigín. Some eight years later a certain Mustaufí 'Azíz-ul-Dín built 'a school for orphans which he provided with a perpetual endowment by which the orphans, until they reached maturity, were assured of their expenditure, their clothing, and their food. There they were taught their letters, learned the Qur'án by heart, and acquired knowledge of what is lawful and unlawful.'[1]

In 1160 Benjamin of Tudela, the Jew, found no fewer than sixty well organized medical institutions in Baghdad:

> All well provided from the king's stores with spices and other necessaries. Every patient who claims assistance, is fed at the king's expense until his cure is completed. There is further the large building called the Dár-ul-Maraphtan in which are locked up all those insane persons who are met with during the hot season, everyone of whom is secured by iron chains until his reason returns, when he is allowed to return to his home. For this purpose they are regularly examined once a month by the king's officers appointed for that purpose, and, when they are found to be possessed of reason, they are immediately liberated. All this is done by the king in pure charity towards all who come to Baghdad, either ill or insane, for the king is a pious man and his intention is excellent in this respect.[2]

The hospital system of Baghdad was repeated in the provincial cities through the generosity of rich citizens who lived there. 'Aẓud-ul-Doula founded a hospital in Shiraz which formed part of a university in which were taught philosophy, astrology, medicine, chemistry and mathematics. Abu Sa'íd Kúkubúri, lord of Arbela, was another famed for his public spirit. He is said to have built in Arbela four asylums for the blind and for persons suffering from chronic diseases. He also supplied all their wants. In addition he also built a house for the reception of widows, another for orphan children, and a third for foundlings. In this

1 Al-Bundari quoted by Levy in *A Baghdad Chronicle*, p. 212.
2 Rabbi Benjamin of Tudela, *Itinerary* (Asher's translation), vol. 1, p. 99.

last a number of nurses were always in waiting, ready to suckle whatever child might be brought in.[1]

In Jurjan there was the hospital of Bahá'-ul-Doula over which al-Jurjání for some time presided. It was here that he complained bitterly that as soon as he took office the number of patients so increased that he could not find time to complete his writings.[2] The small township of Biriz, a few miles south of Shiraz, is another example. It was famed throughout Persia in medieval times for its school of civil law, astrology, and medicine. Herbert found the school still flourishing when he passed through in 1628.[3]

Even in the Mongol days the building of hospitals was not neglected, although after the fall of Baghdad first Tabriz and then Samarqand, being the capital cities, boasted the finest hospitals. Tamerlane, indeed, decreed that each city of his realm was to contain at least one mosque, one school, one *serai*, and one hospital. The lethargy of the later Safavids allowed this excellent ordinance to be forgotten and the buildings to decay. It was, I imagine, the Afghan invasion in the first half of the eighteenth century that put an end to all these pious and learned foundations.

To a very large extent the credit for the whole hospital system must be given to Persia. The hospitals of the Mohammedan period were built very largely upon the ideals and traditions of the Sassanian hospital of Jundí Shápúr. At first Christians and Jews were predominant in the Baghdad hospitals; Jundí Shápúr was called upon for many years to provide the staffs of the new Arab foundations. It is no exaggeration to say that Sassanian tradition was bled to death to infuse life into the recently born child of Islam. Asad bin Jání shows how strong was public feeling in favour of non-Muslim medical tradition when he complains of his failure to build up a clientele, even in times of excess of sickness:

> In the first place I am a Muslim, and before I studied medicine, nay, before ever I was created, the people held the view that Muslims are not successful physicians. Further my name is Asad, and it should have

1 Ibn Khallikán, vol. II, p. 537. 2 Al-Jurjání, *Thesaurus*, Appendix I.
3 Herbert, *A Relation of some Yeares Travaile*, p. 63.

been Saliba, Mara'il, Yúḥanná or Bira (i.e. a Syriac or Aramaic name); and my *kunya* is Abu ul-Ḥáris̤, and it should have been Abú 'Ísá, Abú Zakaríyyá or Abú Ibráhím (i.e. Christian or Jewish instead of Mohammedan); and I wear a cloak of white cotton and it should have been of black silk; and my speech is Arabic and it should have been the speech of the people of Jundí Shápúr.[1]

Even the word for 'hospital' is a Persian word, which was taken into Arabic and adopted far beyond the Baghdad caliphate. For in Egypt and Syria also these institutions are called Bímáristán or Máristán, which means in Persian 'a place for sick people'.

The Bímáristáns were of two sorts—the fixed and the moving. The moving hospitals were transported upon beasts of burden and were erected from time to time as required. The practitioners who travelled with the moving hospitals were of the same standing as those who served the fixed hospitals. Sinán bin S̤ábit was a travelling physician during part of his life. So was al-Báhali, who had with him as phlebotomist and assistant physician al-Sadíd abu ul-Wafa, better known as al-Murakhkhim, who in middle life forsook medicine and became chief justice of Baghdad. Abú ul-Ḥakam al-Báhali was a man skilled in all the branches of learning which the fashions of the day demanded of an educated man. But more especially he excelled in poetry and medicine. He was born in Yemen in the year 1093. Because his family came originally from Spain he was also known as al-Maghribi or al-Andalusí, that is, the Westerner or the Andalusian. When he reached manhood he moved to Baghdad and opened a school for boys. Among his more tiresome customs was his habit of lampooning his friends and of writing scurrilous epitaphs upon them before their death. A more serious vice was his intemperance. In his later days he was rarely sober and possibly on this account he was compelled to give up his post in Baghdad and move on to Damascus. Here he made a fresh start and again he was placed in charge of a hospital. But his drinking bouts continued and he gradually lost the best part of his practice and was finally

1 Browne, *Arabian Medicine*, p. 7.

reduced to keeping a drug store. It would point a moral to say that he died in poverty, but in truth he did not. For his wit was much appreciated and his shop was frequented by many of the leading men of Damascus. He died in 1154, leaving behind a son named Abú ul-Majd, a far greater physician than his father and famed for ever as the teacher of Ibn abí Uṣaybiʻa. He also left to posterity several medical works and a collection of verses of different sorts.[1]

Of course similar moving hospitals accompanied the armies in the field. The first of which there is any detailed record is the field hospital which accompanied the Seljúq Sulṭán Maḥmúd.[2] Its organization is ascribed to Mustaufí ʻAzíz-ul-Dín (the same that founded the school for orphans), who well equipped it with medicaments, instruments, tents and a staff of doctors and orderlies. These hospitals were also used by prisoners and by the general public, above all in times of epidemics.

The rudiments of a poor law system are to be found in some letters which Sinán bin Ṣ̈ábit received from the Minister ʻAlí ibn ʻÍsá ibn ul-Jarráḥ:

> May God prolong your life [runs one]. I have been thinking of the lot of the prisoners who on account of the greatness of their number and the poorness of their lodging are exposed to innumerable diseases. Besides which, because of their state of life they are prevented from bettering their condition and from applying to the doctors whom they would like to consult. There is thus an opportunity for you—and may God reward you—to set aside for them certain physicians who may visit them every day and provide for them remedies, medicine and all medical requirements. Such physicians should have free access to all prisons, should treat all the sick, and should assure their cure by the treatment which they will give under the Will of God.[3]

On another occasion it was a question not of prisoners but of outlying villages which could not support a doctor:

> I have considered the case of the inhabitants of the village of al-Sawád and others which are without a doctor and may have need of one if the

1 *I.A.U.* vol. II, p. 145; Ibn Khallikán, vol. II, p. 82.
2 Al-Bundárí, p. 137; quoted by Levy in *A Baghdad Chronicle*, p. 212.
3 *I.A.U.* vol. I, p. 221.

inhabitants are ill. Take steps therefore—and may God prolong your life—to delegate certain physicians, equipped with a supply of medicine, to go to al-Sawád, and bid them stay there as long as may be necessary for the treatment of the sick in each village.

The correspondence showed that Sinán carried out his orders, for a little later he wrote back to the minister saying that the travelling hospital had reached a village called Saurah. As the majority of the inhabitants of this village were Jews, he asked whether the hospital should stop there or should move on to a Mussulman village. The minister replied:

I have taken note of what you have written—and may God honour you—and I agree with you about the necessity of treating non-Muslims and animals. But you must always give priority to men over animals and to Muslims over non-Muslims. If then, when you have treated all the Muslims, there remain over any medical supplies, treat the non-Muslims in due order. Act always upon these principles which you should impart to your colleagues. Tell them to go out with their transport to villages and localities where epidemics are raging. If the doctors cannot find guides, tell them to halt when the road becomes impassable. Thus by the grace of God your work will be crowned with success.

The fixed Bímáristáns correspond to the modern hospital. They varied in size and equipment according to the wealth and social position of the founder, the importance of the town in which they were placed, and the value of the endowments set aside for their upkeep. One of the finest Islamic hospitals was that at Marrakesh in North Africa, which was built about 1200 and of which 'Abd-ul-Wáḥid al-Marrakhshí has left a description.

Here was constructed a hospital, which I think is unequalled in the world. First there was selected a large open space in the most level part of the town. Orders were given to architects to construct a hospital as well as possible. So the workmen embellished it with a beauty of sculpture and ornamentation even beyond what was demanded of them. All sorts of suitable trees and fruit trees were planted there. Water there was in abundance, flowing through all the rooms. In addition there were four large pools in the centre of the building, one of which was lined with white marble. The hospital was furnished with valuable carpets of wool, cotton, silk and leather, so wonderful that I cannot even describe them.

A daily allowance of thirty dinars was assigned for the daily ration of food, exclusive of the drugs and chemicals which were on hand for the preparation of draughts, unguents, and collyria. For the use of the patients there were provided day-dresses and night-dresses, thick for winter, thin for summer.

After he was cured, a poor patient received on leaving the hospital a sum of money sufficient to keep him for a time. Rich patients received back their money and clothes. In short, the Founder did not confine the use of the hospital to the poor or to the rich. On the contrary, every stranger who fell ill at Marrakesh, was carried there and treated until he either recovered or died. Every Friday the Prince after the mid-day prayer mounted his horse to go and visit the patients and to learn about each of them. He used to ask how they were and how they were being treated. This was his use until the day of his death.[1]

Like the Prince of Marrakesh, Aḥmad ibn Ṭúlún, the founder of the oldest hospital in Cairo, used to visit it daily until a lunatic begged a pomegranate of him, and then, instead of eating it, threw it at him with such violence that it burst and spoilt his clothes. After this he would never again visit the hospital.

It would appear from this that not only was the treatment in the large hospitals gratuitous, but that the poor were actually given some financial assistance on their discharge. The medical staff certainly did not give their services gratis, for a salary of 300 dirhams a month was appointed for each physician when the ʻAẓudí Hospital was first founded.[2]

Every hospital was divided into two completely separate sections. This was required by the laws of a religion which forbade a woman to appear unveiled before the opposite sex. Each section was furnished with a nursing staff and porters of the sex of the patients to be treated therein. The medical and surgical staff was male. There is no mention of any woman

1 *Bul. Soc. Fr. Hist. Med.* (1922), vol. XVI, p. 145.

2 *I.A.U.* vol. I, p. 145.

practising on the staff of any of the Baghdad hospitals, although there appear to have been plenty of female charlatans and quacks outside.[1]

Each of the two main sections of the hospital was divided up into several smaller halls. The biggest hall served for general medical cases and was itself subdivided into separate cubicles for the segregation of cases of fever, mania, cold diseases and diarrhoea. Other halls were devoted to surgical cases, diseases of the eyes and orthopaedic cases. There was even in those days an attempt to confine diseases to special clinics, so that the visiting staff might become specially skilful in whatever branch their fancy lay.[2]

From the point of view of treatment the hospital was divided into two main sections—the Out-patient Department and the In-patient Department. The reception of Out-patients took place at fixed hours and on regular days. The favourite days for the visits of the senior members of the staff were Mondays and Thursdays. Each patient was examined and given a prescription which he took to the pharmacy to have dispensed.[3] The Arab system can be seen in practice any day of the week in any large London hospital to-day.

The system of the In-patient Department differed only slightly from that of to-day. Patients who were too sick for out-patient treatment were admitted to the ward which specialized in their particular disease. Each ward had one, two or three physicians attached to it, depending upon the importance and the number of cases which it contained. When a difficulty was met with, a physician was called from one ward to another for consultation. The visiting staff also took their turns of duty and during their turn were obliged to stay within the hospital walls. Thus, Jibrá'íl ibn 'Ubayd Ulláh ibn Bukht Yishú' had to spend two days and two nights in every week on duty within the hospital.[4]

1 *I.A.U.* vol. II, p. 155.

2 Ibid. vol. I, pp. 254 and 310; vol. II, p. 243.

3 Ibid. vol. II, p. 243.

4 Ibid. p. 242; al-Qifṭí, p. 148.

Cases of acute mania were interned in the asylum known as the Dár-ul-Maraftán or 'Abode of those who require to be Chained', in a special ward of a hospital, or even in a prison as a temporary measure.[1] Hence an escaped felon was apt to be mistaken for an escaped lunatic. Certification of acute insanity was pronounced by a civil judge. Normally the insane remained a prisoner for life, but it was possible for him to be liberated by the orders of a commissioner who inspected lunatics from time to time. These commissioners were medical men.[2] Judging from the frequency of cases of madness which occur in the stories of the *Arabian Nights* the number of lunatics in Baghdad in 'Abbásid times must have been high.

Cases of acute poisoning were frequently diagnosed as mania and help to swell these figures. For it was generally held that certain drugs had the power of making the eater insane. Chief among these was *ḥashísh*, a drug which 'is composed of hemp leaves, whereto they add aromatic roots and somewhat of sugar: then they cook it and prepare a kind of confection which they eat'.[3] This was the drug which the head of the Order of the Assassins administered to the neophytes. While under its influence they were set in a garden, complete with houris and wine. On waking they thought themselves in Paradise. A second dose again drugged them and they were returned to their everyday world. On returning to consciousness for the second time, they remembered what they had seen and thought that they had been given this glimpse of Paradise in advance by the power of their chief. Thus they were ready to give their lives at his bidding, for there could be no doubt of his ability to give them the joys he promised. The very name of the Order is a derivation from the Arabic word *al-Ḥashashín* or the 'Eaters of Hashish'.

There is a vivid account of the treatment of a case of acute mania in one of the stories of the *Arabian Nights*.

1 *Arabian Nights* (Suppl.), no. 399; *Siyásatnáma*, p. 107.
2 *Contes du Cheykh el-Mohdy*, vol. 1, p. 402.
3 *Arabian Nights* (Suppl.), no. 395.

When the people heard his words, they said: 'This man hath become mad.' And not doubting his insanity, they came in and laid hold upon him, bound his hands behind him, and conveyed him to the mad-house. There every day they punished him, dosing him with abominalbe medicines and flogging him with whips making him a madman in spite of himself. Thus he continued, stripped of his clothing, and chained to a high window by his neck, for the space of ten days.[1]

This description of the current method of treatment is by no means exaggerated. Al-Jurjání[2] recommends that a lunatic be severely beaten about the head if other methods of treatment fail. Bahá'-ul-Doula orders the patient to be shut up and so terrified that he dare not open his mouth. The soles of the feet should be beaten after every meal and the head shaved, branded, and beaten with a strap.[3] Others recommend the drawing of the patient's teeth and the branding of the temples. Beating with the penis of an ox, a method that was revived in Nazi Germany, is often mentioned in the *Arabian Nights*. Al-Rúmí writes:

He has gone into the mad-house and taken refuge from the wickedness of the vulgar. He has become mad on account of the infamy of the sane.

From feeling the disgrace of the dull, body-serving intellect he has purposely gone and become mad.

Saying: Bind me fast with the penis of a bull: smite me on the head and back and do not dispute this (matter),

That from the stroke of the part of a cow I may gain life, as the murdered man (gained life) from the cow of Moses, O trusty ones.[4]

The lot of the chronic lunatic was much happier. Apparently he was often interned in a monastery, for Badí'-ul-Zamán in one of his Assemblies uses the phrase 'like a madman escaped from a monastery'. Near Al-Nu'máníyya was a monastery called Dayr Kizkil which used to receive the insane. During the days of the caliphs there were a large number of monasteries in Baghdad and no doubt one or more served as the asylum of the city.

1 *Arabian Nights*, Nights 271–290 (Lane's translation), vol. II, p. 362.
2 Al-Jurjání, *Thesaurus*, bk. vi, ch. 2, 2.
3 Bahá'-ul-Doula, *Khulásat-ul-Tajárib*, ch. viii.
4 Masnaví, bk. ii. v. 1434 (Nicholson's translation). See also v. 3500.

Harmless lunatics wandered about the streets at large. Rhazes one day, when walking with a party of his pupils, met a madman who would look at no one but him and stood staring and smiling at him. On returning home Rhazes ordered his druggist to prepare for him a draught of dodder of thyme, a popular remedy against insanity. This he at once drank off. When his pupils asked him why he found it necessary to take this medicine, he replied that the lunatic would not so fixedly have stared upon him had he not perceived in his face some sign of his own disease. And he quoted the Arab proverb about birds of a feather flocking together.[1] The same story, even to the quotation of the proverb, is told of Galen by Al-Rúmí.[2]

These thoughts naturally lead on to a consideration of the dispensary which played such an important part in the scientific life of the hospital. The hall in which the medicines were dispensed was called the *Khazánah-ul-Sharáb* or *Sharábkhána*, that is, the Treasury or Place of Draughts. The first phrase is Arabic, the second Persian. Here were to be found every type of remedy. The Arab pharmacopoeia contained simple drugs, which might be of animal, vegetable or mineral origin, and compound drugs, such as ointments, salves, boluses, sternutatories, and many other kinds whose names have passed out of modern use. A list of the diets and drugs in use at the 'Azudí Hospital is to be found in a manuscript now in the British Museum.[3]

The hospital dispensary was also of the nature of a treasure house, for many were enriched with objects of art, porcelain vases, pitchers, and so forth, so that it was said that some of the bigger pharmacies rivalled the royal palaces. In Egypt, and probably also in Persia, the pharmacy was also the strong room of the hospital where were kept the title-deeds and all other documents relative to the foundation and endowment. The chief officer of the dispensary was called by the high-sounding title

1 Qábusnáma, ch. vi, anecdote 4.
2 Masnaví, bk. ii, v. 2095.
3 Brit. Mus. Or. 8293.

of Shaykh Ṣaydalání.[1] This title was also given by courtesy to all druggists. Junior officers were called by the Persian title of Mehtar or 'Prince'; those engaged in more menial tasks, such as washers-up, porters, and others who were employed in the dispensary, were called Sharábdár.

The governor of the hospital (and modern practice follows this precedent) was a layman and not a qualified man. His post was a sinecure and was an office of honour. It was generally given only to princes and generals. Ibn Iyás writing of Cairo in 1495 said: 'To-day the Atabeg generalissimo Timraz had the singular honour of being nominated governor of the al-Manṣúrí Hospital. He proceeded thither with a large retinue.' It was the same in Damascus, where a son of the reigning sultan usually held the post. For all practical purposes the governor delegated his duties to another. This delegate, too, was held in extreme honour and the post was considered one of the highest offices of the State. The deputy governor was known by the title of Savar-ul-Bímáristán. He was assisted in all administrative acts by the heads of the three main clinical branches of the hospital—the physician-in-chief, the ophthalmologist-in-chief, and the surgeon-in-chief.

The actual director of the hospital—*mutawallí* the Arabs called him, dean would be the modern equivalent—was a medical man. Rhazes was *mutawallí* of the hospital at Ray and later took over the same position in the old hospital in Baghdad. Al-Jurjání, as I have already said, held this post at Khwárazm. The director in that city was known as the *taymardár*.

The director was assisted by two junior officers, known as *mushrif* or superintendant and *qawám* or administrator. These formed the almoner's staff. It was their duty to collect all legacies due to the hospital and any voluntary offerings which might be made from time to time. Such a one was Abu Saqar al-Kávdání, whom Ṣábit bin Qurra was obliged to report for his mismanagement of the monies entrusted to him. This money was being diverted to other uses and the patients of the hospital were in

1 *I.A.U.* vol. 1, p. 309.

consequence suffering from a lack of charcoal, food and bed coverings.[1]

In spite of this apparently elaborate organization the hospitals were not popular. I have nowhere come across in Persian or Arabic writers any eulogy such as modern patients so often give when they are discharged. On the contrary it was generally considered a very grave misfortune to be taken into hospital and kept there. 'They had already unbound him', says the Merchant in the Story of Ganem as related in the *Arabian Nights*, 'and were carrying him into hospital, when I happened to pass by....I took pity on him, and being used to sick people perceived that he had need to have particular care taken of him. I would not permit him to be put into hospital; for I am too well acquainted with their way of managing the sick and am sensible of the incapacity of the physicians.'[2]

1 Ibid. p. 221.

2 *Arabian Nights*, Nights 36–44 (Burton's translation). Lane's version is even stronger: 'The Sheykh of the market came and repelled them from him, and said, I will gain Paradise by means of this poor person; for if they take him into hospital they will kill him in one day.' *The Thousand and One Nights*, vol. 1, p. 509.

CHAPTER VII

AVICENNA[1] AND RHAZES

AT this point there walks into the story one of the greatest men that this world has ever seen. It is not the court of the caliphs nor one of the noble families of Baghdad that produces this prodigy. He is the son of a middle-class countryman in a far-away trans-Caspian province, the son of a tax-collector it is said. Here is a man who starting with none of the advantages of life (except perhaps an appreciative father) becomes, while still a youth, the adviser and confident of his ruler, who, change his city though he may, yet always becomes the leading citizen within a few months, and whose writings influenced all Europe, although he died before he was sixty and never travelled outside the semi-desert of central Asia. He was hailed by his countrymen as the Second Teacher, the Chief Master; he has been set by Dante in Paradise along with the greatest intellects of the non-Christian world; and William Harvey will say 600 years after his death to his friend Aubrey: 'Go to the fountain-head and read Aristotle, Cicero and Avicenna.'

Ḥusayn bin 'Abd-Ulláh Ḥasan bin 'Alí bin Síná was the son of a citizen of Balkh. The name of his mother has been preserved; she was one Satára, the daughter of a householder in Afsháneh, a village not very far from the modern town of Bukhara. Avicenna himself (to use his latinized and more familiar name) was probably born in the village of Kharmesan, also in the province of Balkh, being the elder of two sons. His brother's name was Maḥmúd.

In A.D. 985, when the elder child was but five, his father moved the family to Bukhara, and Avicenna started his education. First

1 For a detailed account of Avicenna see: al-Qifṭí, pp. 413–426; *I.A.U.* vol. II, pp. 1–20; *Hyst. Dynst.* vol. IX, p. 229; Ibn Khallikán, vol. I, p. 440; Brockelmann, *Gesch. d. arab. litt.* vol. I, p. 452; Leclerc, *Hist. Méd. Arabe*, vol. I, p. 466; Soubiran, *Avicenne* (Paris, 1935).

he was instructed in the Qur'án. His extraordinary memory at once displayed itself. He was one of those remarkable children, who learn to recite the whole of the Mohammedan scriptures by heart. His next subject was rhetoric. He was then sent to Maḥmúd the geometrician, from whom he also learnt algebra and arithmetic, and to Abú ul-Ḥasan Kóshyár under whom he studied astronomy. Within a few years he was considered fit to start theology under Isma'íl the Ṣúfí, and logic under the physician Abú 'Abd-Ulláh al-Nátalí. When he reached the age of sixteen, on the advice of Abú Sahl 'Ísá bin Yaḥyá al-Masíḥí, a Christian physician of Jurján, he started medicine and took as his tutor Abú Manṣúr Ḥassan bin Núḥ al-Qamarí. Abú Sahl, besides the glory that is rightly his as the adviser and companion of Avicenna, was himself no mean physician. His knowledge of medicine was acquired chiefly at Baghdad. Later he left the court of the caliph for that of Ma'mún ibn Muḥammad Khwárazmsháh and here he became acquainted with the young Avicenna. His book, the *Ṣad Báb* or *Kitáb-ul-Mi'a fi Ṭibb* or 'The Book of the Hundred Chapters on Medicine', was one of the standard text-books for medical students for many years after his death.[1]

Of Abú Manṣúr Ḥassan bin Núḥ al-Qamarí al-Bukhárí much less is known. He was a court physician to Manṣúr Samání. Several works are ascribed to him of which the best known is the *Kitáb-ul-Ghaní wa ul-Maní* or 'Book of Life and Death'. This has come down to us. It is a general treatise on medicine and mentions Rhazes by name. Another of his works[2] is entitled *Kitáb 'Ilal-il-'Ilal* and it is interesting to note that Rhazes quotes in the *Continens* from this.

Avicenna in his autobiography states that at first he treated patients not for fees, but for his own instruction. During this period of his studies he never passed a whole night in sleep nor passed a whole day in any other occupation but study. Whenever he met with an obscure point, it was his custom to perform the

1 *I.A.U.* vol. 1, p. 327; *Chahár Maqála*, p. 79.
2 *I.A.U.* vol. 1, p. 327; *Maṭraḥ-ul-Anẓár*, p. 160.

total ablution and then proceed to a mosque where he would pray to God to grant him comprehension and unlock for him the gates of difficulty. He says that he found medicine an easy subject. But that he composed the *Canon* at this early age, as al-Haraví states, is ridiculous. To such a length will flattery go.[1]

The early days of his practice were not uneventful, for the ruler of Bukhara, Núr bin Manṣúr Samání, fell ill, and the regular doctors having failed to bring about a cure, Avicenna was called in. He effected a cure to the intense delight of the *amír*. He was given a place of honour in the court and was further rewarded by being granted the right of access at any time to the royal library. Apparently he utilized this permission to the full. Núr bin Manṣúr was the seventh of a successful line of Sámánid rulers and by this time the library was well stocked with useful and rare manuscripts, including many Greek volumes. 'I went there', Avicenna writes, 'and found a great number of rooms filled with books packed up in trunks. I then read the catalogue of the primitive authors and found therein all that I required. I saw many books, the very titles of which were unknown to most people, and others which I never met with before or since.' Avicenna was then just eighteen. Some little time after he had received this permission the library was destroyed by fire and in the fire most of the manuscripts perished. Avicenna according to later writers had a hand in the outbreak, being desirous that his rivals in the medical world should have no access to the texts which he had studied there. But this is probably mere slander, although a Persian historian, Mas'úd Aurráq, states that the story was related of him also by contemporary writers.

Whatever the truth of the story, very soon after he had finished his medical education he was to be found at the court of the king of Khwárazm and he never returned to his native land. His departure from Bukhara was probably due to the death of his father, which occurred in 1002. Avicenna writes in his diary that necessity forced him to leave, but he does not add what

1 *Baḥr-ul-Jawáhir*, p. 7.

the nature of this necessity was. Some think that it was the need to earn his own living. Viewed in the light of his later career, I am inclined to think that he was so unpopular that he found it preferable to live and practise in other surroundings. At that time Abú ul-Ḥusayn Aḥmad ibn Muḥammad al-Suhaylí, a man of scholarly tastes, was prime minister at Khwárazm. Here Avicenna turned and was treated with the greatest respect. It is clear that his genius was even then recognized to be of no common order, for already his fame had reached that liberal tyrant Maḥmúd Ghaznaví. Maḥmúd, who in the art of war had been so completely successful, was determined to make his court as brilliant in intellect as it was rich in spoils. The court of Khwárazm, far inferior in power, was yet vastly superior in art and science, for Abú ul-'Abbás Ma'mún, the Khwárazmsháh, was himself a philosopher and a friend of scholars. Maḥmúd sent an imperious summons to the Khwárazmsháh, bidding him send to Ghazna certain of his leading scientists and men of learning. Abú ul-'Abbás heard of this before the arrival of the ambassador. He called his philosophers, his astronomers and his physicians into his presence and with a pathetic courage explained that he dare not resist Maḥmúd, but that he would shut his eyes to any who might wish to escape before he was officially informed of Maḥmúd's command. For 'Maḥmúd hath a strong hand and a large army: he hath annexed Khorasan and India and covets Iraq, and I cannot refuse to obey his order or execute his mandate. What say ye on this matter?'

Among the physicians who preferred liberty to the court of the tyrant were Avicenna and his old master Abú Sahl and the physician Abú 'Alí bin Miskawayhí. Perhaps, too, they had heard how Maḥmúd had treated the poet Firdausi, breaking his word and robbing the poet of the reward of the work of a lifetime. Unlike al-Bírúní, who obeyed the summons, these preferred not to serve a low-born Turk. So the little band of refugees set out for Jurjan. On the way Abú Sahl died and Avicenna after suffering much from the winds, dust and thirst reached Tus and eventually made his way to Nishapur. But the hue and cry was raised throughout the land and Avicenna thought it more prudent to push on to Jurjan, where Qábús ibn Washmgír was reigning.

For a while Avicenna remained in hiding living in a caravanserai and earning his daily keep by treating the sick around him. His success led to his downfall, for he was called in to treat a member of the reigning house. Now, among those who had obeyed Maḥmúd's summons was a young man named Abú Naṣr-i-'Arraq, a nephew of the Khwárazmsháh. He was summoned because of his fame as a physician, but it seems that his skill as an artist was the greater and more useful gift. For Maḥmúd, finding that Avicenna had eluded him, bade Abú Naṣr draw his portrait, and, having forty copies of it painted by lesser artists, had these distributed in all districts together with a proclamation, which ran: 'There is a man after this likeness, whom they call Abú 'Alí ibn Síná. Seek him out and send him to me.'

By this portrait Avicenna was recognized. According to Niẓámí, Qábús sent for Avicenna and loaded him with honours. But Avicenna himself relates that he reached Jurjan just too late to see Qábús, who had been deposed and cast into prison a short while before. Niẓámí's tale bears such a resemblance to the first cure, when Avicenna had the good fortune to treat Núḥ bin Manṣúr, that it may well be false and that Avicenna's own version is the correct one.

While still at Jurjan Avicenna met Abú 'Ubayd 'Abd-ul-Wáḥid ibn Muḥammad al-Júzjání. Mírzá Muḥammad, the great Persian collaborator with Professor Browne, has been able to fix the date of their meeting to the year 1012, when Avicenna was thirty-two. It is to Abú 'Ubayd that the world owes the detailed information that it now has of the life of Avicenna and also of his many works. For Avicenna was careless. His time was much taken up with statecraft and less creditable occupations. Without Abú 'Ubayd's spur much that he wrote would have been left unwritten and without Abú 'Ubayd's industry and prudence much that was written would have been lost. For Avicenna was in the habit of giving away his manuscripts without keeping any copy. Not only did Abú 'Ubayd complete Avicenna's autobiography from the time of their meeting until the day of his death, but he also completed his most important Persian work, the *Dánishnáma-i-'Alá' í*, and collected and edited the minor works which his friend had scattered about so liberally during his lifetime.

Either the death of Qábús or undesirable publicity caused Avicenna to flee once more. This time he turned west and passing through the forests of Mazanderan made his way across the Elburz Mountains and came to Ray, the capital of 'Iráq-i-'Ajamí. Here he found himself in that great mountain plain which embraced the three great cities of Persia of those days—Ray, Ispahan and Hamadan. All these were under the rule of a member of the Buwayhid family. In Ray a woman, named Sayyida, the widow of Fakhr-ul-Doula, was ruling on behalf of her infant son, Majad-ul-Doula Daylamí. Avicenna was received with all marks of respect. It is said that the young prince took Avicenna as his minister and that this became the cause of an open war between him and the queen mother. When the latter was victorious Avicenna was obliged to flee from Ray. Whatever may have been the cause, again necessity made him pass on to Qazvin, less than 100 miles away; and from there he moved on to Hamadan.

At that time Shams-ul-Doula, another son of Sayyida, was ruler of Hamadan. Following the example of his mother, he welcomed Avicenna and soon gave him ministerial rank. But his rule was troubled. A revolt among the underpaid and underfed soldiery broke out and Avicenna's house was attacked and looted. He was forced into retirement, from which, however, he was soon summoned to undertake the treatment of Shams-ul-Doula, who was attacked by severe colic, which baffled his doctors. Again Avicenna triumphed and he was restored to his high office of state.

It was now that Abú 'Ubayd asked the Shaykh to write a

general commentary on Aristotle. Avicenna refused to take up so large a task, but consented to set out on paper a refutation of certain points in Aristotle's teaching. It was thus that the work now known as *al-Shifá*, or 'The Healing', was commenced. This work is to be regarded as a treatise on philosophy and not on medicine. Persian writers class it along with Ptolemy's *Almagest* as a work devoted to a branch of astronomy. The sections on the medical properties of stones and other chemical chapters are included only because those subjects were in his day considered an integral part of philosophy. Ibn abí Uṣaybi'a states that this book was written in 20 days while Avicenna was living at Hamadan. But Niẓámí says that it was written with great deliberation page by page while he was at Ispahan. The work as a whole lies outside the limits of a chapter that deals only with Avicenna the physician. His greatest medical work, the *Canon*, had already been started at Ray. Here it was finished.

The death of his patron lead to trouble. Táj-ul-Doula, who succeeded, preferred another to Avicenna and Avicenna was forced to hide in the house of a druggist Abú Ghálib. But he could not remain concealed for long. His flight gave rise to suspicions and, search being made, he was found and condemned to imprisonment. He was lodged in the fortress called Faraján, but after four months escaped in disguise and fled to Ispahan, where another member of the Daylamí family was reigning. This was 'Alá'-ul-Doula Hasam-ul-Dín, often known as Ibn Kákúyá or Son of Kákúyá, because his father was the *kákú* or uncle of the famous queen Sayyida.

Again Avicenna rose triumphant over his misfortunes. He was received with the greatest respect by 'Alá'-ul-Doula who placed at his disposal a palace with gardens and a guard, such as he merited, as he himself said. He had now no further desire to meddle in politics and was the prince's confidential adviser without assuming the obligations of the wazirate. Thus affairs of State had not robbed him of his scientific tastes nor now did they occupy too much of his time. It was his custom to rise before dawn and every day write a couple of pages of his *al-Shifá*. At daybreak he would receive his pupils and friends. With them he would study until the hour for the morning prayers. He would then attend to matters of State. A large escort, sometimes amounting to 2000 men, would ride behind him to the ruler's apartments. There he would deal with claims, dispense justice and receive foreign ambassadors. At midday he would take his meal in his office and there he would take his afternoon siesta. On rising he attended upon the ruler, and stayed until the call to the sunset prayer warned him that it was time to return home. The evenings were spent in a very different manner. The great doctor now relaxed with women and wine, often carrying on his carousals long into the night.

It was impossible, even for Avicenna, thus to burn the candle at both ends. Weakened by overwork and probably also by over-indulgence in the pleasures of the flesh, he was taken with severe abdominal pain. In his desire to be well without delay he administered to himself eight enemas in one day. This set up an ulcerative diarrhoea. But Avicenna declared himself better and resumed his old habits of work and play. He made his condition worse by innumerable draughts of infusion of celery; and a servant, who had deceived him and feared his punishment, nearly poisoned him with opium. It has been suggested that the cause of all this trouble[1] was a cancer of the stomach. Nevertheless, he felt himself well enough to accompany his patron on a journey to Hamadan. On the road he was again struck down with colic, never regained his health, and entered Hamadan only to die a few days later. During the last fortnight of his life he refused all medical treatment. He gave alms to the poor, freed his slaves and read through the entire Qur'án once every three days. His tomb is shown in Hamadan to this day. It lies in the centre of the modern city, just off the main road. There are two stones in the floor of the little shrine. One covers the remains of Avicenna, the *Shaykh-ul-Ra'ís*, the *Mu'allim-ul-Ṣáni*, that is, Chief of Lords,

1 Ducastel, *La Vie Médicale*, 1929.

the Second Teacher, as he is here called, and the other covers the body of Shaykh Abú Sa'íd, the son of a druggist and a mystical poet. He was a contemporary of Avicenna, and said to have been acquainted with him. These two once met. Avicenna, speaking of the poet said: 'All I know, he sees.' But the poet capped the remark by saying: 'What I see, he knows.' A modern inscription records that the tomb had fallen into disrepair, a fact noted by al-Kashmírí when he passed through Hamadan in 1741, and that it was restored by Princess Nigar Khánum of the Qájár family in the year A.H. 1294, that is A.D. 1877. It has since been restored again, thanks to the interest which the late Sir William Osler showed in Avicenna and all connected with him.

The exact year of the birth of Avicenna is uncertain. The author of the *Ṭabaqát-il-Aṭibbá* gives on the authority of Abú 'Ubayd Juzjání 375 as his birth and 428 as his death, that is A.D. 985 and 1036 respectively.[1] But it is generally agreed that Ibn Khallikán, who makes the date of his birth five years earlier, is the more correct. He agrees in the date of his death, adding that it was on a Friday in the month of Ramazan, for Avicenna's first recorded case is said to have been his attendance at the death-bed of Núḥ bin Manṣúr. This prince reigned from A.D. 976 to 997. In al-Qifṭí's *Ta'ríkh-ul-Ḥukamá* is found an extract of Avicenna's autobiography. He there states that he was seventeen when he was called in to attend upon the prince. This would therefore fix A.D. 980 as the date of his birth.

A wit of the day wrote the following epitaph upon him (I use Professor Browne's translation and explanation):

> 'I saw Ibn Síná contending with men, but he died in prison (or, of constipation) the most ignoble death;
>
> 'What he attained by the *Shifá* (or, by Healing) did not secure his health, nor did he escape death by his *Naját* (or, Deliverance).'
>
> In this verse there are three ingenious word-plays, for *ḥabs* means both 'imprisonment' and 'constipation', while two of his most famous works are entitled *Shifá* ('Healing') and *Naját* ('Deliverance').

1 *I.A.U.* vol. II, p. 9.

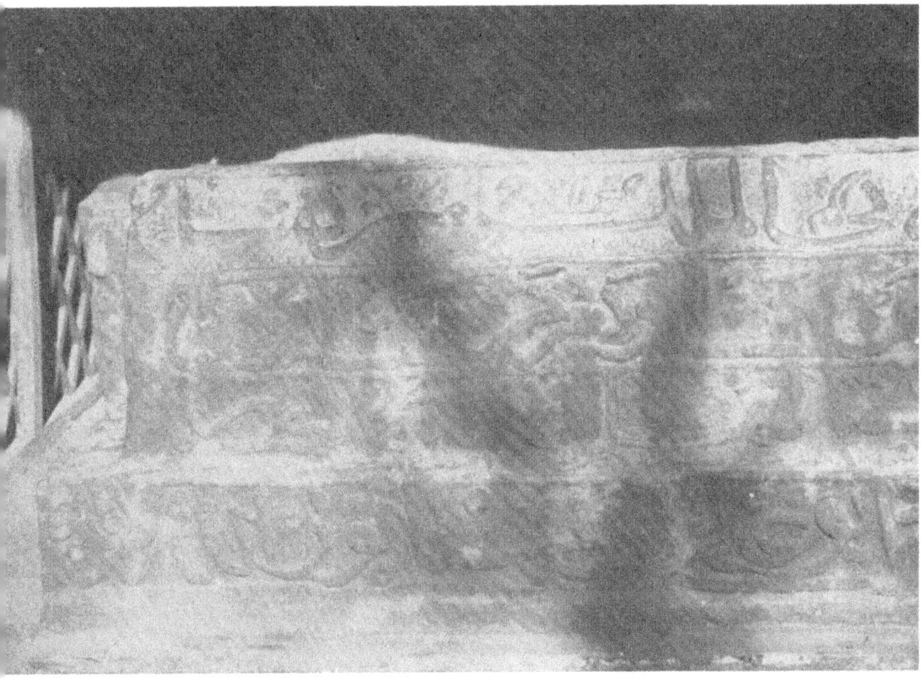

PLATE II. Interior of the tomb of Avicenna at Hamadan

The written works of Avicenna differ considerably in value. There are but few subjects on which he did not write—music, mathematics, astrology, logic, medicine, and even love and wine. Some of his works are of outstanding importance, others are valueless. He began to write at a very early age, for two of his works were written while he was still at Bukhara and a third is dedicated to Núḥ bin Manṣúr. All three must therefore have been written before he was seventeen. He wrote mainly in Arabic; but two works in Persian are ascribed to him. Of these the more important is the *Dánishnáma-i-'Alá'í* or 'The Book of Wisdom of 'Alá'í'. This is a large manual of philosophy, dedicated to his master at Ispahan. It was designed to treat of logic, metaphysics, natural science, mathematics, astronomy, music and arithmetic. But after his death only the first three sections could be found. The missing portions were therefore compiled and translated by ul-Juzjání from the *Shifá* and other Arabic works of his master and the lacuna thus filled. It has been lithographed in India, but never printed in Europe.

The other Persian work is a small treatise on the pulse. Browne considers this to be a genuine work of Avicenna, but the opening words, if correct, show that this is impossible. 'There came to me a command from 'Aẓud-ul-Doula Daylamí that I should write a book on the pulse. So I have written the following work on the knowledge of the blood vessels.' 'Aẓud-ul-Doula died in 982 when Avicenna was only two years old. It was two other members of the Daylamí family whom he served in Hamadan and Ispahan. The author of the *Maṭraḥ*, a modern Persian collection of medical biographies, suggests that the authorship of this treatise would be more rightly ascribed either to Abú 'Alí bin Miskawayhí or Abú 'Alí bin Mandúyah. Avicenna also wrote a certain amount of poetry in Persian.

A large part of his work in Arabic is of no interest to a medical historian. Browne has translated in his *Literary History of Persia* (vol. II, pp. 110, 111) his most celebrated poem. His philosophical works have received the attention of Baron Carra de Vaux in his

Les Grands Philosophes: Avicenna (Paris, 1900). His works on music are still the subject of discussion in the *Journal of the Royal Asiatic Society of London*. But by far the most important part of his literary output, his medical works, these, although the most accessible, have received the least notice from modern writers. He wrote at least eight large medical treatises which together are of the utmost importance in the story of medicine, for by means of these he rivalled, if indeed he did not actually displace, the medical works of Galen and Hippocrates which had been the foundations of the study of medicine ever since they were written.

The first of these is his sequel to Ḥunayn's 'System of Medicine', which exists only in manuscript. Next comes his work on colic, a subject upon which he might almost claim to be a specialist, for it was a complaint to which he owed his temporal supremacy. Two other minor medical works are the *Qawánín* or 'The Laws' and the *Ḥadúd-ul-Ṭibb* or 'Medical Definitions'. His treatise on cardiac drugs lies third in importance to the *Qánún* and the *S͟hifá*, while another called *Kitáb-ul-Mabda' wa ul-Ma'ád* or 'The Book of the Origin and the Return', which he dedicated to Abú Muḥammad S͟hírází, contains a chapter on 'the possibility of the production of exceptional psychical phenomena' which Jámí borrowed for his poem *The Chain of Gold*.

A curious anecdote hath reached me which I have heard related. A certain physician was attached to the court of one of the House of Sámán, and there attained so high a position of trust that he used to enter the women's apartments and feel the pulses of its carefully guarded and closely veiled inmates.

One day he was sitting with the King in the women's apartments in a place where it was impossible for any other male creature to penetrate. The King demanded food, and it was brought by the hand-maidens. One of these who was laying the table took the tray off her head, bent down, and placed it on the ground. When she desired to stand upright again, she was unable to do so, but remained as she was, by reason of a rheumatic swelling of the joints. The King turned to the physician and said 'You must cure her at once in whatever way you can.' Here was no opportunity for any physical method of treatment, for which no appliances were available, no drugs being at hand. So the physician bethought himself of a psychical treatment, and bade them remove the veil from her head and expose her hair, so that she might be ashamed and make some movement, this condition being displeasing to her, to wit that all her head and face should thus be exposed. As, however, she underwent no change, he proceeded to something still more shameful, and ordered her trousers to be removed. She was overcome with shame, and a warmth was produced within her such that it dissolved that thick rheum and she stood up straight and sound, and regained her normal condition.[1]

Finally we come to the *Qánún*, the 'Canon or Laws of Medicine', upon which Avicenna's reputation is for the most part built. In spite of contrary opinions it is safer to agree with those writers who hold that this great work was the result of careful examination and much thought. The book was started when Avicenna was in Jurjan and finished at Ray. When it became known to the medical world, it at once superseded all previous works on medicine. Bar Hebraeus says that before the composition and diffusion of the *Canon* all aspirants to medicine were used to study al-Majúsí's *Kámil-ul-Ṣaná'at*, the *Liber Regius*, but that after the *Canon* of Avicenna was made known, the study of the *Liber Regius* was completely abandoned. But he admits that, although the *Canon* excels in the theoretical parts, it is still excelled by the *Liber Regius* in the practical. Niẓámí, after narrating the various works which it was essential for a medical student to read, concludes by saying that 'whoever has mastered the first volume of the *Qánún*, to him nothing will be hidden of the general and fundamental principles of medicine, for could Hippocrates and Galen return to life, it were meet that they should do reverence to this book'.[2]

The *Canon*, unlike so many books of this period contains no elaborate opening or dedication. The first book, considered by the ancients to be the most distinguished part of the work, is

1 Niẓámí, *Chahár Maqála*, p. 82. 2 Ibid. p. 79.

confined to a discussion of general principles, physiological and pathological. It has recently been translated into English by Dr O. C. Gruner (London, 1930) with the exception, unfortunately, of the anatomical section, and has been commented on by him and by Dr Soubiran (Paris, 1935). The second book deals with simple drugs, each described and listed under the initial letter. It is notable that Avicenna does not arrange them in the Persian alphabetical order, but in the order of the letters of the Abjad system. This was an arrangement of the letters in the order of their numerical values. A was the equivalent of 1, B of 2, J of 3, D of 4, and so on through the alphabet. This section of the *Canon*, compared with other pharmacopoeias of the early Arab school, is marked neither by its completeness nor by its originality.

Of all the great Arabian or Persian physicians there is only one who is worthy to be compared with Avicenna. This is Muḥammad ibn Z̲akariyyá. To the West he is known as Rhazes; to his fellow countrymen he is sometimes called Ibn Z̲akariyyá, sometimes Abú Bakr, and sometimes al-Rází. Chronologically I should have dealt with him before Avicenna, for he was born on 27 August, A.D. 865, 115 years before Avicenna.

In his early life his interest was chiefly in music. He wrote an encyclopaedia on this subject, which he entitled *Fi Jamál-il-Músiqí* or 'On the Beauty of Music' and was a skilful player on the lute as well as a singer. He is said to have abandoned music on the grounds that it 'proceeded from between the moustachio and the beard' and had no claims to recommend it. At the same time he was studying philosophy under Aḥmad bin Sahl al-Balk̲h̲í and was writing poetry on metaphysical subjects. He earned his living apparently as a banker, for Ibn abí Uṣaybi'a says that he possessed a copy of one of Rhazes' works inside which was written in the handwriting of Rhazes himself: 'A Compendium of the Manṣúrí, written by Muḥammad bin Z̲akariyyá al-Rází the Money Changer.'[1]

1 *I.A.U.* vol. 1, p. 314.

About the age of thirty Rhazes made his first visit to Baghdad and there he had an experience which changed the whole of his life. He visited in a spirit of mere curiosity the Muqtadirí Hospital and became interested in a conversation with the old pharmacist. He returned on the following day and happened to meet a physician to the hospital who showed him a human foetus with two heads. So interested was he in this and in what he heard from the druggist that he determined to study medicine for himself.

He probably stayed in Baghdad some time and there received a thorough grounding in his new profession. It is usually asserted that he made his medical studies in Ray under ‘Alí bin Sahl al-Ṭabarí. This was the view of al-Qifṭí. All medical historians have been contented to accept this statement until Max Meyerhof showed how unlikely it was, seeing that al-Ṭabarí was at least 75 years of age when Rhazes began to read medicine. On his return to Ray, Rhazes became the *mutawallí* or administrator of the hospital of that city. He did not hold this post for long, for some time between A.D. 902 and 907 he returned to Baghdad and took charge of the Muqtadirí Hospital. During these years he lived in the Darb-ul-Nafal or the Street of Lucerne. This street was almost certainly in the al-Karkh quarter of Baghdad. For here were also to be found streets with similar names, such as the Myrtle Wharf, the Barley Street, and the Pomegranate Bridge. His hospital, too, was situated in this quarter, near the bridge over the Karkhiya Canal.

As chief physician of Baghdad the fame of Rhazes spread through the lands of the caliph and his services were in constant demand even in distant cities. Being a Persian he had a very warm corner in his heart for his Persian clients. He attended most of the nobles and princes of the minor Persian courts. For them he composed many of his works on medicine. Towards the end of his life, he was considerably hindered by a slowly increasing blindness. Some asserted that this was caused by a blow on the head. But it is not at all improbable that he ruined his sight by excessive study, for he seldom left his books and was always to be found copying manuscripts or writing out fair copies of his lectures. He admitted that he sorely overtried his powers and used to spend many a night with a friend reading Hippocrates and Galen.

Both the place and date of his death are uncertain. The earliest that any authority gives is A.D. 912. Ibn Khallikán made it occur in A.D. 923, while Ibn Juljul and Ḥájjí Khalífa place it as late as A.D. 932. Al-Bírúní, who was a very exact chronologist, asserts that it happened on 26 October 925 at Ray. There the matter must rest.

Seeing that Rhazes at the most cannot have practised medicine for more than 35 years and that during those years he was travelling about a great deal and engaged in many duties, clinical and administrative, his literary output on medical subjects was enormous. With the possible exception of music and chemistry, his writings on other subjects besides medicine did not enhance his reputation. Qáẓí Sa'íd, for instance, says that he failed ever to understand the real purport of theology, that his philosophical beliefs were unsound, and that his criticism was ill-founded.

As a practical chemist he was a tragic failure. He seems to have spent his time in the quest of the transmutation of base metals into gold. His reputation for this power brought him the beating which may have been the cause of his blindness, caused him to be strangled by a disappointed minister, and gained for him the name of a swindler among some travellers from Europe. His less speculative work does him more credit, for he attempted to classify chemical substances and carried on original investigations on specific gravity by means of an hydrostatic balance.

His medical works are among the most important of the Arabian school of medicine. Among these works priority in importance and in interest must be given to his *al-Ḥáwí* or *Continens*. Of this the complete Arabic text has never been published. In its Latin form it is available in the edition translated by Faraj ibn Salem or Farraguth for King Charles of Anjou in 1279 and printed at Brescia in 1486. Portions of the original text can be seen in various libraries. One day, perhaps, they will be collected, edited and printed. This is highly desirable for the *Continens* must be regarded as more important, even than the *Canon* of Avicenna, to the historian of Arab medicine. Access to the complete, original text is essential for the full history and appreciation of the part that the Arabs and Persians played in the progress of medicine. But, as Professor Browne wrote years ago, who can find a patron who will finance the editing and the printing, not to mention the journeying from library to library, of a book on a science that is dead, obsolete, and despised even in its own country?

Perhaps it is fitting, though it is a great pity, that there is no Arabic edition of the work, for Rhazes himself apparently never intended it to appear as one complete book. It is to be looked upon rather as an *aide-mémoire* or as a foundation for smaller works. It represents the thoughts, the reading, and the clinical notes of Rhazes' entire medical life. When he died, the whole of this disorderly matter, the original observations, and the extracts from other people's works, was sold by Rhazes' sister for a large sum to Ibn ul-'Amíd, the *wazír* of Rukn-ul-Doula. He, being not only a statesman but also a scholar, summoned Rhazes' pupils and the best doctors of Ray to draft these rough notes into book form. Their united efforts produced the book which was known thereafter as *Kitáb-ul-Ḥáwí fí il-Ṭibb* or 'System of Medicine'. The work was enormous and not many copies were made. In fact, 50 years later, Haly Abbas thought that there were only two copies in existence. Professor Browne has translated a few of the clinical notes into English and Max Meyerhof has recently published the text and translation of thirty-three more. Apart from these few extracts there is no means by which an ordinary reader can form any judgement about this, the greatest work of the Arab school. Perhaps in these circumstances it is best to accept the criticism of Haly Abbas:

> As to his book which is known as *al-Ḥáwí*, I found that he mentions in it everything the knowledge of which is necessary to the medical man, concerning hygiene and medical and dietetical treatment of

diseases and their symptoms. He did not neglect the smallest thing required by the student of this art concerning treatment of diseases and illnesses. But he made no mention at all of natural matters, such as the elements, the temperaments and the mixtures of the humours. Nor did he speak of anatomy and surgery. He wrote, moreover, without order and method, neglecting the side of scholastic learning. He omitted to subdivide his book into discourses, sections and chapters, as might have been expected from his vast knowledge of the medical art and from his talent as a writer. Far be it from me to contest his excellence or to deny his knowledge of the medical art or his eminence as an author. Considering this condition or imagining the causes of it by comparison with the vast knowledge shown in this book, I think there are two possibilities; either he composed it and collected in it the entire field of Medicine as a special memorandum of reference for himself, comprising hygiene and therapeutics, for his old age and time of forgetfulness: or being afraid of damage which might occur to his library, which was to be made good in this case by the book in question. Likewise in order to relieve his writing from bulkiness and in order to be useful to the people and to create for himself a good memorial for coming generations he provided reference notes for his entire text, put them in order and compared each one with its like and fitted it in its chapter according to his knowledge of appropriateness in this art. In this way the book should be complete and perfect.

He was, however, prevented from continuing it by hindrances and death befell him before its completion. If such was his aim, he treated his subject at too great length and made his book too voluminous without any urgent necessity to claim in his favour. This was the reason why most scholars were not able to order and purchase copies of the book, except a few wealthy literary men, and so copies are scarce. He proceeded in such a manner that for each disease, its causes, symptoms and treatment, he mentioned the sayings of every ancient and modern physician on the disease in question from Hippocrates and Galen down to Isḥáq bin Ḥunayn, and all the physicians, ancient and modern, who lived in between them, without omitting the sayings of any one of them and reference to them in this book, so that the entirety of medical literature was comprised in this book. You must know, however, that skilful and experienced physicians agree about the nature of diseases, their causes, symptoms and medical treatment, and that there exists no marked difference between their opinions, except that they treat more or less of the matter and that they speak in different terms, because the rules and the schools they follow in the knowledge of diseases, their causes and treatment, are obviously the same. If this is so, it was not necessary to record the sayings of all the ancient and modern physicians and the reiteration of their utterances, since they all repeat the same things.[1]

Rhazes' second most important work is the *Kitáb-ul-Manṣúrí* or *Liber ad Almansorem*. The Manṣúr to whom this book is dedicated, was certainly Manṣúr ibn Isḥáq, who was appointed governor of Ray in A.D. 903. On all sides mistakes as to the identity of this Manṣúr have been made. None of the oriental biographers, with the exception of Yáqút in his *Mu'jam-ul-Buldán*, have successfully identified him. The work must have been one of the early works of Rhazes, for it lacks the originality of the *Continens* and is merely a sort of summary or reproduction of Greek medicine. There is no evidence in it of the clinical acumen which his later works display. Like the *Continens*, the Arabic text has never been published as a whole, but a Latin translation by Gerard of Cremona was printed in 1489. The importance of this work in the eyes of medical professors in medieval Europe was enormous. Above all the ninth book under the title of *Nonus Almansuris* was the subject of numerous commentaries and formed part of the regular medical curriculum of almost every medieval university. This ninth book dealt with disease *a capite usque ad pedes*. According to Haly Abbas the fault of the *al-Manṣúrí* lay in its brevity.

Of his many minor works the majority are known only by their titles. His *Barr'-ul-Sá'at* or 'Cure within the Hour' has received more notice than most, even more notice than it deserves. It was translated into Persian under the title of *Tuḥfa-i-Sh̲áhí* by Sh̲ayk̲h̲ Ḥusayn Jabírí al-'Anṣárí about A.D. 1700 for the use of Sulṭán Muḥammad 'A'ẓamsh̲áh of Delhi and again by Mír Muḥammad Ḥusayn ibn Karam 'Alí under the name of *Dastúr-ul-Ṭibb*. In more modern times it has been translated into French by Dr P. Guigues of Beirut under the title of '*La Guérison en une*

1 *Liber Regius*, vol. I, p. 5.

Heure' par Rhazes; and the contents of a modern edition, which still circulates among the more old-fashioned practitioners of Persia, was summarized by me in the *Royal Asiatic Society's Journal* for October 1932. Rhazes also wrote a pamphlet which he called 'Of Habit which becomes natural', thus anticipating Sherrington's conditioned reflex theory. By writing a monograph on 'Diseases in Children' he may also be looked upon as the father of paediatrics. Several of his minor works were translated into Latin in medieval times and collected together and printed under the title of *Opera Parva Abubetri*.

Perhaps a word more is due about the most important of these minor works, his treatise on small-pox and measles. This, translated into Latin, was printed in Venice in 1489, in Basle in 1549, in London in 1747, and in Göttingen in 1781. In addition to these a Greek translation was printed in Paris in 1762 and an English translation was made in 1848. The importance of the work is that it is the first definite description of small-pox as a clinical entity and thus, as Neuburger says: 'On every hand and with justice it is regarded as an ornament to the medical tradition of the Arabs.' Whether it is equally true to say, as so many assert, that in this work Rhazes was also the first to distinguish small-pox from measles, I have grave doubts. I have read the book many times and cannot come to any conclusion. Rhazes himself says in his preface that his work deals with small-pox because 'there has not appeared up to this present time either among the ancients or the moderns an accurate and satisfactory account of it'. He nowhere says that he is about to deal with a second and separate disease. Yet in his mind he clearly distinguished between the two, for in his *Taqsím-ul-'Ilal* or 'Division of Diseases' he states that the premonitory symptoms of small-pox are fever and pain in the back, while in measles the heat is greater and there is marked mental distress. Again, in the *Continens*, he states that the rash of measles comes out all at once, whereas the rash of small-pox comes out gradually. Whatever he himself may have held, his successors certainly did not consider that he made out a successful case for the separation of these diseases into two. Avicenna must have had in mind these two passages that I have just quoted, when he wrote:

> Know, then, that measles is a bilious small-pox. In most respects there is no difference between them, save only that measles is derived from the bilious humour. And again, the rash of measles is smaller, does not penetrate the skin, is not appreciably elevated, at least not in the beginning, whereas the rash of small-pox at the onset is appreciable to the touch and is elevated. The individual spot of measles is smaller than that of small-pox and less rarely erupts on the eye. The physical signs of measles are nearly the same as those of small-pox, but the nausea is greater, the mental disturbance and inflammation is more severe, though the pains in the back are less. The rash of measles usually appears all at once, but the rash of small-pox spot after spot.[1]

It is not unnatural to ask which of these two outstanding figures is the greater, Rhazes or Avicenna. In many ways they are singularly alike. Their work and life are marked by a catholicity of interests, in both cases only equalled by the craftsmen of the Italian renaissance. Avicenna started medicine when a mere boy and in manhood took up other subjects. Rhazes, having gained a mastery of non-medical subjects, was in middle life attracted to medicine. Thus each by the time he was forty was a master of medicine and an authority on music, chemistry, geology, and philosophy. The original contributions which these two made to medicine and to non-medical subjects would entitle each of them to a high place among the thinkers in either category. The originality of Rhazes lay rather in the practice of medicine, that of Avicenna in its theory. Thus, to Rhazes is to be ascribed the first use of mercury as a purgative. White lead ointment was introduced into the pharmacopoeia by him, so that it became known in the Middle Ages as 'Album Rhasis'. Certain trochisci for application to the eye were known as 'Arab Soap' or 'Trochiscus Rhasis'. He also introduced the use of animal gut as a ligature for surgical operations and was the first to recognize the reaction of the pupil to light. To Avicenna, on the other hand,

1 *Canon*, Bk. iv, pp. 1, 4.

is to be ascribed the championing of the unorthodox views of Alhazen on the cause of vision, views which we now know to be correct. He also seems to have understood the difference between obstructive and haemolytic jaundice and was the first to give a good description of meningitis.

Both men are loud in the scorn of quacks and charlatans. Nor apparently had they very much use for the ugly sister of medicine, astrology. Rhazes was so indignant at the pretentions of the ignorant that he denounced them at length in the *Liber Almansuris*[1] and was moved to write three pamphlets on the subject. In one of these he discusses the reason why most people prefer quacks to orthodox practitioners and why they make even the ablest of the regular physicians the butt of their sarcasm and scorn. In a letter he attempted to explain why in some cases 'inexperienced physicians and even women in certain cities are more successful in their treatment than the most learned of physicians'.

Among their own countrymen these two were and are almost equally famous. They were not, however, without their critics. Of Rhazes a certain al-K'abí complained that he was a threefold impostor. He claimed to be an alchemist, yet once he could not raise 10 dirhams to save himself from prison. He claimed to be a physician, yet he could not cure his own blindness. And he claimed to be an astrologer, yet he could not foresee his own fate. Of Avicenna 'Abd-ul-Laṭíf of Baghdad wrote that the majority of men were drawn to perdition by no other cause than his writings and that his works added nothing to philosophy, but rather derogated from it.

But these are voices crying in the wilderness. The vast majority of their compatriots flatter them with a praise which outruns discretion and certainly justification.

During these fifteen centuries [wrote Niẓámí][2] which have elapsed since the time of Aristotle, no philosopher hath won to the inmost essence of his doctrine, nor travelled the high-road of his method, save that most excellent of the moderns, the Philosopher of the East, the

1 *Lib. Alman.* bk. vii, p. 27.

2 *C͟habár Maqála*, p. 80.

Proof of God unto his creatures, abú 'Alí al-Ḥusayn ibn 'Abd Ulláh ibn Síná. He who finds fault with these two great men will have cut himself off from the company of the wise, placed himself in the category of madmen, and exhibited himself in the ranks of the feeble-minded. May God (blessed and exalted is He) keep us from such stumbling and vain desires by His favour and His Grace.

A more moderate judgement summed up their merits by saying that Rhazes excelled all others in the clinical side of medicine, Avicenna in the theoretical.

The influence of Rhazes and Avicenna upon Western thought was equally great. This is not to deny that other Arabian physicians, especially some of those who lived under the caliphs of Spain, also contributed largely to the renaissance of learning in Europe. None, however, excelled these two. Scarcely more than a century elapsed after the death of Avicenna before manuscripts of his works found their way into Europe and began to be translated. The success of Arab arms favoured the spread of Arab science. There was also a constant contact between the eastern caliphs and the powers of Europe. Hárún-ul-Ras͟hid sent an ambassador to the court of the emperor of the Holy Roman Empire. Courtesies were frequently exchanged between the emperor of Arabic East and of the Latin West. It is even said that Charlemagne paid an incognito visit to Palestine in order to consult Arab physicians about his health. There was therefore every reason why Arab learning should be well received by men of learning in Europe. On the other hand, after the death of Charlemagne in A.D. 814 Latin Europe sank to the lowest depths of barbarism that history records. It was only in those parts which were under Moslem domination, that is to say, Sicily and Spain, that Roman civilization survived. It was to these centres that Arabic manuscripts first travelled, and it was from these centres that Arabic science was propagated among a people who were very ready to accept it.

Of these two centres of diffusion Sicily was the less important. There the period of greatest energy was when Frederick II, having quarrelled with the Pope, drew to his court scholars whose investigations were discouraged by the clergy. The most famous of these was Michael Scot (*c.* 1175–*c.* 1232), who, aided by Andrew the Jew, translated Avicenna into Latin. The last of the great translators of the Sicilian School was the Jew Farraguth who died in 1285 and who translated into Latin not only the *Continens* of Rhazes, but also the *Tacuini Aegritudinem* of Ibn Jazlá, a work on surgery by Mesue Junior, and a pseudo-Galenic work to which Ḥunayn had given an Arabic form.

The school of Toledo was of far greater importance. Here a Society of Translators, comparable to the Bayt-ul-Ḥikmat of Baghdad, was founded by the Archbishop Raymond. Toledo was by this time nominally Christian once more. Internal dissensions among the Arab aristocracy of the western caliphate allowed the rulers of Castile to reassert the supremacy of Christianity and Toledo was rescued from the Moors in 1085. But the city remained Moorish at heart. The Spanish Jews retained Arabic as their medium of expression long after Islam had yielded its temporal supremacy. Spanish Jews, too, formed the bulk of the physician-philosophers of those times. Speaking and writing the language of the Qur'án and *Canon* they were ready interpreters of Arabic medicine to the rest of the Latin-reading world. It was to them, therefore, that Raymond turned, and from their pens during the twelfth century a deluge of Latin translations was offered to the rest of Europe.

Another patron of the Society of Translators was Frederick Barbarossa, and in the encouragement of the translating movement at Toledo he found an outlet for his pro-Arabian sympathies. Some time between 1170 and his death in 1187 Gerard of Cremona, the greatest of the Toledo translators, made the first translation into Latin of the *Canon* of Avicenna, at the command, it is said, of Frederick Barbarossa. A good knowledge of Arabic and the assistance of a native Christian writer, Ibn G͟hálib, allowed Gerard to put forth in his own lifetime an enormous number of translations. Leclerc, in his *Histoire de la médecine arabe*, gives a list of these works. They include Rhazes' *Liber ad Almansorem*, Ibn

Serapion's works, and the *Canon*. His translation of the *Canon* formed the prototype upon which most other translations were based.

The lesser works of Avicenna now received notice. Gundisalvus translated his *Sufficientia*, Armengaud his *Canticum* with the Commentary of Averroes on it, and Arnold of Villanova his *De Viribus Cordis*. The popularity of the Arabs was thus established and among them Rhazes and Avicenna were considered pre-eminent. So great was their popularity and so long did it endure that we find Montagna, Gentile da Fabriano and other artists decorating the edge of the Madonna's robe with Arabic lettering and two Arab doctors, Cosmas and Damian, raised to the altars of the Church.

In 1285 Farraguth the Jew died. That year may be taken as the date when the era of Latin translations ceased and the Arab scholastic revival entered into its full glory. Two universities of Europe specialized in Arab letters and became identified in their medical schools with the propagation of the teaching of Rhazes and Avicenna. The interest of the university being speculative rather than practical Avicenna was preferred to Rhazes. The medical students, however, read both. Of these universities, one was Montpellier, the other Bologna. Montpellier was the protagonist of Arab culture. Its library was immense. All the translations of Arab writers made by Constantine the African and by Gerard of Cremona were housed in its library and that at a time when the medical library of Paris University contained less than a score of works. From these two centres the teaching and influence of the Arabs spread to every medical school in Europe. From the twelfth to the seventeenth century Rhazes and Avicenna were held superior even to Hippocrates and Galen.

At the height of this Asiatic domination of Europe a new spirit began to stir. Certain Greek works had come to light. They were translated into Latin and found not to be in complete agreement with the Latin translations of their Arabic versions. The first reaction was to criticize the Arabs as traducers of the Greek texts. The second reaction was a determination to explore further and to see to what extent the Arabs had misrepresented Greek thought. Thus, research in literature, like experiment in other fields, began to shake the supremacy of the Arabs. It was not long before the universities were divided into four schools of thought. First came the Arabists, who were safely enthroned with many years of tradition behind them and represented the conservative opinion. Immediately opposed to them were the Humanists or neo-Hellenists, who claimed to go behind the Arabs and who appealed to the sources from which the Arabs had themselves drawn. The Arabists they dubbed Neoterics or 'newfangled'. Between these two was the School of the Conciliators, who attempted to reconcile the doctrines of the Greeks and the Arabs and to explain away such difficulties as were manifest. Finally, there were those who had no use either for Greeks or for Arabs, the Experimenters, who would listen to none of the old school, whose eyes were on the future, and who refused to hold themselves bound by either Greek or Arab tradition.

The first three parties were, of course, doomed from the moment that experiment and research began. In vain did Mundinus of Bologna (d. 1325) attempt to retain Arab supremacy over anatomy by using only Arabic names in his practical dissection classes. In vain did Guy de Chauliac (d. 1368) win for himself the title of 'The Restorer' by his vigorous propagation of Arab terms and doctrines. The combined opposition of the Hellenists and the Experimentalists was too strong, although it was a long time before the fortress, founded upon Avicenna, fell. Lectures at Montpellier up to 1555 continued to be given upon the text-books of Rhazes, Avicenna and the two Mesues. In 1558 Saporta, the doyen of the Faculty of Medicine of that university, was still lecturing upon the *Liber Nonus ad Almansorem*. In the University of Brussels by some curious oversight the lectures upon Avicenna survived until 1909.

The Humanists fared no better. Their attempt to put the clock back to the age of Galen was as idle and as retrograde as the attempt of the Arabists to make it stand still at the age of the caliphs of Baghdad. Greek medical texts formed no inspiration for scientists as Greek statues did for artists. Even in letters the attempt to stereotype literature upon Greek models must be considered harmful in both prose and verse. In medicine it was definitely so, for it meant an interest philological rather than scientific and made medicine owe more to erudition than to observation.

The death-blow to Arabic medicine came from many quarters. In Italy Leonardo da Vinci (d. 1519), though he used Arabic terms, did as much to overthrow the Avicennan system of anatomy as did any medical anatomist. Nor did he even pay lip-service to the system in which he was reared. 'They scorn me who am a discoverer', he wrote. 'Yet how much more do they deserve censure who have never found out anything, but recite and blazon forth other people's works.... Those who study old authors and not the works of Nature are the stepsons not the sons of Nature, who is the mother of all good authors.' In Basle so great was Paracelsus' (d. 1541) dislike of the Arabs that he publicly burnt the *Canon* of Avicenna as a protest. In France Champier (d. 1535) printed his *Contra Arabum Traditionem* and Rabelais (d. 1553) wrote of 'badauds médecins, ceux qui ont été herselès en l'officine des Arabes'. Finally, Harvey of Padua and London published his *De Motu Cordis* in 1628 and drove the last nail into their coffin.

During the Stuart period to study the Arabs was the mark of a charlatan and a quack. Shakespeare is a little too early to show the truth of this sad decline. The satirists of the Restoration, however, are filled with cheap jokes on this subject. The *Quacks Academy*, written in the reign of Charles II, and printed in 1678, shows with what ingratitude the world of that time looked upon the great masters who had rescued Greek science from oblivion and who had now become the stock-in-trade of impostors. 'Further, let your table be never without some old musty Greek or Arabic author and the Fourth Book of Cornelius Agrippa's *Occult Philosophy*, wide open, to amuse the spectators; with half a dozen of gilt shillings, as so many guineas received that morning for fees.'

CHAPTER VIII

THE SELJÚQS AND THE LAST OF THE CALIPHS[1]

IN Baghdad Buwayhid rule was not a great success. It is true that they maintained their supremacy for just over 100 years, but it was weakened by family quarrels and the religious antipathies which the family faith aroused in the orthodox Baghdadis. The material position of the caliphs could not have been lower. Al-Muṭí', a son of al-Muqtadir, was the first to be allowed to assume the office under the new *amír*. After reigning for nearly 30 years and now a sufferer from paralysis, he was deposed in favour of his son al-Ṭái'. He in turn held office for 17 years and was finally deposed and cast into prison so that Bahá'-ul-Doula, the Buwayhid *amír*, could take possession of his property over which he had long cast eyes of envy. In his place al-Qádir received the office of caliph and reigned for 40 years, dying a natural death at the age of eighty-seven and while still on the throne. It was during his caliphate that the power of Maḥmúd of Ghazna arose. His son al-Qá'im succeeded him, but found his position even more difficult than had his predecessors. The hold over the city by the Buwayhid family was becoming looser. Scarcely a day passed without tumult and bloodshed. Frequently the city was left without a ruler at all. For the Daylamite general and the *wazír* were at loggerheads. The former accused the latter of making overtures to the rising power of the Seljúqs, while the *wazír* accused the general of attempting to supplant the reigning caliph by the Egyptian anti-caliph. So violent were the passions that at times Malik-ul-Raḥím, the Buwayhid prince, was obliged to flee the city in order to save his life. With Baghdad in this state of political confusion Ṭughril Bég of the house of

1 Much of the non-medical part of this chapter is taken from Muir's *Rise and Fall of the 'Abbasid Caliphate*, pp. 579 et seqq.

Seljúq thought fit to enter Iraq with a large army on the pretence of performing the pilgrimage to Mecca. The Turks and the Buwayhids were averse to allowing him to approach Baghdad: the caliph was only too glad to invite him. Accordingly, in the year A.D. 1055, Ṭughril Bég entered the city at the head of his army, cast Malik-ul-Raḥím into prison, and disbanding the Daylamite forces replaced the house of Buwayhid by the house of Seljúq as virtual ruler of the empire of the caliphs.

Ṭughril had two famous *wazírs*, 'Amíd-ul-Mulk and Niẓám-ul-Mulk. Both were citizens of Nishapur. The less famous of the two was 'Amíd-ul-Mulk al-Kundurí, of whom it is said that falling sick of colic one day he sent for the most famous physician of that city, a certain Abú ul-Qásim 'Abd-ul-Raḥmán bin 'Alí bin Aḥmad, usually known as Ibn abí Ṣádiq. Unfortunately for 'Amíd-ul-Mulk, by the time that he had need of his services, Ibn abí Ṣádiq had already retired from active practice and had taken up his abode in a hermit's cell. From this he refused to come and the *wazír* had to content himself with the treatment of one of his pupils.

On the death of Ṭughril 'Amíd-ul-Mulk continued to act as *wazír* to Alp Arslán, his successor. When that monarch wished to ally himself by marriage with the Khwárazmsháh, it was 'Amíd-ul-Mulk that he sent to negotiate the match. In his absence his enemies spread the report that he had asked the shah for the hand of his daughter for himself. Alp Arslán believed the report and deposed him from office. In his place he appointed Niẓám-ul-Mulk. 'Amíd-ul-Mulk saved his life for the moment by self-castration, but on his return from Khiva he was imprisoned and soon after murdered. His body was cut up into pieces, so that it was said that his testicles were buried in Khwárazm, his blood was shed at Merv, his body was interred at Kundur, his skull and his brain at Nishapur, and his scrotum, stuffed with straw and sent as a trophy to Niẓám-ul-Mulk, was buried at Kerman.[1]

1 Ibn Khallikán, vol. III, p. 294.

In addition to this claim to fame Niẓám-ul-Mulk is well known to English readers because he is said to have been one of the Three Friends (the others being the poet Omar Khayyam and the chief of the assassins, Ḥasan-i-Ṣabbáh), who made a pact of friendship and mutual support. Actually, as Professor Browne has shown, it was probably 'Amíd-ul-Mulk and not Niẓám-ul-Mulk, who was the fellow-student of the Old Man of the Sea. In the college which Niẓám-ul-Mulk founded in Baghdad he left a more tangible and less debatable memorial than the stories which have been weaved around his name. His college lay on the eastern side of the Tigris, three or four miles below the old Khuld Palace. It formed no part of the medical school, however, and was purely concerned with the teaching of Sháfi'ite Law. Niẓám-ul-Mulk also founded colleges at Ispahan and Nishapur to which were attached libraries containing scientific works.[1]

Hospital building was not altogether neglected in this age. A little further east and on the other side of the main road was another college, called the Baháíyya College, also concerned with the teaching of the Law. Beyond this was the Báb-ul-Ázaj or Gate of the Gallery which led to the Tutushí Market. Here stood the Tutushí Hospital. Both hospital and market were built by Khamártagín, a man who had originally been a slave of Táj-ul-Doula Tutush, one of the sons of Alp Arslán. The hospital must have been built some time just prior to 1114, for in that year Khamártagín died. A century later Yáqút states that the buildings were in a good state of repair.[2]

About this time died the last of the great family of Bukht Yishú's, Abú Sa'íd 'Ubayd-Ulláh bin Jibrá'íl, a great-great-grandson of the famous Bukht Yishú' II. Strangely enough, it is a work from his pen, the last of the line, which must represent the writings of the whole family. Of all that the other members of the family wrote—and all apparently composed one or more

1 Those interested in fuller details of the Baghdad Niẓámiyya may consult *La Madrasa Niẓamiyya* of Asad Talas (Paris, 1939).

2 Yáqút, *Mu'jam-ul-Buldán*, vol. 1, p. 826.

books—nothing has survived with the possible exception of a treatise on the eye by his father. Fortunately a few manuscript relics from the hand of 'Ubayd-Ulláh exist of which the text of one, though not a translation, has been published.[1]

'Ubayd Ullah was a contemporary and friend of Ibn Buṭlán. He lived for the greater part of his life in the town of Mayáfáriqín, near the modern Diarbekr. He was a convinced Christian, showing how nobly the Bukht Yishú's kept the Faith for three centuries, and was, as his Arabic biographer says 'excellent in the medical profession, renowned for his prominent activity in it, perfect in its principles and branches, and distinguished above all the nobles attached to this profession'. Apparently he never entered the service of the caliph and he died in A.D. 1058 honoured if not distinguished.[2]

According to the biographers his written works are many. He wrote a description of the various kinds of milk, a panegyric on his profession, and a work on eugenics which he called 'On the Right Way to preserve Descent', a book on Natural History, and several open letters on medical subjects. All these are lost except two. His work on natural history, called 'On the Nature, the Properties and the Utility of the Organs of Animals', composed for the Prince Naṣír-ul-Doula, a governor of Damascus, survives in a copy now in Paris. It is an interesting manuscript because it is illustrated.[3] Of his other surviving work there are several manuscripts. This is entitled *Al-Rauẓat-ul-Ṭibb* or 'The Medical Garden' and is apparently an abbreviation of his longer work entitled *Taẕkirat-ul-Ḥáẓir wa Zád-ul-Musáfir* or 'Memorial of the Resident and Provision of the Traveller'. Brockelmann claims to have discovered yet another of his works at Leyden and states that it is a treatise called 'On Love as a Disease'.

The 'Medical Garden' is an interesting little book. A glance at the headings of the chapters shows at once that the work is

1 P. Paul Sbath, *Ar-Raoudat at-Tibbiyya*. Cairo, 1927.

2 *I.A.U.* vol. 1, p. 148.

3 *Bibl. Nat.* no. 1077, ancien fond.

more metaphysical than medical. Physiology, represented by chapters on the temperaments, sleep, the pulse and vision, occupies a very small space. Pure medicine even less. The thoughts expressed are purely Greek, though the language of the book is Arabic. It is very evident that the author had not studied the Greek texts first-hand and that he had made use of Arabic translations of the philosophers and their Greek commentators. In other words, Arab love of speculation and Greek learning were still standing in the way of practical medical research.

A minor but interesting point is the twenty-first chapter 'On Love', for here he quotes a work by his own father, which he calls *Al-Káfí* or 'The Sufficiency', which according to Ibn abí Uṣaybi'a was a large treatise in five volumes. The original is lost; all that has survived of this great work of Jibrá'íl is the little paragraph quoted here where he says that Love is a corruption caused by the influence of the senses, especially the sight, on the rational soul which is subdued to the morbid passion like a great king when he becomes an instrument in the hands of a vile slave.

Contemporary with 'Ubayd-Ulláh was another famous physician named Ibn abí Ṣádiq, whom I have just mentioned in connection with the *wazír* 'Amíd-ul-Mulk. He was for a time a pupil of Avicenna. In turn he won great fame as a clinician and as a writer, but chiefly as an anatomist. Some of his anatomical writings have survived. His most famous work is a commentary on the *Manáfi'-ul-A'ẓa'* of Galen which he finished in the year 1066 and which was studied as a text-book of anatomy for many years after.[1]

To Ibn abí Ṣádiq in his old age came a young man of Jurjan, who sought to learn from him the methods of the great Avicenna. This was a certain Isma'íl bin Ḥasan bin Muḥammad bin Maḥmúd bin Aḥmad al-Ḥusayní, whose *kunya* was Abú Ibráhím and whose *laqab* was Sharaf-ul-Dín or Zayn-ul-Dín. His is a name almost unknown in Europe; his works did not reach the medieval schoolmen. In consequence he has no latinized name. The

1 *I.A.U.* vol. II, p. 22.

Persians themselves refer to him as al-Jurjání or as Sayyid Isma'íl or occasionally as Zayn-ul-Dín. Whenever I wish to make mention of him, I shall call him al-Jurjání.

The date of his birth is unknown. From the fact that he was a pupil of Ibn abí Ṣádiq, who died between 1066 and 1077, it is clear that al-Jurjání was born about the middle of the eleventh century. This century was marked by the general decline of medicine, the rise of philosophy, and the development of a vernacular medical literature. Until the days of al-Jurjání the vastly greater part of all scientific writing was in Arabic, even by Persian, Christian and Jewish authors. It is true that there are notable exceptions. By the dawn of the twelfth century the waning political power of the caliphs of Baghdad and the rising power of the petty kingdoms of Persia were reflected in a change of mind towards things Arab, and more especially towards the Arabic language. Al-Jurjání was the first physician of the highest class to shake off these traditional shackles and write all his scientific works in his own tongue.

In spite of his great importance in the history of the development of medicine in Persia extremely little is known about his personal career. No anecdotes surround his life as they do the lives of other prominent physicians. Ibn abí Uṣaybi'a devotes only a few lines to him. He was, he says, in the service of the Sulṭán 'Alá'-ul-Dín Muḥammad Kh̲wárazmsh̲áh. In this he makes a mistake, for Sulṭán 'Alá'-ul-Dín was the fifth of the line of the House of Anúsh̲tigín, and it is certain from other evidence that it was in the time of Quṭb-ul-Dín, the first of the line, that al-Jurjání became court physician. It was more probably in the court of 'Alá'-ul-Doula Atsiz, son of Quṭb-ul-Dín, that al-Jurjání took service.

Unlike most of the great physicians of those times he did not travel much during his youth. Yet he found opportunity to study in 'Iráq-i-'Ajam and in Fars, as well as in his own Jurjan. He was not therefore quite unknown when in the year 1110 he reached the court of the Kh̲wárazmsh̲áh and offered him his services. The biographers add no further details about his life and are contented with stating that he died at Merv in the year 1136 or 1140.[1]

Al-Jurjání wrote five books of which by far the most important is the *Zakhíra-i-Khwárazmsháhí* or 'Thesaurus of the Shah of Khwárazm'. The importance of this work lies not merely in its contents, which are themselves a masterful, concise and easily understood exposition of the whole system of medicine as it was taught in his day, but rather in the language in which it is written. Al-Jurjání did for Persian science what the Bible did for English prose. By this great encyclopaedia of medicine he standardized medical technical terms. The phrases which he borrowed from the Arabic text-books of Rhazes and Avicenna, became thereafter incorporated in the scientific language of the Persians for the use of later writers. After Rhazes and Avicenna this work became the most consulted and the most frequently quoted of all the text-books of medicine which the Arabian school produced. The rapidity with which it gained favour almost rivals that of the *Canon*. For al-Niẓámí, writing only 20 years after the death of al-Jurjání, classes the *Thesaurus* with the sixteen treatises of Galen, the *Continens* of Rhazes, the *Liber Regius* of Haly Abbas, the *Ṣad Báb* of Abú Sahl al-Masíḥí and the *Canon* of Avicenna as one of the standard works which the student of medicine should read in order to complete his education.[2]

The *Thesaurus* is a large book, smaller than the *Continens*, of course, but about the same size as the *Canon* of Avicenna. It is divided into nine books. The contents of each book have been briefly analysed by Professor Browne in his *Arabian Medicine* and by Fonahn in his *Zur Quellenkunde der persischen Medizin*. The first book is devoted to physiology and anatomy. The second book treats of general pathology and returns to discuss the physiology of infancy. The third book deals with treatment in the broadest sense of the word. It contains an interesting chapter on alcohol in which he gives suggestions as to the manner of conducting a

1 *I.A.U.* vol. II, p. 31.

2 *Chahár Maqála*, vol. IV, p. 32.

successful wine party. He warns the host against having pictures in the room, because 'the sight of these, when in a state of drunkenness, renders the mouth bitter'.

The fourth book is devoted to the importance of diagnosis in general. The fifth book deals with fevers, the sixth with medical diseases. In these two books are to be found an enormous number of interesting observations and several clinical cases which he himself saw and treated. In his chapter on 'Diseases of the Throat' he is the first to mention, so far as I am aware, the connection between exophthalmos and goitre, a sign which Parry rediscovered in 1825.[1]

The seventh book deals with various surgical conditions, with the exception of obstetrics which had already been discussed in the sixth book under the heading of diseases of the pelvis. This book concludes by two most excellent chapters on fractures, dislocations, and bone-setting. The detail with which this subject is here treated and the enormous number of technical terms which this speciality employs would alone be sufficient to show, even were other evidence wanting, that orthopaedics was a well-developed branch of Arab surgery.

The ninth book is a short one and deals with poisons, animal, vegetable and mineral, and their antidotes. The work concludes with three appendices. The first is the author's apology for his delay in completing the work, the second is his apology for its defects, and the third is his defence of all those physicians who died of the diseases which they had been treating in others.

These nine books completed the *Thesaurus*. Al-Jurjání himself states that it was his original intention to omit any special chapters on drugs. A sense of incompleteness, however, prompted him to add three more chapters. This postscript he dignified with the name of the tenth book. The first chapter he calls the 'Uses of the Parts of Animals' and is a forerunner of the lengthier treatises on natural history, as exemplified by the *Nuzhat-ul-Qulúb* of al-Qazvíní. The second chapter classifies drugs according

1 *Thesaurus*, bk. vi, 6.

to the part of the body upon which they act. The third chapter is perhaps the most interesting of the three and deals with compound drugs. It includes descriptions of the methods of preparing the elaborate prescriptions which were in use in his day, a discourse on ancient Greek measures, and a page of explanation of some of the difficult terms which were commonly employed in medicine.

In style the *Thesaurus* falls between the *Canon* and the *Continens*. It is not without plenty of physiology and pathology, scattered throughout every book. It is also enlivened by a considerable number of personal clinical notes. It must be admitted that the *Canon* is very dull reading. The *Thesaurus* never is. It is surprising that it never became popular in Europe. It was translated into Hebrew. An incomplete copy of this translation exists in Paris.[1] The catalogue claims that it is the only known Persian work to be translated from Persian into Hebrew. It was also translated into Urdu and still circulates among the old-fashioned *ḥakíms* of India. The tenth book was translated into Turkish by Abu ul-Faẓal al-Daftarí in 1574. Finally, Professor Browne called attention to its great merits in his Fitzpatrick Lectures[2] and Dr Abbas Naficy made it the foundation of his short work on Persian medicine.[3]

The other works of al-Jurjání, all of which are written in Persian, are only abbreviated editions of his *Thesaurus*. The *Ag͟hráẓ-ul-Ṭibb* or 'Aims of Medicine' was written at the command of Majd-ul-Dín al-Buk͟hárí, the *waẓír* of Atsiz K͟hwárazms͟háh. The *Yádgár-i-Ṭibb* or 'Medical Memoranda' and the *Muk͟htaṣar-i-K͟huffi-i-'Alá'í* are the names of two more of his works. The latter was composed for 'Alá'-ul-Doula Atsiz S͟háh and was written in two volumes, to be carried in either riding-boot: hence the name 'An Abridgement for the Boots of 'Alá''. His fifth work, according to Dr Naficy, is a treatise on public health which was written in 1101 before he went to live at K͟hwárazm.

1 *Bibl. Nat.* no. 1169.
2 Browne, *Arabian Medicine*, p. 110.
3 Naficy, *La Médecine en Perse.* Paris, 1933.

A few years after the death of al-Jurjání there was born at Ray Fa<u>kh</u>r-ul-Dín, who in middle-life also received the patronage of the court of <u>Kh</u>wárazm. Just as al-Jurjání is the glory of the Persian school of medicine, so Fa<u>kh</u>r-ul-Dín is the glory of the Persian school of philosophy. Islamic tradition holds that God will raise up one great theologian in each century to strengthen and defend Islam. In the fifth century after the flight al-<u>Gh</u>azálí Ḥujjat-ul-Islám fulfilled this office: in the sixth Abú 'Abd-Ulláh Muḥammad Fa<u>kh</u>r-ul-Dín.

With his merits as a philosopher and a theologian I have no concern. It is by virtue of the minor role that he played as a physician that his name must be recalled.

He was born in the year 1149. His father was a famous preacher and hence he himself was often called Ibn-ul-<u>Kh</u>áṭib or the Son of the Preacher. The professors under whom he studied philosophy and theology are named in his biography. Who taught him his medicine is not known. In middle life he left Ray and set out for Bukhara. On the way he was compelled to stop at the town of Sarakhs. Here he took the opportunity of visiting the physician 'Abd-ul-Raḥmán, usually known as al-Sara<u>kh</u>sí. In gratitude for his entertainment he wrote a commentary on the *Canon* of Avicenna, which he dedicated to al-Sara<u>kh</u>sí, filling the preface with his praise.[1]

His stay in Bukhara was not a success and he found himself poor and without resources. So he turned to the hospitable court of Quṭb-ul-Dín bin 'Alá'-ul-Dín bin Taka<u>sh</u>, the second of that name to reign at <u>Kh</u>wárazm. With traditional generosity the court received the stranger and gave him honour and all that he needed. Ultimately the <u>Kh</u>wárazm<u>sh</u>áh presented him with a house in Herat and here he practised the profession of a preacher, wrote his books, and begat his children. And here he died in the year 1209.

His children remained in Herat after his death and a daughter married 'Alá'-ul-Mulk, a minister of the <u>Kh</u>wárazm<u>sh</u>áh. In 1222

1 *I.A.U.* vol. II, p. 23; *Hist. Dynst.* vol. IX, p. 299.

the Mongols under <u>Ch</u>ing<u>h</u>íz <u>Kh</u>án attacked Herat. 'Alá'-ul-Mulk, seeing that the cause of his master was hopeless, deserted to the enemy and secured a guarantee of safety for the whole of the family of Fa<u>kh</u>r-ul-Dín. Herat fell and the Mongols kept their word. In the midst of the general massacre the children of Fa<u>kh</u>r-ul-Dín were spared.

The greater part of the literary work of Fa<u>kh</u>r-ul-Dín is, of course, theological. He did, however, write half a dozen works on purely medical subjects. One of these, called the *Ḥifaẓ-ul-Saḥḥat* or 'Preservation of Health', has been summarized and partly translated by Professor Nicholson.[1] Whether it is to be accepted as a genuine work of Fa<u>kh</u>r-ul-Dín, I am doubtful, for Ibn abi Uṣaybi'a does not include it in his list of his works. Besides this book he wrote another on the pulse, the Commentary on the *Canon* which I have already mentioned, a manual of anatomy, and an epitome of medicine. The last is written in Persian, the others in Arabic. Finally, he also began, but did not finish a large text-book of medicine, which he called *al-Jámi'-ul-Kabír* or *al-Ṭibb-ul-Kabír*, that is, 'The Great Collection' or 'The Great Medicine'.

His general attitude towards his own achievements is summed up in a quatrain that he composed at the end of his life.

> Never was I without knowledge;
> Few were the mysteries that passed my comprehension.
> Now have I lived to a ripe old age
> And now have I learnt that I know nothing.

In spite of the teaching of such eminent theologians as Fa<u>kh</u>r-ul-Dín, and of the complete predominance in all walks of life of the followers of the faith of Islam and in spite of numerous conversions from Christianity to Mohammedanism the greatest and most learned physicians of these times continued to be Christians. In the medical school of Baghdad the Christians had their own college to the lectures of which members of other faiths

---

1 *Jour. Roy. Asiatic Soc.* (1899), p. 424.

were not admitted. One of the greatest of the teachers in this college was Abú ul-Faraj ʻAbd-Ulláh bin ul-Ṭayyib, a Nestorian priest and secretary to the primate of Baghdad. He was well versed in theology, philosophy and medicine, and wrote a prodigious number of books. Most of these were commentaries. Avicenna was well acquainted with him and valued him more as a physician than as a philosopher, as might be expected when a Moslem criticizes a Christian. Ibn Buṭlán, his most famous pupil, states that it was over-study which brought about his death, which occurred in Baghdad in the year 1043.[1]

Ibn Buṭlán, as Abú ul-Ḥasan al-Mukhtár bin ul-Ḥasan bin ʻAbdún is usually called, was also a Christian of Baghdad. After receiving his education under Abú-ul-Faraj he began a friendly, if critical, correspondence with the famous physician of Cairo, ʻAlí bin Riẓván. After a few years Ibn Buṭlán left Baghdad and in the year 1049 had the pleasure of reaching Cairo and meeting him face to face. Though he was impressed by his learning, he was repelled by his ugliness and referred to him in his *Waqʻát-ul-Aṭibba* or 'Battle of the Physicians' as the Devil's Crocodile. He even wrote the following scurrilous verse of him:

> When his face appeared to the midwives
> They recoiled in perplexity;
> And said, keeping their words to themselves:
> 'Alas, had we only left him in the uterus!'

ʻAlí bin Riẓván answered his vulgarity with an equally rude and discourteous reply, and a coldness sprang up between the two. After staying only three years in Egypt Ibn Buṭlán moved on to Constantinople and from there fled to Antioch at the time of the great plague, in which so many learned men lost their lives. Here at the very end of his life he was asked to construct a new hospital and, while engaged on that task, he wrote a book on medicine, fragments of which have been preserved by Ibn abí Uṣaybiʻa. His theme in this book was the change in the methods

1 *I.A.U.* vol. II, p. 141; *Hist. Dynst.* vol. IX, p. 233.

of treatment which he had seen gaining popularity within his own lifetime. Thus, he says that Sa'íd bin Bishr bin 'Abdus of Baghdad replaced the usual 'hot' electuaries in the pharmacopoeia of the great hospital of Baghdad by diet, venesection, barley water and infusion of seeds and 'this treatment worked miracles'. He also had a new method of treating paralysis which was very successful.

Finally, wearied with travel and overwork, having quarrelled with everybody he met, Ibn Buṭlán died in a monastery at Antioch in the year 1063. A monk of that city said that even inanimate objects showed their dislike for him and that a lamp hanging over the spot where he was wont to say his prayers, would never burn, no matter how many times it was lit.[1]

Ibn Buṭlán was the author of numerous works on medical subjects, of which the manuscripts of several have survived. Five of the treatises in the medico-philosophical controversy in which he engaged with 'Alí bin Riẓván, have recently been published in Cairo together with critical notes and a translation into English.[2] His most famous work is the *Taqwím-ul-Saḥḥat* or 'Calendar of Health'. It was printed in Strasbourg in 1531 under the title of *Tacuini Sanitatis Eluchasem Elimithar medici de Baldath*. This work, although not remarkable for its contents, deserves a notice for the novelty of its form and arrangement. Instead of consisting of straightforward descriptions of diseases, as is found in most medical works, it is written in the form of a series of parallel tables, common enough nowadays, but new in those times. The work treats of foods and drugs and other matters which affect health, such as exercise, baths and music. The nature, the effects, the indications and so forth of each are set out in tabular form.

This method of writing a text-book was copied in the *Taqwím-ul-Buldán* or 'Calendar of Cities' by Abu ul-Faydá, the geographist, and by Ibn Jazlá, the physician, in his *Taqwím-ul-Abdán*, or

1 *I.A.U.* vol. I, pp. 227 et seq.; al-Qifṭí, p. 315. See also Meyerhof, *Med. Phil. Cont.* pp. 59 et seqq.

2 Meyerhof and Schacht, 'Une controverse médico-philosophique au Caire.' *Bull. Inst. Egypt*, no. XIX, 1937, and *Faculty of Arts Publication*, no. 13.

'Calendar of Bodies'. Ibn Jazlá, whose name was Abú ul-Ḥasan Yaḥyá bin 'Ísá bin 'Alí was also a citizen of Baghdad and was slightly younger than Ibn Buṭlán. He made his medical studies at Baghdad under Sa'íd bin Hibat Ulláh, and then went on to study philosophy under a Mussulman. In this school he was so impressed with the arguments of his master that he forsook Christianity for Islam and wrote an apologia for his action in an open letter addressed to a Christian priest of the city.

Ibn Jazlá was a man of means. His intellectual powers, his social standing, and above all his skill in handwriting and his new-found faith fitted him for the post of secretary to the chief justice of the Caliph al-Muqtadí. Although holding a political office he did not altogether give up medicine, but continued to see patients, although he now gave his services without accepting any fee. Among the many medical works which he composed, two are of primary importance. One is the *Taqwím-ul-Abdán*, to which I have already referred, which was, like its prototype, translated into Latin at Strasbourg and given the title of *Tacuini Egritudinum et Morborum Buhv Hylyha byn Gezla autore.* The material of the *Taqwím* of Ibn Jazlá is superior to that of Ibn Buṭlán. Here are discussed fevers, diseases of the skin and questions of prognosis, as well as disease *capite ad calcem.* It is interesting to notice that in discussing the diseases of women he takes a view on the subject of birth-control contrary to the majority of Persian and Arab writers.

His other important work is the *Minháj-ul-Bayán fí má yast'amalahu ul-Insán* or 'The Detailed Description of all that Man uses'. This is a treatise in alphabetical form of remedies and foods, simple and compound. It was the source of inspiration of Ibn Bayṭár's great work three centuries later and formed the basis upon which most of the later Persian pharmacologists built.

A third and far less important work on foods and simples was translated into Latin by Jambolinus.

According to Abú ul-Faraj and to the author of the *Kitáb-ul-Ḥukamá*, Ibn Jazlá died in A.D. 1080, according to Ḥájjí Khalífa and Ibn Khallikán he died in 1099. This later date is the more likely, for many of his written works are dedicated to the Caliph al-Muqtadí, who did not ascend the throne until 1075.

The Seljúq rule over Baghdad, thus peaceably established, lasted from 1055 to 1180. Ṭughril Bég, the founder of their prosperity, was succeeded by his son, Alp Arslán, who extended the spiritual dominion of the caliph and gave to Baghdad a security which it had long forgotten how to enjoy. With this came an encouragement of the arts of commerce, peace and learning. Alp Arslán and al-Qá'im, the caliph, died about the same time. The former was succeeded by Maliksháh, the latter by al-Muqtadí. Under the beneficent rule of Maliksháh the empire remained at peace. Successful in his frontier wars, he laboured also to spread the benefits of civilization. He dug canals, built bridges and constructed great caravanserais. His daughter he married to the reigning caliph and a second daughter after his death married the caliph's son, who succeeded to the throne under the name of al-Mustaẓhir. The death of Maliksháh was sudden. Taken ill while out hunting, after eating too freely of antelope's flesh, he was bled. His medical advisers did not consider that they had removed enough blood and hurried him back to Baghdad for a second operation. He died on the following day, 18 November 1092. Other writers have ascribed his death to a prick from a poisoned tooth-pick.

The end of his reign saw once again the clash between Western and Eastern civilizations. In 1099 the Crusaders captured Jerusalem and an attempt was launched to attack Baghdad. In the realm of medicine the position is now the reverse of what had formerly been the case. Western physicians could now teach nothing to their Eastern colleagues. Among the chronicles of these times have been preserved the memoirs of a Saracen *amír*, named Usáma ibn Munqiz. In these memoirs are several stories of Arab and Frank medical practice. Among them he relates that a certain Frank governor requested his uncle for the loan of a doctor. He therefore sent a Christian physician named Ṣábit.

He returned after a very few days and told the Arabs what he had seen of Frank medicine. He had been introduced to two patients, one a man with an abscess of the leg and the other a woman with consumption. The former he treated with poultices, the latter with a suitable diet and drugs. Both cases were making good progress until a Frank doctor arrived. He denounced Ṣábit's treatment as useless in both cases. Of the man he asked whether he would prefer to live with one leg or to die with two and, when the man replied that living with one was decidedly preferable, he called up a servant and bade him hew off the diseased leg. The servant so damaged the leg in the operation that shortly after the man expired. The case of the woman the Frank doctor diagnosed as one of possession by devils and bade the attendants carve a cross in her scalp and rub the wound with salt. As a result of this treatment the woman died. 'So after this', said Ṣábit, 'I asked if my services were any longer required and, being told that they were not, I returned home, having learnt of their medical practice what had hitherto been unknown to me.'[1]

A similar contrast between the learning of the Arabs and the proud ignorance of the European doctors is well portrayed by Sir Walter Scott in *The Talisman*. Here a physician whom he names Adonbec el-Hakim is introduced into the camp of King Richard Cœur de Lion. His imaginary conversation with the king, with the archbishop of Tyre, and with other noblemen, show very accurately the difference of level between Arab and European learning in those days.

Al-Mustaẓhir was succeeded in the caliphate by his son, al-Mustarshid, who made a fresh bid for temporal power. Indeed, he was very near success when he attacked the Seljúq Sulṭán Mas'úd near Hamadan. But there he was defeated and soon after murdered in his tent. Had he held his hand, as Muir remarks, from the temptation to arms (for him a dangerous anachronism), he might have built up the caliphate by the peaceful arts he was better fitted to employ.

1 Quoted in Browne's *Arabian Medicine*, p. 69.

His successor reigned only one year and continued to struggle against the Seljúqs. But defeat and an assassin's dagger put a stop to his scheme. Al-Muqtafí, his successor, had better fortune and reigned for 25 years. He was in many respects the best of the later caliphs. He possessed great abilities, though scarcely great virtues. During the first two-thirds of his reign he sowed in silence, during the last third he reaped in triumph. For he drove the Seljúq sultans away from Baghdad, and while the advancing Crusaders kept all the petty princes in fear for their own independency, he raised the caliphate once more to a power that could rule itself. He died in 1160 in the sixty-fifth year of his life.

The reign of his son al-Mustanjid, who succeeded him, was peaceful. The sword that he wielded was directed rather against those who disturbed the peace at home than against external enemies of the state. To one who offered him 2000 gold dinars for the liberation of a criminal he replied that he could not accede to his request but that he would willingly give him 10,000 gold coins if he would deliver up to justice a second similar malefactor.

After only 11 years of reign he perished at the hands of one of his own confidential servants Ibn Ṣafiya abú Gh̲álib ibn Ṣafiya the Christian, who was both his personal physician and his secretary. In the court of al-Mustanjid there had been considerable rivalry between the followers of Sh̲araf-ul-Dín the *wazír* and those of another nobleman named Quṭb-ul-Dín Qáímáz. The caliph happening to fall ill, the *wazír* used his influence over the sick man to persuade him to commit Quṭb-ul-Dín to prison. Ibn Ṣafiya the physician was a personal friend of Quṭb-ul-Dín and therefore warned him of the order which the sick caliph had just issued. Quṭb-ul-Dín went into hiding. Fortunately for him the caliph grew worse and the sentence of imprisonment was forgotten. In the meantime Ibn Ṣafiya had determined that Quṭb-ul-Dín should be revenged to the full. He had the hot Turkish bath, which the caliph was accustomed to frequent, heated to the greatest heat that could be obtained. The caliph was wont to go to the bath alone. That day Ibn Ṣafiya accompanied him and shut and fastened the door from the outside. An hour later when the door was opened, the unfortunate caliph was found lying dead upon the floor. Quṭb-ul-Dín and his followers, assuming an air of grief, approached al-Mustaẓí, a son of the late caliph, and begged him to accept the vacant throne. In justice to Ibn Ṣafiya it should be added that the version which Bar Hebraeus gives of the story makes Quṭb-ul-Dín himself and not Ibn Ṣafiya the villain of the piece.[1]

Al-Mustaẓí, therefore, took up the vacant caliphate and, though fully aware of the part which Ibn Ṣafiya had played in the death of his father, for the time being retained him as his personal physician. At length, finding his position more secure, he determined to punish the murderers of his father. Ibn Ṣafiya in his capacity as secretary soon became acquainted with the caliph's plans and again gave warning to Quṭb-ul-Dín. But the new caliph was a match for him. He was summoned late one night and bidden prepare a deadly poison for one of the royal enemies. Unlike Ḥunayn of old, the physician forgot his oath and his faith and returned next day with a draught which he guaranteed would prove fatal to anyone within an hour. Instead of the expected reward and robe of honour he received from the caliph the order to drink at once the draught himself. His supplications were in vain. He was given the choice of death by his own poison or by execution with the sword. He chose to die by his own hand. After drinking off the cup he just had time to make his way to Quṭb-ul-Dín to warn him of what had happened and to make known to him that through excess of zeal in his friendship he was thus condemned to die. Within an hour, as he had boasted, the poison worked. 'It is not fitting', wrote Ibn Tilmíẕ of him, 'for a physician to enter into the secrets of kings. Nor should he go beyond barley water, infusions and syrups. For verily when he exceeded these, he perished.'

It is with al-Náṣir, who reigned from A.D. 1180 to 1225, that the lamp of the fortunes of the 'Abbásid caliphs burned

1 *I.A.U.* vol. I, p. 258; *Hist. Dynst.* vol. IX, p. 254.

bright, flickered, and expired, as Muir so aptly describes it. During the early part of his reign he had as his chief physician a Christian named Abú ul-Khayr bin abí il-Baqa, often referred to as Ibn ul-'Aṭṭár or more simply as al-Masíḥí or 'The Christian'. His services are said to have been much sought after by the wives and concubines of the caliph. He had a son named Abú 'Alí, who was also a distinguished physician and for a time the director of the 'Azudí Hospital. On the death of his father in 1211 the young man found himself possessed of considerable wealth. It proved his ruin, for he abandoned medicine in favour of a life devoted to women, wine, and song. The scandal of his behaviour reached such a pitch that he was arrested together with two of his ladyloves. The women were condemned to imprisonment; Abú 'Alí saved himself by paying a fine of 6000 dinars.

It was fortunate that al-Masíḥí did not live to see the downfall of his son, for in his old age he had misfortunes enough of his own. It happened that the caliph showed symptoms of stone. Try as he might, al-Masíḥí could not disperse the stone or give relief to the caliph, whose symptoms grew more and more painful every day. At length al-Masíḥí announced that an operation was the only means of cure and suggested that Ibn 'Akásha, a surgeon who lived in the Karakh quarter of Baghdad, should be called. The caliph had him summoned at once. Ibn 'Akásha heard the caliph's story, but requested to be allowed to summon his colleagues for further consultation before undertaking any operation. His request was allowed and he summoned to the palace a hitherto unknown physician, called Abú Naṣr, who was also a Christian. Again the caliph recounted in detail all his symptoms and all the treatment which he had received. At the finish Abú Naṣr, as medical etiquette demanded, pronounced that the diagnosis and treatment already prescribed were perfectly correct. The caliph was infuriated at this answer and shouted at Abu Naṣr that he had been summoned to the palace not to justify his colleagues, but to point out their errors

Abu Naṣr then changed his manner of speech and so pleased the caliph that he was appointed physician in charge of the case. The unfortunate al-Masíḥí was accordingly banished from the court and in fact never regained the royal favour. Abu Naṣr then expressed himself against immediate operation and suggested a fresh trial of medical treatment. His star was in the ascendant, for on the third day after he had assumed charge the caliph passed the stone which had caused all the trouble. He was overcome with joy. He bade Abu Naṣr take as his fee as much gold as he could carry away from the treasury, bade all members of the court make presents to him, and promoted him to the highest medical post in the kingdom, left vacant by the unfortunate al-Masíḥí. He was still physician-in-chief when the caliph died.

Abú Naṣr is said to have written a book on medicine in the form of question and answer, which he called *Kitáb-ul-Iqtiẓáb* or 'The Book of Amputation'. A book of the same name was written by al-Masíḥí, who had as a brother a well-known physician named Abú ul-Ḥusayn Sa'd bin ul-Mu'ammul. This Abú ul-Ḥusayn, whose *kunya* appears in some writers as Abú ul-Ḥasan, was also a personal physician to the Caliph al-Náṣir. The two brothers were Christians and were usually known as Ibn al-Masíḥí or 'The Sons of the Christian'. For two things Abú ul-Ḥusayn was famous. One was his overweening pride which earned for him the nickname of 'The Fool'. The other was his book on medicine in which he incorporated a chapter on trees which was looked upon as a very novel theme. He died in A.D. 1194.

The object of al-Náṣir's policy was to crush the Seljúq power which was already weakened by quarrels among members of the family, and to build up anew on the ruins of that house the old traditions of the caliphate. At his instigation the Shah of Khwárazm attacked the Seljúq forces and defeated them, leaving Ṭughril, the last of the race, dead upon the field. The Khwárazm-sháh now became recognized as the supreme Islamic power. The caliph having used him for his own ends now foolishly picked a quarrel with him. In reply the shah marched upon Baghdad. The caliph in despair appealed to the Mongol chief, Chinghíz Khán sometimes written Janghíz Khán), who, setting in motion his pagan hordes, left central Asia for the rich towns of Persia. The Khwárazmsháh was put to flight and died in exile. But Chinghíz Khán did not return to his steppes. Al-Náṣir, indeed, was well satisfied. He held uninterrupted possession of a large empire. Peace reigned at Baghdad; learning flourished; schools and libraries were patronized; refuges for the poor and other works of public interest were encouraged. He could not foresee the terrible result of the movement that he had thus set on foot.

In his later days the caliph became afflicted with a failing vision and a failing memory. Much of the direction of affairs of State was left to his womenfolk, at times even the signing of official documents. In consequence a certain amount of disorder became apparent. It was said that those who now had the supreme direction were looking after their own interests rather than those of the empire and the caliphate. So patent did this at last become that Abú ul-Faraj bin Yaḥyá, also known as Amín-ul-Doula, the royal physician, stepped in and bade the *wazír* delay carrying out some of these orders on the grounds that the caliph was incapable of determining such matters. This considerably annoyed the little clique who had succeeded in getting the management of affairs into their own hands. They determined upon the murder of the physician who stood between them and their ends. One night they lay in ambush for him and as he left the house of the *wazír*, two military officers set upon him and murdered him.

There was no more opposition. The State drifted along. Al-Náṣir died and was succeeded by his son al-Ẓáhir and his grandson al-Mustanṣir. The former only ruled for a year. The latter in pathetic ignorance of the fate which was about to overwhelm all Baghdad, spent his 16 years of power in beautifying his city. Among his building efforts was a small hospital and a school of law which he built to rival the college which Niẓám-ul-Mulk, the *wazír* of the Seljúq monarchs, had founded nearly two centuries before. In al-Mustanṣir's day the caliph resided on the eastern side of the river in a large walled-in compound, known as the Ḥarím or 'Sanctuary'. The first building to be erected on this site was the palace of Ja'far the Barmecide, which he built on the riverside at some distance from the Baghdad of his days in order that he might indulge in his orgies without exciting either his father's wrath or the mob's indignation. On his death the caliph took possession. The Caliph al-Ma'mún enlarged the palace and added a polo ground. It continued to be the abode of distinguished people. On the return of the government from Sámarra it became the official residence of the caliphs. The Caliph al-Mu'taẓid built four more palaces close to Ja'far's palace, and it was probably he who surrounded the whole Sanctuary with a wall.

Here the caliphs were wont to live until their destruction. Ruler after ruler continued to adorn the Sanctuary. Al-Mustanṣir was the last to add any notable building. His hospital and school which he founded within the walls are usually known as the Mustanṣiriyya College. In its magnificence, its external appearance, its ornamentation and its luxurious furniture it is said to have surpassed anything that Baghdad had ever seen before. The foundation stone was laid by the caliph himself in the year A.D. 1227. The college lay up against the northern wall of the Sanctuary. On one side ran the river; its walls in fact are said to have been washed by the waters of the Tigris. Adjoining, but outside the walls of the Sanctuary, was the Wharf of the Needlemakers and the bridge of boats which connected the eastern with the western half of Baghdad. On the other side of the college was the Gate of the Willow Tree which, piercing the walls, allowed the populace to enter the Sanctuary.

The college was furnished with a great kitchen which provided food daily for all the students, with a large bath for the use of the inmates, and with a library in which were kept rare scientific books and where copying by students was allowed, pens and paper being supplied by the authorities. The hospital was provided with its own staff, special store chambers, and its own dispensary. In the great entrance hall of the college stood a clock (a Chest of Hours is the Arabic name), which announced the times of prayer and showed the passage of the hours.

The college was completed in 1234. Apparently it escaped destruction by Húlágú, for Ibn Baṭúṭa describes it in 1327 as being much frequented by law students. A few years later the Persian Mustaufí al-Qazvíní describes it as the most beautiful building of Baghdad in his day.[1] Ruins of the college still exist.

A comparison between the Mustanṣiriyya College and the Niẓámiyya enforces the conclusion that the conception of the former was much the wider and more elevated. Whereas Niẓám-ul-Mulk was concerned only with propagating the doctrines of one sect of Islam, al-Mustanṣir aimed at restoring the cultural heritage of the early caliphs. Niẓám-ul-Mulk planned a theological college, al-Mustanṣir a university. Niẓám-ul-Mulk demanded no intellectual test for admission to his foundation: a profession of the correct form of Islam was enough. Al-Mustanṣir set a very high standard. Admission was competitive. His college would take no more than 308 students of which only ten were accepted for medicine. In the eyes of al-Mustanṣir poverty was no bar. Lodging and food were to be gratuitous within the college. There was even a monthly payment of one gold dinar to poor students. Whether this charity was also found in the Niẓámiyya College, I am not sure. It is, however, quite evident that the conception of al-Mustanṣir was an enormous advance not only in the teaching of medicine, but also in education in general.

During all these years the Mongols had not ceased to gaze with envy at the rich prizes which the expedition of Chinghíz Khán had laid before their eyes. Húlágú had now succeeded to the headship of the race, and, after receiving a satisfactory answer from the astrologers who accompanied him, he marched on Baghdad. The impotent caliph could do nothing, and meeting with scarcely any resistance Húlágú entered Baghdad in A.D. 1258 and gave the city

1 *Nuzhat-ul-Qulúb*, p. 42.

over to be looted. As it was against the faith of the Mongols to shed royal blood, the caliph, now al-Musta'ṣim, was placed in a sack and trampled to death by horses. The valuable libraries were destroyed and the rare manuscripts, which the caliphs of old had spent so much time and money in amassing, were thrown into the Tigris so that for three days, so the chronicler says, the water of the river ran black, red and green from the ink of the illuminations. Another writer says that so many manuscripts were thrown into the river that it was possible to walk upon them from one bank to the other.

Thus came to an abrupt end the 'Abbásid caliphate and with it the only period of Arabian medicine which has any claim to the title of Arab. Greek medicine, as interpreted by the Arabs, now becomes completely Persian.

CHAPTER IX

ARABIAN MEDICINE IN THEORY

A PHYSICIAN should be of tender disposition and wise nature, excelling in acumen, this being a nimbleness of mind in forming correct views, that is to say, a rapid transition to the unknown from the known. And no physician can be of tender disposition if he fails to recognize the nobility of the human soul; nor of wise nature unless he is acquainted with Logic, nor can he excel in acumen unless he be strengthened by God's aid; and he who is not acute in conjecture will not arrive at a correct understanding of any ailment.[1]

In such words did Aḥmad ibn 'Umar ibn 'Alí of Samarqand, poetically named Niẓámí and 'Arúḍí, poet, courtier, astrologer, and in case of need physician, sum up in the twelfth century of the Christian era his ideal of a physician. And in truth the majority of the physicians of Islamic times came very near to this ideal. For never was there a time when the physician himself was more worthy of honour and trust.

The fall of Baghdad meant the end of a chapter. The caliphate and the centralizing influences, with all that they meant to medicine and science, came to an abrupt end. The effect upon Persian medicine, it is true, is not so great as was the effect upon it of the successful invasion of the Arabs and the founding of Baghdad. But it compels a pause; and, as it does indeed mark the end of an era, it is fitting to cast a glance backward and a glance forward upon medicine in Persia as a whole during Islamic times. For Persia did not suffer much change between A.D. 800 and 1800. Within a few years the barbarian Mongols were completely Islamized and Persianized.

The profession of a physician maintained the lofty standard which the early Greeks had set in the Achaemenian courts. As has already been pointed out, the first physicians of Islamic days were

1 *C̲hahár Maqála*, p. 76.

almost all Christians or Jews. This position was maintained throughout the days of the caliphate and with certain notable exceptions in independent Persia. The gradual disappearance of Christianity in the Middle East reduced the number of Christian physicians. The persecution of the Jews, though to a lesser degree, reduced the number of Jewish practitioners.

In the early days of the caliphate the influence of Jundí Sh̲ápúr was sufficient to ensure that all the leaders of medical thought should be Christians. The foundation of hospitals in Baghdad meant the entry of Moslems into the realm of medicine. Yet the caliphs continued to show a preference for Christian and Jewish physicians. This was reflected in the conduct of the court and lower classes. When Faẓal ibn Yaḥyá̲ the Barmecide asked who was the most skilful physician in Iraq, Khorasan, Syria, and Fars, at once came back the answer 'Paul, the Christian Patriarch in Shiraz'. The stories in the *Arabian Nights* show that, though he was often disliked and mocked, it was nearly always to a Jewish physician that the poor of Baghdad took their troubles.

Medical training in those days began very young. Ḥunayn, for example, came to Baghdad to make his studies when he was seventeen and by then he had already finished his medical training at Jundí Sh̲ápúr. Avicenna began his about his eleventh year. Rhazes was a notable exception. The same custom prevailed throughout the Islamic world. Maimonides, the Spanish Jew, began at the age of thirteen. Even as late as 60 years ago medical students were enrolled at the al-Azhar University in Cairo at the age of twelve and were transferred to the Kasr-ul-'Aini Hospital two or three years later.

In addition to the purely medical knowledge it was held desirable, though not essential, that the medical student should also have studied geometry in order that he might know the shapes of wounds, 'for round wounds heal with difficulty, polygonal with ease', astronomy so that he might know the lucky and the unlucky quarters of the moon, and music in order that he might appreciate the subtleties of the human pulse.

The young student began his purely medical studies by apprenticing himself to some senior practitioner. Those who had a close relation in practice usually made their studies under him; a father or an uncle made an excellent master. Others apprenticed themselves to anyone who was willing to take them. Some moved from teacher to teacher. Thus, Avicenna, in addition to his teachers in non-medical subjects, studied in turn under Abú Sahl, Abú Manṣúr al-Qamarí, and under a certain Kó<u>sh</u>yár. With this exception the method of learning the art of medicine differed in no respect from the methods by which the modern student graduates.

The most important part of the training was the clinical instruction in hospital. Haly Abbas writes:

And of those things which are incumbent upon the student of this Art are that he should constantly attend the hospitals and sick-houses; pay unremitting attention to the conditions and circumstances of their inmates, in company with the most acute professors of Medicine; and enquire frequently as to the state of the patients and the symptoms apparent in them, bearing in mind what he has read about these variations, and what they indicate of good and evil. If he does this, he will reach a high degree in this Art. Therefore it behoves him who desires to be an accomplished physician to follow closely these injunctions, to form his character in accordance with what we have mentioned therein, and not to neglect them. If he does this, his treatment of the sick will be successful; people will have confidence in him and be favourably disposed towards him, and he will win their affection and respect and a good reputation; nor will he lack profit and advantage from them. And God most high knoweth best.[1]

Those who wished to practise surgery were bidden also to attend at a hospital where well-known surgeons operated and to be constant in their reading and in their attendances at operations. The classes were not very large, I think. ‘Ammár bin ‘Alí of Mosul says that he was accompanied by only two or three students when he operated. But he was referring to private cases and possibly in hospital he had more onlookers.

1 *Liber Regius* of Haly Abbas, vol. 1, p. 2, quoted by Browne, *Arabian Medicine*, p. 56.

In the general hospitals the method of instruction was the same as is found to-day. Students attached themselves to a teacher and followed him round the wards in his daily visits. Ibn abí Uṣaybi'a says that he used first to assist in the treatment of In-patients and then 'go and look for Shaykh Raẓí-ul-Dín al-Raḥabí, to watch how he diagnosed his cases and to see his methods of treatment and the prescriptions which he would give to his patients. Then I used to discuss with him many of the cases and the best method of treating them'.[1] Rhazes apparently only used the more difficult cases for teaching purposes, for a contemporary of his states that it was his custom to call first upon the beginners to examine a patient. If they failed to diagnose the condition, he called upon a higher class and 'only if it had eluded the knowledge of all the disciples did it come to the attention of the Master'. Of Abú ul-Majd ibn abí il-Ḥakam, Ibn abi Uṣaybi'a says that he

> used to examine the patients at the hospital, take note of their condition and listen to their complaints in the presence of the nurses and porters, who were charged with looking after them. All methods of treatment and prescriptions which he gave were carried out to the letter. After finishing his ward round, he would pass on to a magnificently furnished hall to consult there various scientific works. For the Sultan had created a special endowment for this hospital so that it contained a large number of medical works, arranged in two book-cases, which graced the centre of the hall. There all the physicians and students gathered round him in order to discuss medical points. When he had asked questions of his pupils and had worked for about three hours in the wards and in the library, he would return to his home.[2]

Some physicians even held public courses in medicine, which were attended by anyone interested in the subject. Others apparently held private classes in their own houses, for Ibn abí Uṣaybi'a speaks of a certain al-Ḥasan, physician to al-Muqtadir, who 'was a physician at Baghdad, very learned in the medical science, and his house was a House of Medicine'. Alternatively this may be a reference to a private nursing home.[3]

1 *I.A.U.* vol. II, p. 243. 2 Ibid. p. 155. 3 Ibid. vol. I, p. 318.

Apparently the utmost freedom was allowed to the young students. They could question their teachers and even attempt to prove them wrong. Rhazes recalls in the opening section of his *Barr'-ul-Sá'at* that he was once heckled by a class, containing both qualified and unqualified men, because he had said that it was possible to disperse the *materies morbi* of certain diseases within an hour. To justify himself he was compelled to write a small treatise which he called 'The Cure within an Hour', wherein he enumerated those diseases which judicious treatment could drive out within that time.

The bedside teaching was supplemented by set lectures. Where no special school of medicine existed, these lectures were delivered in the local mosque. The seat of a student in the lecture theatre depended upon his progress, all who had reached the same stage being seated together. The system was not quite the same as that which prevails to-day. Part of a text-book or a written lecture was read out to the class by a 'Reading-out Physician'. The professor then answered any doubtful points and explained any difficulties that the class might raise. At the lectures of Ibn ul-Tilmíz̲ two skilled Arabic grammarians also assisted, whose duty it was to explain to the students the meaning of the scientific terms and to correct their pronunciation. Frequently the lectures were given during the night or late hours of the evening, especially during the summer and the month of Ramaẓán. Rhazes was often so tired that he would put his lantern into a niche and stand resting his book upon the wall beneath. When he fell asleep, the book would drop and wake him up. Famous lecturers attracted students from all over the empire. Abú ul-Faraj 'Abd-Ulláh bin al-Ṭabíb, a Christian and a scribe to the patriarch of Baghdad, who was also a physician on the staff of the 'Aẓudí Hospital, was one such. Avicenna said of him that his books upon medicine were faultless, but that the opposite was true of his works on logic and physics. The fame of his lectures upon Galen drew to Baghdad disciples from all parts of Persia.[1]

1 Ibn K̲h̲allikán, vol. III, p. 602.

The classes of Ibn ul-Tilmíz̲ used to average about fifty. In the case of Rhazes, so great was the demand for attendance at his lectures that the more distant students could not even hear what he said. Those near at hand passed on his words to an outer circle, who in turn passed them on to a circle yet more remote.[1]

Of the text-books of medicine which were most popular, the 'Aphorisms' of Hippocrates,[2] the 'Questions' of Ḥunayn, and the 'Guide' of Rhazes were looked upon as elementary and suitable for the first year of study. Abú Sahl Sa'íd ibn 'Abd-ul-'Azíz of Nishapur, also called al-Nílí, wrote a commentary on these three works and this was read by most young students. Professor Browne suggests that he was given this title from some connection with the indigo trade. But I think he is wrong in this deduction and that more probably he was a native of al-Níl, a town on the Euphrates between Baghdad and Kufa. Although a small town, it is said to have produced many famous men.[3] The next year's course included the 'Treasury' of Ṣ̈ábit ibn Qurra, the *Liber Almansoris* of Rhazes, and the 'Aims' of Sayyid Isma'íl al-Jurjání. To these were added the *Ḥidaya* or 'Direction' of Abu Bakr Ajwíní or else the *Kifáya* or 'Sufficiency' of Aḥmad ibn Faraj. This formidable list of works sufficed, and more than sufficed, for the greater number of students. Those who wished to study yet more deeply the philosophy and theory of disease were recommended to read during their leisure hours one or more of the following—the 'Sixteen Treatises' of Galen, the *Continens* of Rhazes, the *Liber Regius* of Haly Abbas, the 'Hundred Chapters' of Abú Sahl, the *Canon* of Avicenna, or the *Thesaurus* of Sayyid Isma'íl al-Jurjání. All these are gigantic works. Their cost alone would have made it impossible for the ordinary student to buy more than one or two. The *Continens* of Rhazes, although recommended, can scarcely ever have found a place in any practitioner's library. For within 50 years of the death of the author only two complete copies were known to exist. Of the

1 *I.A.U.* vol. 1, p. 239.
2 *C̲h̲ahár Maqála*, p. 78.
3 Ibn K̲h̲allikán, vol. 1, p. 449.

large text-books the *Canon* of Avicenna was by far the most popular and, judging from the number of quotations found in later writers and the number of manuscripts which have survived, the *Thesaurus* of al-Jurjání was second favourite. When the student had completed the study of any work, it was usual for his teacher to sign the book, an act which also gave him permission to teach to others its contents. This also served as a recommendation of the work itself, so that it was said that students and scholars avoided any manuscript which did not bear the impression of the signatures of many masters.

The question whether the student had to take some form of examination before beginning to practise is difficult to answer. Previous to the year 931 (at least, as far as Baghdad is concerned) it is clear that there was no such check upon anyone wishing to enter the profession, for in that year the Caliph al-Muqtadir learnt that the mistake of a private practitioner had resulted in the death of a subject. He therefore gave orders to the inspector-general Ibráhím Muḥammad ibn abí Baṭiḥá to prevent the practice of medicine by any person who had not been previously examined by Sinán bin Ṣ̈ábit bin Qurra. The caliph wrote out this order with his own hand, and after that, thanks to the powers thus given to him, Sinán only authorized those persons to practise medicine whom he had previously examined. In addition he suggested to each in which branch of medicine he ought to work. The total number of physicians examined in the first year exceeded 860 for Baghdad alone.[1]

The examinations were not, however, of a very severe nature. There may well have been a similar examination in Khiva. For Ibn ul-K͟hammár is said to have been commanded by K͟hwárazm-s͟háh to write a special treatise on the examination of doctors.[2] Two viva voce examinations are on record, although their similarity suggests a common origin. One is a tale told of Sinán when the Board of Examiners was first instituted. I borrow Professor Browne's translation from al-Qifṭí.[3]

1 *I.A.U.* vol. I, p. 222; al-Qifṭí, p. 191.
2 *I.A.U.* vol. I, p. 323. 3 Browne, *Arabian Medicine*, p. 40.

Amongst the practitioners who presented themselves before Sinán, was a dignified and well-dressed old man of imposing appearance. Sinán accordingly treated him with consideration and respect, and addressed to him various remarks upon the cases before him. When the other candidates had been dismissed, he said: 'I should like to hear from the Shaykh something which I may remember from him, and that he should mention who was his Teacher in the profession.' Thereupon the old gentleman laid a packet of money before Sinán and said: 'I cannot read or write well, nor have I read anything systematically, but I have a family which I maintain by my professional labours, which therefore, I beg you not to interrupt.' Sinán laughed and replied: 'On condition that you do not treat any patient with what you know nothing about and that you do not prescribe phlebotomy or any purgative drug save for simple ailments.' 'This,' said the old man, 'has been my practice all my life, nor have I ever ventured beyond oxymel and rose-water.' Next day, among those who presented themselves before Sinán was a well dressed young man of pleasing and intelligent appearance. 'With whom did you study?' enquired Sinán. 'With my father', answered the youth. 'And who is your father?' asked Sinán. 'The old gentleman who was with you yesterday', replied the other. 'A fine old gentleman', exclaimed Sinán: 'and do you follow his methods? Yes? Then see to it that you do not go beyond them.'

The examination system seems to have been enforced only during the lifetime of Sinán, for within a few years of his death there were again to be found many ignorant physicians in Baghdad, practising to the danger of the public. His son Ibráhím, who had become the chief physician of Baghdad, grew alarmed at the state of affairs and determined to reinstitute the test. It was his duty to act as chief examiner, but this task he deputed to Abu Sa'íd Yamání of Basra and bade him again put all doctors of the city through a test. The examination took six months to complete. The result was that 700 were allowed to continue to practise: the remainder, unfortunately an unspecified number, were forbidden.

If a popular story is authentic, after this revival the board continued to exist for the next 300 years. In these later days Ibn ul-Tilmíz̲, court physician to the Caliph al-Mustaẓí, occupied the presidential chair. The story, however, bears rather too close a resemblance to the anecdote I have just related for its evidence to carry much weight. It is said that once when all the practitioners of Baghdad had collected together at the house of the new chief to be examined by him, he saw among them a remarkable old man of an imposing appearance and a tranquil mean. Ibn ul-Tilmíẕ, wishing to show him honour, was deceived by his appearance. For this old man, although much experienced, had no scientific knowledge whatsoever on the subject which he claimed to have studied so profoundly. When his turn arrived, Ibn ul-Tilmíẕ said to him: 'Why, honourable Sir, do you take no part in the discussion, so that we may have the benefit of your learning?' To which the old man replied: 'I know well all the subjects about which you have been speaking, for my knowledge is yet deeper.' Ibn ul-Tilmíẕ then asked him who his teacher had been. To which he replied: 'At my age it is not fitting that I should be questioned about my teachers, but rather about the number of my pupils and about their distinctions. As for my teachers, they are all dead long ago.' To this the president of the board could but say: 'Honoured Sir, it has always been the custom to put such questions and there is no shame in replying to them. But, however that may be, let us pass on. Would you care to tell me what works on medicine you have read?'

In putting this question Ibn ul-Tilmíẕ wished indirectly to be able to judge the degree of knowledge to which the old man had attained. But he protested violently, saying: 'Allah, Allah, this is strange. Have we arrived at such a point that we are treated like children? A man such as I, and you demand what works I have read instead of asking what works on medicine I have written and what commentaries I have composed. Now therefore it is my duty to introduce myself to you.' Then the old man got up and sitting himself beside the president said in a low voice: 'Know, then, O my Master, that I am now an old man and that of the science of medicine I know nothing except a few expressions and some technical terms. But I have practised it all my life and, as

I have a family dependent upon me, I trust that you will not take away my means of existence and that you will not make me an object of derision before the world.'

Said Ibn ul-Tilmíz to him: 'So be it, but only on condition that you never give to your patients any remedy of whose actions you are ignorant and that you only prescribe bleeding and purging in diseases which are easy to recognize.' 'Yes, yes,' said the old man, 'that is what I have always done. I have never administered anything except oxymel and rose-water.' 'Then', said Ibn ul-Tilmíz in a loud voice so that he could be heard by all present: 'Excuse me, honoured Sir, I did not recognize you. But now that we have become acquainted to-day, continue your work. No one shall in future oppose you.' Seeing him thus honoured, several of the more ignorant examinees named him as the tutor under whom they had learned their medicine. Ibn ul-Tilmíz having accepted the old man felt also obliged to accept the claims of the younger.

Whether this board survived until the caliphate came to an end and whether any similar board was set up in Persia, I believe there is no evidence to prove or disprove. Dr Ahmed Issa Bey, in his *Histoire des Bimaristans*, quotes in full two diplomas which were given in Cairo at the beginning of the seventeenth century of our era, one to a phlebotomist and one to a surgeon. Though therefore the practice survived in Egypt, it does not follow that there was any formal initiation in Persia. Persia was only rarely under a single ruler; the capital of the country was frequently changed. Unless, therefore, each big city had its own examining board, it is improbable that the Persian student had to face any test before starting practice. There was certainly no such board in Ispahan in the days of the Sháh 'Abbás the Great, for Fryer,[1] who visited Ispahan in 1677, wrote that there was 'such a strange itch of Learning that before they are half-way instructed in one Book, they are desirous to be perfected in another; and before they have read Philosophy, Morality, or any other Science to qualify them, they leap into the Alcoran; for here are neither Public Professors

1 Fryer, *New Account*, p. 361; *Travels*, vol. III, p. 66.

to examine or Publick Acts to be kept, either in Divinity, Law, or Physick'. Fryer, however, is a poor authority, for we know from other sources that a licence of some sort was required from all doctors before they could practise. The granting or withholding of this rested with the *ḥakím-báshí*. Fr. Raphael du Mans estimated that in his days in Ispahan there were about 1500 physicians, 200 druggists, a few surgeons, and phlebotomists innumerable.[1] The population of the city was then something between three-quarters of a million and a million souls.

In addition to some form of qualifying test or central licensing there was another method of checking grossly ignorant practitioners. In Baghdad the caliph himself exercised a general control over all the faculty. For the most part he delegated his powers to his chief physician and to an official known as the *muḥtasib* or inspector-general. Both these offices formed part of the Persian Safavid system. Among the *muḥtasib's* duties was the administration of the Hippocratic Oath, which required physicians to swear that they would administer no poisonous draughts to their patients nor prepare any poison for them to use nor entrust poisons to any unauthorized persons: that they would not prescribe abortefacients for women or contraceptives for men: that they would avoid looking upon womenfolk within a sick household: and that they would never reveal to a third person anything said in confidence by a patient. Ḥunayn reminded the caliph of this oath when asked to prepare a deadly poison for one of his enemies. It was also the *muḥtasib's* duty to see that practitioners were possessed of such instruments as were necessary and suitable for the particular branch of medicine that they were practising. He could further, if he wished, examine them on the work of Ḥunayn called 'The Examination of the Doctors'.[2]

The majority of well-born students took up general medicine, aiming at becoming physician to a governor or a local grandee or even to the caliph or shah himself. The Safavid shahs retained

1 du Mans, *Éstat de la Perse*, pp. 175, 178.

2 Ibn al-Ukhuwwa, *Ma'álim al-Qurba*, ch. 45 (Gibb Memorial edition).

many physicians-in-ordinary and a great many extra-ordinary physicians. The chief physician was known as the *ḥakím-báshí*. To hold this office was a gamble, for on the death of the sovereign he not only suffered banishment but was also despoiled of his goods and might even lose his life. Anyone who failed to get one of these fairly lucrative appointments settled himself for preference where competition was least. Here he joined himself to an apothecary who would not only make up his medicines, but also act as a herald of his skill.

There was no formal specialization in the different branches of medicine, as there is to-day. But some approximated to a modern specialist by acquiring a proficiency in the treatment of certain diseases or in the use of certain drugs. Avicenna, for example, was held to be more proficient than most in his treatment of nervous diseases and hence a large number of psychological cases were brought to him. Abú ul-Barqát is said to have introduced the method of treatment by suggestion and may therefore be looked upon as another psychologist. Possibly the reason why Faẓal ibn Yaḥyá the Barmecide preferred Paul of Shiraz to Jibrá'íl, his family doctor, was because he was suffering from a skin disease and Paul had made a greater study of diseases of this type than had Jibrá'íl. 'Imád-ul-Dín in later times popularized the use of sarsaparilla and gained a great reputation in his treatment of diseases for which this drug was commonly employed.

A few, but far fewer, took up surgery. The Persians in general agreed that European surgeons were more skilled than their own, though they held exactly the opposite view about physicians. Those few Persians who became highly proficient in surgery were entitled to prefix the title *Ustád* to their name (though a few physicians also used the title). This exactly corresponds to the old English term Master Surgeon. Physicians were frequently addressed as *Rabbán*. Their official title was *Ṭabíb*, a title never applied to a surgeon. This implied one who had not only studied the practice of medicine, but also knew the theory and underlying principles of the art and was widely read in the ancillary arts of natural philosophy, theology and logic. A practitioner who had not the same theoretical knowledge was known as *Mutaṭabbib*, and was considered to be of an inferior status. Ibn Riẓván once scoffed at Ibn Buṭlán on the ground that he was a mere *mutaṭabbib*. Thus the *Ṭabib* corresponds very roughly to the modern consulting physician, the *mutaṭabbib* to the general practitioner. The quack, the lowest class of physician, was known as a *mudáwí*.

Besides the general qualifying examination surgeons had to undergo a further examination. Before they could practise they were compelled to know the first part of Galen's *De Medicamentorum Compositione secundum locos et genera*, which had been translated into Arabic by Ḥubaysh. They were also examined in anatomy. Orthopaedic surgeons had a further examination in the sixth book of the *Pandect* of Paul of Aegina, which Ḥunayn had translated, and were compelled to have a special knowledge of bones. All surgeons had to possess a case of rounded bistouris, a case of curved bistouris, a scalpel, a bone-saw, and ear-curette, and a special knife for the opening of cysts. This was the minimum. More complicated instruments were kept by richer practitioners. All surgeons were also compelled to possess a set of leeches, a box of dressings and of ointments and a remedy called al-Kundur, which was a composition of frankincense, acacia, and white of egg, and which had the reputation of being a powerful styptic for the control of haemorrhage.

Like the surgeons, the ophthalmologists had to undergo a further examination. They had to know the 'Ten Treatises on the Eye' of Ḥunayn ibn Isḥáq and were forbidden to practise unless they knew the gross anatomy of the eyeball. It is said that Rhazes, when about to undergo an operation to relieve his blindness, first examined his surgeon on the anatomy of the eye and finding him wanting refused to submit to the operation. Ophthalmologists had also to satisfy the examiner that they knew the three principal diseases of the eye and their complications. Besides this, they had to be able to demonstrate to him that they could prepare collyria and ophthalmic ointments. They had to swear not to lend out to unauthorized persons their surgical instruments, such as the lancet used for cases of pannus and pterygium and the curette used in cases of trachoma. Even when qualified, they were despised and thought nothing of unless they were on the staff of a hospital, for the number of ignorant and fraudulent eye-quacks was legion.

A certain number of physicians gave up practice and took to tutoring or possibly added tutoring of the sons of their patron to their duty of treating the household. Such was Ibn Durayd, who, born in 838, came to Baghdad in 920 and at this advanced age became the tutor to the young son of 'Alí bin 'Ísá, the *wazír*. Although addicted to wine and music even in his old age, Ibn Durayd was much sought after on account of his vast knowledge of Arabic. His surviving works are all poetical and philological, none medical.

Another type of low class, though orthodox, practitioner was the phlebotomist, who also added to his income by practising as a barber. In Safavid days, the Shah had his own special barber who was granted the title of *Kara Setashe*. It was his duty to let blood and shave the royal head. Under no circumstances could he give over his duties to another. The ordinary rank and file were wont to ply their trade in a regular shop in the bazaar, settling as a rule in the quarter known as the Druggists' Bazaar. Both in their training and in their discipline the phlebotomists followed the physicians. They were supposed to have a fair knowledge of anatomy, to know the surface markings of the principal internal organs, muscles and arteries, and to be able to recognize the named superficial veins. They were bidden to learn their art on the veins of beet-root leaves before attending any human subject. On setting up in practice all blood-letters had to swear before the *muḥtasib* that they would not, except after consultation with a physician, let blood from children, the aged, the anaemic, those suffering from extreme leanness, dryness or emaciation, sufferers from chronic diseases, those possessed of an extremely cold temperament, or from persons in great pain. In any case venesection was not to be performed in public. They had also to swear that they would never let blood from two veins in the head, known as *waswaq*, for these, if incised, were held to prevent procreation.

It was the duty of the *muḥtasib* to see that every phlebotomist possessed the proper instruments of his calling. These were lancets for breathing the vein, a tourniquet to tie round the arm in order to make the vein stand out, musk and pastilles to restore a fainting patient, a ball of silk or thread for ligatures, an instrument to excite vomiting in case of syncope, rabbit hair to use as a styptic, and oil to rub on the tip of the lancet in order that the pain of the incision might be less. As phlebotomists usually practised the art of circumcision together with the trade of blood-letting they were also obliged to possess a pair of scissors and a razor. These, no doubt, they also used in their humbler practice as a barber. On the whole the profession was looked upon with anything but respect, in fact, to call a man a barber or cupper was a form of abuse.

Strictly speaking, the medical business of the phlebotomist was limited to the letting of blood. Nevertheless, on the quiet, he often prescribed for his clients.[1] In his box of lancets he usually carried some simple remedies and was not averse to performing a minor operation, such as opening an abscess or removing a fish-bone from the throat. Not that they were all the equal of that garrulous blood-letter described in the *Arabian Nights*, who wearied his clients by the long catalogue of his merits.

> I have brought my razors and lancets. Do you wish to be shaved or bled? You do not know that all barbers are not like me. You only sent for a barber. But here in my person you have the best barber in Baghdad, an experienced physician, a very profound chemist, an infallible astrologer, a finished grammarian, a complete orator, a subtle logician, and mathematician perfectly versed in geometry, arithmetic, astronomy, and all the refinements of algebra: an historian fully master of the histories of all the kingdoms of the universe. Besides I know all parts of philosophy. I have all our law traditions at my fingers ends. I am a poet: I am an architect. What is there that I am not? There is nothing in Nature that is hidden from me.[2]

1 *Arabian Nights*, Night 184.

2 Ibid. Nights 160, 161.

The only form of minor surgery that apparently the barber-surgeons did not practise was dentistry. This was left to the regular physicians and surgeons. 'The physician extracts bad teeth', wrote al-Rúmí, 'in order that the beloved (patient) may be saved from pain and sickness.'[1] As a speciality dentistry came into fashion much later.

The lowest type of physician, a class peopled by the unsuccessful, the drunken and the ignorant, was the wandering leech. It was the custom of these low-class physicians to wander from town to town, hawking their pills and their knowledge and trading upon the superstition and ignorance of the villagers. Ḥáfiẓ scathingly remarks that the roadside physician cannot even diagnose the wounds which Love inflicts. Such was the recourse of Másawayh when Jibrá'íl drove him out of the dispensary at Jundí Sh͟ápúr. At first he took refuge in a monastery in Baghdad and asked permission to beg from the Christians who came to worship. By the advice of a priest he decided to become a roadside doctor and took up his station outside the door of the harem of al-Faẓal the *waẓír*. I have already related the happy sequel.

This practice, of course, led to unlimited abuse. It was open to any one to assume the dress of a physician and to defraud the people of the villages. So scandalous was the conduct of these ignorant doctors that it was declared the duty of the *muḥtasib* to see that such men performed no operation upon the eyes and never gave to their patients any preparation which was intended to be applied within the lids. Their very existence harmed the dignity of the profession as a whole. The regular physicians who adopted such a mode of living were indistinguishable from the out-and-out quacks, the class upon whom Rhazes poured out his wrath. For often it was more profitable to be a quack than an orthodox physician. The people of Persia, not unlike many people of England to-day, often turned first to the quack and only when he failed did they come to consult a regular doctor.

1 Al-Rúmí, *Maṣnaví*, bk. i, v. 3870.

Perhaps for this reason many forms of quackery were adopted by physicians who ought to have known better. The best known and the widest spread of such quackery was that of the uroscopists. Uroscopy was the art of diagnosing from an inspection of the urine alone. The claim to such powers is an extremely ancient one. Firdausi says that Alexander made a successful uroscopist his chief physician. Some of the greatest men in the days of the caliphate laid claim to these powers. Jurjís I, physician to al-Manṣúr, was greatly opposed to such claims, but his son Bukht Yishú' II apparently pretended to them.

They say that there was once in Herat a certain philosopher, who also practised medicine, named Khwájá Adíb Isma'íl. A Shaykh named 'Abd-Ulláh Anṣárí conceived a great hatred for the doctor because his great skill led many people to believe that he could even bring the dead back to life. And this is heresy. So the holy Shaykh burned the doctor's books and tried by every means to harm him. One day the Shaykh fell ill with a severe hiccough which was resistant to all treatment. Finally, in despair, a sample of his urine was sent to Khwájá Isma'íl for diagnosis and suggested treatment. The cunning men of Herat, however, knowing well the enmity between the two men, sent it under a false name. But Khwájá Isma'íl was not thus to be deceived. So great was his power of uroscopy that he recognized whose urine it was. He then made a diagnosis and recommended an appropriate treatment. In conclusion he added: 'Give him also this message, that he should study science and not burn books.'[1]

Among the more peculiar of the quack specialists were the healers of jaundice, known technically as *ṣafrá-band*. This power was apparently the monopoly of a tribe who lived in the hills around Ray. All members of this tribe are said to have been of an olive complexion with yellow sclerotics and of a markedly bilious temperament. Strangers afflicted with jaundice were cured by eating their bread or by washing in water from their vessels, especially in water which had stood some time in their

1 *Chahár Maqála*, p. 94.

family brass jars. If these measures were not sufficient, the tribesmen knew incantations which would cure the most obstinate of cases.[1]

Another strange speciality was that claimed by the chiefs of a tribe who lived in the neighbourhood of Kerind, a village well known to all those who have travelled on the Baghdad-Kermanshah road. They claimed to be able to cure the ague by the bastinado. It was their habit to tie the patient up by the heels when the rigor began and then to beat and abuse him most unmercifully, the theory being that the heat thus inspired would drive out the cold. Apparently the faculty of cure was hereditary to the chief of the tribe and resided in him alone.[2]

Holy men, such as jogis and dervishes, were at all times held to be skilful curers. Even their descendants retained something of their power.[3] It is said that the water in which the Safavid monarchs had washed was held to be a panacea by the common people, such was the holiness of the sainted ancestor. Snake-charmers, in most cases the very reverse of holy men, were also held to be able to cure various diseases by virtue of the magical powers which had been implanted in them by the Imams or by God himself. Perhaps too the almost universal belief in the efficacy of vipers' venom and vipers' flesh in the cure of disease was an additional reason why these men who had such a mastery over living serpents, could perform the same function as the snakes.

The lengthy description by Rhazes of the quacks who plagued the Baghdad of his day is perhaps not too well known to be quoted once more:[4]

There are so many little Arts used by Mountebanks and pretenders to physic, that an entire treatise, had I a mind to write one, would not contain them: but their impudence, and daring boldness is equal to the guilt and inward conviction they have of tormenting and putting

1 Bahá'-ul-Doula, *Khulásat-ul-Tajárib*, f. 515.
2 Malcolm, *History of Persia*, vol. II, p. 535.
3 Ibid. p. 427 n.
4 *Lib. Alman.* bk. 7, ch. 27.

persons to pain in their last hours, for no reason at all. Now some of them profess to cure the falling sickness, and thereupon make an issue in the hinder part of the head, in the form of a cross, and pretend to take something out of the opening, which they hold all the while in their hands. Others give out that they can draw snakes or lizards out of their patients' noses, which they seem to perform by putting up a pointed iron probe with which they wound the nostril until the blood comes: then they draw out the little artificial animal composed of liver, etc. Some are confident they can take out the white specks in the eye. Before they apply the instrument to that part, they put a piece of fine rag into the eye and taking it out with the instrument, pretend it is drawn immediately from the eye. Some again undertake to suck water out of the ear, which they fill with a tube from their mouth, and hold the other end to the ear; and so spurting the water out of their mouths, pretend it came from the ear. Others pretend to get out worms, which grow in the ear, or roots of the teeth. Others can extract frogs from the under part of the tongue; and by lancing make an incision into which they clap in the frog and so take it out. What shall I say of bones inserted into wounds and ulcers, which after remaining there for some time they take out again? Some, when they have taken out a stone from the bladder, persuade their patients that there is still another left; they do this for this reason to have it believed that they have taken out another. Sometimes they probe the bladder, being altogether ignorant and uncertain whether there be a stone or no. But if they do not find it, they pretend at least to take out one they have in readiness before, and show that to them. Sometimes they make an incision into the anus for piles, and by repeating the operation bring it to a fistula or an ulcer, when there was neither before. Some say they take phlegm, of a substance like unto glass, out of the penis or other part of the body, by the conveyance of a pipe which they hold with water in their mouths. Some pretend that they can contract and collect all the floating humours of the body to one place by rubbing it with winter cherries; which causes a burning or inflammation; and then they expect to be rewarded as if they had cured the distemper; and after they have suppled the place with oil, the pain presently goes off. Some make their patients believe they have swallowed glass; so, taking a feather, which they force down the throat, they throw them into a vomiting which brings up the stuff they themselves had put in with that very feather. Many things of this nature do they get out, which these imposters with great dexterity have put in, tending many times to endangering the health of their patients, and often ending in the death of them. Such counterfeits could not pass with discerning men, but that they did not dream of any fallacies, and made no doubt of the skill of those whom they employed; till at last when they suspect, or rather look more narrowly into their operations, the cheat is discovered.

Among the quacks must certainly be classed the female practitioners of medieval Baghdad. It is true that a certain Zeenab of the tribe of Baní 'Aud is mentioned with respect and is said to have treated with success the wounds and eye diseases, even of men. There was also the Shaykhah Rájihab 'to whom they present whoso hath any ailment and he passeth a single night in her house and awaketh on the morrow whole and ailing nothing'.[1] Usually this Shaykhah was screened by a curtain from the sight of male patients, but at times she allowed them to pass into her full presence. Women seem at times even to have entered into a loose partnership with male doctors. Al-Ṭabarí relates how a woman with a wounded shoulder attended in error the clinic of an eye-doctor, who asked her to wait until a woman practitioner arrived, whose duty it was to attend to female patients and dress their wounds.[2] For the most part the women doctors were of the witch type. They were frequented by young girls requiring love potions, by men requiring poisons for a rival, and by neurotics of all ages and classes who demanded relief from headaches, rheumatics, and the nervous diseases of which orthodox medicine had failed to rid them.

The success of these women prompted Rhazes to write a special pamphlet which he entitled 'Why unskilled Doctors, common People, and even Women in certain Cities are more successful in their treatment than the most learned Physicians'. He relates the story of how an official of his own hospital once complained to him of difficulty in moving some of his finger-joints on account of a small but very hard sore. When Rhazes was unable to restore to him full movement, he openly reviled him, asking him how he

1 *Arabian Nights*, Night 989.

2 Al-Tabarí, vol. III, p. 2226.

could hope to treat broken ribs and arms when he could not even cure a small sore on the finger. He then sought treatment, Rhazes concludes, 'from women and the vulgar'.

The retailers of drugs, too, should really be included in any survey of the cheap and ignorant quacks. While they confined themselves to their own profession, there is no class of men who deserve more praise than the Baghdad druggists. The science of pharmacy was nowhere more highly developed or more exact than in the city of the caliphs. Meyerhof has shown that the druggists could, if need, measure out their wares to the fraction of a grain.

But most of them also maintained an irregular medical practice. The dividing line between the druggist and the physician was in those times not so definite as it is to-day. I am inclined to think that the poorer classes habitually consulted the druggists and that only the upper classes went to the physicians. In other words, the druggists functioned as second-class doctors. If this is so, once again Europe is indebted to the Arabs, for it was certainly the system that prevailed in England until the passing of the Apothecaries Act in 1815. The granting of two grades of diploma in London to-day, the one by the Royal Colleges of Physicians and Surgeons (with which I class the Universities), the other by the Society of Apothecaries (with which I class the qualifying diploma issued jointly by the two Royal Colleges), represents the regularizing of this state of affairs. Modern practitioners who hold a Fellowship of the College of Surgeons or a Membership or Fellowship of the College of Physicians are the descendants of the Physicians and Surgeons; those who content themselves with the Conjoint Diploma of the Royal Colleges or the diploma of the Society of Apothecaries are the lineal heirs of the druggists, pedlars and quacks. This may also be the explanation of why the Royal College of Physicians forbids its Fellows to dispense their own physic.

The druggists were for the most part low-class people, ranking far below a merchant in the social scale. Occasionally one of them, sharper of wits than the rest, would rise from the ranks of his fellows and enter the preserves of the orthodox physicians. The newcomers were not popular. Such a one was Abú Quraysh 'Ísá al-Ṣaydalání, who at first kept a drugstore before the main door of the Caliph al-Mahdí's palace. One day Khayzurán, the wife of the caliph, felt ill and indisposed. As was usual in those times, she sent out a slave girl with a specimen of her urine and instructed her to take it to a learned physician and to find out the cause of her distress and its correct treatment. Abú Quraysh saw the girl passing in front of his shop and called to her, advising her to go no further because he was just the person to deal with her case. The girl consented and entered his shop. Abú Quraysh guessed what was the desired diagnosis and gave it. He announced that the urine was that of a member of the royal harem and that the indisposition was due to pregnancy and moreover that the child in the womb was a male. Khayzurán was delighted and informed the caliph. Weeks passed and the diagnosis was confirmed. Músá was born to the caliph.

Khayzurán then informed her lord of the wonderful skill in diagnosis of the druggist Abú Quraysh. Al-Mahdí was, of course, astonished and recounted the story to his chief physician Jurjís. Jurjís refused to believe and declared that it was impossible to diagnose either pregnancy or the sex of an unborn child from an inspection of the maternal urine. Khayzurán was furious at his narrow orthodox scepticism and to spite Jurjís increased Abú Quraysh's fee a hundredfold and had him appointed a physician to the royal household. Abú Quraysh accordingly closed his drugstore and took up the office of chief of the physicians in attendance upon the royal harem.

Some months later Khayzurán again became pregnant. Jurjís seized this opportunity and begged the caliph to put Abú Quraysh's powers of diagnosis to a fresh test. Again he diagnosed a son and again he was right, for Hárún was the result of the pregnancy. Abú Quraysh's triumph was complete. He was rewarded by being elevated to the rank of personal physician to the caliph and by an immense present of money, and finally, as the Persian chronicler says: 'Although he had but slight knowledge of medicine, except that which he had gained by experience, he was set over all the physicians of the court.'

Hárún-ul-Rashíd once remarked to a courtier that he had no faith in Abú Quraysh and only kept him at the court on account of his position under his parents. Yet he, when he in turn became caliph, elevated a druggist of Baghdad by name Abú Ḥasan ibn Ṭáhir, to a high rank in his household. This man was described as 'having more wit and politeness than people of his profession ordinarily have and his integrity, wit and jovial humour made him beloved and sought after by all sorts of people'. The caliph thought so highly of him that 'he entrusted him with the care to provide his favourite ladies with all the things they stood in need of'.

A word on the matter of the dress of a physician of this period may well conclude this brief summary of medieval Arab medicine.

Physicians of the 'Abbásid period wore a distinctive dress whatever their social standing might be. In the *Arabian Nights*[1] is the story of 'how the Prince of Persia let his beard grow and putting on the habit of a physician passed for a leech' and so entered the royal apartments of the princess, his beloved. When the Devil visited Abu Isḥáq Ibráhím al-Móṣuli, he had no difficulty in gaining admission after assuming the role and dress of a doctor. For this he clothed himself in a white cloak and white shirt with a doctor's turban[2] on his head, all well perfumed. In his hand he carried a silver-headed stick. A distinguishing dress, however, was not customary before the days of Hárún-ul-Rashíd. It was a certain Abú Yúsuf, a chief justice in that reign, who introduced a distinctive habit for men of learning.[3]

The frontispiece of this book shows the typical dress of a physician of the Mongol period. The head was shaved and was covered by a large turban of silk or cotton, wound around a

1 *Arabian Nights*, Night 357. 2 Ibid. Night 687.
3 Ibn Khallikán, vol. IV, p. 273.

support, called a *qalansuwa*. Sometimes the *qalansuwa* was worn alone without any covering. The Persians wore it tall and cone-shaped. Those who did not follow Persian fashions wore theirs short, so that it resembled the modern fez. Hárún-ul-Rashíd disapproved of tall hats, but al-Mu'taṣim reintroduced the fashion. Physicians of the court wore a black turban, except in the reign of al-Ma'mún, who for political reasons commanded a change to green. Others wore whatever suited their taste. One night the Caliph al-Amín in a drunken jest compelled Jibrá'íl bin Bukht Yishú' to change clothes with the captain of the guard. Jibrá'íl states that he was forced to hand over his girdle and his *qalansuwa*.

Shaving of the face was not the fashion, although except among old men the beard was usually trimmed to a neat point. Ibn Riẓván maintained that the perfect physician had no need of a beautiful face. In this respect Ibn Buṭlán agreed with him, only adding that it should not be so ugly as to frighten children or disgust adults.

On ceremonial occasions physicians attached to the court and those holding high office of State wore an embroidered jacket, called a *miṭraf* or *muṭraf*. A visitor to Bukht Yishú', the physician, was surprised to find him one day sitting all alone, wearing a heavy *miṭraf* of Yemen silk together with a gown of silk. He explained his unusual attire by pointing out that he suffered from the cold.[1] For to wear a *miṭraf* without proper reason was looked upon as a mark of ostentation. Hence the saying: 'I would rather be respected in a *khamísa* (shirt) than despised in a *miṭraf*', which is almost the equivalent of our saying that the cowl does not make the monk. The *miṭraf*, and in fact all the clothes, of a wealthy physician were scented with rose-water, camphor and sandal wood. Ibn Riẓván used to boast that he himself used a 'delicate perfume'.[2]

The shirt was known as *qamís* or *khamísa*. Over it was worn a tunic, called *durrá'*. Bukht Yishú' is said to have worn a *durrá'*

1 *I.A.U.* vol. I, p. 139.
2 Ibid. vol. II, p. 100.

of embroidered Greek brocade. The tunic was usually worn fastened up across the chest. It was held in position by a girdle, known as the *nayfaq*. To leave the tunic open was the mark of a sloven. When the caliph deliberately undid Bukht Yishú''s tunic, he got a mild reproof when later Bukht Yishú' told him that to undo the tunic of another was one of the first signs of insanity.[1] The sleeves of the tunic according to the curious fashion in the Caliph al-Musta'ín's days were worn very wide. Too narrow a sleeve and too short a coat were evidence of meanness or poverty. Such sleeves were often used as pockets. Bukht Yishú' appeared at a New Year's reception of the caliph, holding within his sleeve his present of a box of gold and ebony. Abú Ma'shar, a doctor of Balkh, is said to have set out to attend a lecture, given by al-Kindí, after concealing within his sleeve a book on astrology within which he had placed a knife in order to murder the lecturer.[2]

The outermost garment or hooded cloak was known as the *ṭaylasán*, and was the distinctive garment of those engaged in the practice of law, medicine and the ritual of Islam.[3] It is recorded that Avicenna, when in the court of the Khwárazmsháh, wore the *ṭaylasán* of a juris consult. It was the custom of the caliph to present to Jibrá'íl bin Bukht Yishú' three new *ṭaylasáns* every year. But this restricted usage was not universal, for by the fourth century A.H. the *ṭaylasán* was part of the costume of the ordinary citizen of Baghdad, was confined to nobles in Ahwaz, and was worn by nobody in Khorasan. It has survived in Egypt until to-day as part of the dress of the Coptic clergy. The special medical hood was the creation of Mongol times.

This outer cloak in the case of doctors of medicine was usually of black silk. Asad ibn Jání said that his wearing of a cloak of white cotton set patients against him. Ibn ul-Tilmíz on the contrary used to say that a prudent man would wear such clothes as may not draw upon him the envy of the lower orders or the contempt of the higher, and accordingly used to wear 'white clothes of

1 *I.A.U.* vol. I, p. 142.
2 *Chahár Maqála*, p. 64.
3 Ibn Khallikán, vol. I, p. 441.

a fine quality'.[1] To wear a cloak of striped Arabian stuff was the mark of a man of renown, but was held to be rather too ostentatious. Abú ul-Taiyyih, who flourished about A.D. 900 and who both taught in an elementary school and lectured in the caliph's palace, held that a man of letters would avoid 'impure' colours, such as yellow or amber, which were only suitable for women and singing girls. Yet such a one might quite properly wear them when being bled or undergoing medical treatment.[2]

Doctors of law apparently wore a green satin cloak, for Dá'úd al-Ẓáhirí, chief professor in the school of law in Baghdad during the latter part of the ninth century, is said to have addressed an audience 'of four hundred wearers of green hoods'. Green, however, was not forbidden to doctors of medicine, for al-Sharísí says that green *ṭaylasáns* were worn by any person of respectability.[3]

Trousers were worn by the wealthy as underclothes, but to allow them to appear was considered by the Baghdadis as Persian or effeminate. Normally they were concealed by the shirt, which reached well below the thighs. So long did some wear their shirts that under the early 'Abbásids it was declared that no garment should be so long as to cover the heels. The lower end of the shirt was hidden by top boots. Boots, called *khuff*, were long and reached above the knees. For use in towns and in fine weather they were red or lacquered and were frequently ornamented with silver or precious stones. Like the sleeve they were used as receptacles for books and documents. Al-Jurjání wrote a treatise on medicine, directing that it should be reproduced in two volumes suitable for placing one in each riding boot. Hence the book was known as the *Khuff-i-'Alá'í* or 'Boots of Exaltation'. In imitation of this another book was written called the *Mújiz-i-Kummí* or 'The Compendium of the Sleeve', since it was intended to be carried within the *kumm* or sleeve.

1 Ibid. vol. III, p. 603.
2 *Kitáb-ul-Muwashsha*, quoted by Levy in *A Baghdad Chronicle*, p. 123.
3 Ibn Khallikán, vol. I, p. 501 and n. 4; Harírí, *Maqáma*, p. 293.

With regard to the material from which clothes were made, it is clear that there was no religious impediment: it was only a question of the wealth of the wearer. Furs were worn by wealthier physicians and formed part, sometimes, of their stipends. The wearing of wool was, however, the mark of poverty, ascetism or Christianity. Ḥammad bin abí Sulaymán, finding his friend robed in a woollen garment, bade him 'put off this Christianity'. Again, some young Persian medical students, coming down to Baghdad to enrol themselves in the classes of Abú ul-Faraj ibn ul-Ṭabíb, the Christian physician of the 'Aẓudí Hospital, found him to their great astonishment in church 'wearing a woollen cloak with nothing on his head, and in his hand a censer'. Having finished his devotions Ibn ul-Ṭabíb put off his wool, put on his physician's dress again, and mounting his mule rode back with his pupils to his house.[1]

1 *I.A.U.* vol. 1, p. 239.

CHAPTER X

ARABIAN MEDICINE IN PRACTICE

PERHAPS the reader will remark that although the subject of this book is Medicine in Persia the phrase Arabian Medicine is constantly recurring. Or alternatively he may ask why the world has given the name Arabian to a science of which the greatest exponents were all non-Arabs. This antithesis has not been unremarked before. Even the ancients were struck with the singular fact that all the greatest men of the Arab regime were themselves non-Arabs.

But apart from poetry and politics, which do not concern us here, the title Arab is not unjust to either side. As applied to the system of medicine which was taught and developed first in Baghdad and then throughout the Middle and Near East, it is entirely suitable; for it was the Arabs who preserved and gave the impetus to the development of Greek medicine at a time when the hold upon this learning in Europe was growing very weak. The energy and enthusiasm was due to the Arab. The language in which the Greek thought was preserved and developed was Arabic. And Arabic remained the language of science long after the destruction of the central authority at Baghdad which had been the influence which decided whether Syriac, Persian or Greek was to be the language of science for the future.

It would seem to be almost an accident, almost due to the chance of racial rivalry, that the Persians became supreme in science among their Arab conquerors. 'It is strange', says Ibn Khaldún, 'that most of the learned men among the Moslems who have excelled in the religious or intellectual sciences are non-Arabs with rare exceptions; and even then savants who claimed Arabian descent spoke a foreign language, grew up in foreign lands, and studied under foreign masters, notwithstanding that the community to which they belonged was Arabian and the author of its religion was an Arab.'[1]

The first Arabs to turn Moslem and to join the standard of the Prophet were all alike ignorant of culture and bookish learning. They were content to carry in their hearts the precepts and unwritten laws of the Qur'án. They knew nothing of the methods of acquiring and imparting knowledge. They neither read books nor did they make books. Chief among their literary men were the Readers who could repeat the Qur'án and the traditions of the Prophet. But it was not until the time of the Caliph Hárún-ul-Rashíd that it was determined to commit these traditions to writing in order to prevent loss and corruption of the original text.

Such a decision required an enormous sifting of evidence with a view to discovering the form of the original tradition and to the settling of the canon. During the 300 years that had intervened between original promulgation of the sayings and the decision to commit them to paper, the Arabic language had undergone certain changes. The purity of the dialect which the Prophet spoke had disappeared when the dialect became the official language of the whole people. To remedy this and to solve various difficulties four sciences arose, the science of quranic exegesis, the science of quranic criticism, the science of apostolic tradition, and the science of grammar. To these were soon added the sciences of jurisprudence, scholastic theology, and lexicography; and as the number of works on these subjects increased, there were also added the science of rhetoric and of literature. These nine sciences, being called into being by the needs of the Qur'án and the Traditions, the Arabs looked upon as their own offspring in a very special manner and therefore called them the nine native sciences.

Opposed to the nine native sciences were the sciences of the foreigner or the ancient sciences. These included philosophy, geometry, astronomy, music, medicine, magic and alchemy. These the Arab scarcely touched: the way was left open to the

1 This and the following page is largely borrowed from Nicholson's *History of Arabian Literature*, p. 277.

Persians, Sabeans, Jews and the mixed races. Thus the Christian Ibn Jazlá studied medicine under a Christian professor. But when he wished to take up logic, he was compelled to seek a Moslem teacher, 'for none of the Christians of those days were enamoured of that science'.[1]

With the overthrow of Yezdegird in A.D. 642 the Arabs found themselves in command of all Persia. This supremacy was not used by them to enforce Islam upon their new subjects. They left their conversion to time and to the advantages which the Persians soon saw followed the profession of faith. Theoretically to embrace the faith of Islam meant to enter the brotherhood of Islam. But in practice, although the Persians were more polished and more refined than the desert Arabs, even after their submission to Islam the Arabs still looked upon them as an inferior class. Just as the Companions of the Prophet were considered superior to all other Arabs, so the Arabs considered themselves of a rank to which no outsider could ever reach. Individuals or families of a subject people could only gain a recognized position by attaching themselves to some Arab chief or clan as *mawálí* or 'clients'. Even in the 'Abbásid times, when Arab dominance had vanished for ever, many Persians produced fictitious genealogical trees to prove that they were of Arab descent, even though in their own line the blood ran bluer.

The Arab despised the *mawálí* and their learning. Accustomed to rule, to hunting and to fighting he kept for the most part the government of his subjects in his own hands. Grudgingly he gave to the *mawálí* a share in the native sciences; for the Persian found the subleties of these sciences peculiarly fitting to his cunning brain. The foreign sciences the Persian assumed as his lawful and normal field, and the Arab did not dispute the claim. Bringing with him from the desert no tradition on these subjects, despising all literary investigation, above all in subjects not connected with his Qur'án, he willingly left them to the conquered people. Thus the Persian, partly because of his innate ability,

1 *Hist. Dynst.* vol. IX, p. 240.

partly because of false Arab pride, and partly because he was already the inheritor of the traditions of occidental learning through Darius, Alexander and Jundí Sh͟ápúr, became the foremost exponent of the foreign sciences, above all of medicine and the sciences allied to it.

As late as 1329 Ibn ul-Uk͟huwwa could write:

Many a town has no physician who is not a *ẓimmí* (that is, Christian, Jew or Zoroastrian), who belongs to a people whose evidence is not accepted in the courts of law, where the laws of Medicine are concerned. No Muslim occupies himself with it: everyone repairs to the study of the Law and more particularly that portion of it which is given over to disputes and litigiousness. The town is full of legists, occupied with granting *fatwas* and giving replies to legal queries on points which arise. Can there be any reason for the Faith's permitting a state of things in which large numbers occupy themselves with one particular duty while another is neglected?

In spite of the cleavage which thus existed between the conqueror and the conquered and which never completely disappeared, the desert Arab became considerably persianized when he became a town-dweller and the Persian flattered the Arab by becoming arabicized. Nowhere is this attitude more clearly marked than in the practice of medicine. The Persian practitioner wrote and thought in Arabic. His approach to the patient was governed by Arab theological prejudices. 'Alí Afẓal of Qazvín bade his son, then a medical student, remember that his first words to his patient should be the Arabic Bismillah: 'In the name of God the all-Mighty, the all-Merciful.' He should then recite the opening verses of the Qur'án and then 'with a cheerful smile and a laying aside of a grave countenance and with an optimịstic spirit' he should begin to elicit the history of the case. Provided that he followed all the proprieties of Islam, he might now show himself in his true colours—Christian, Jew or Zoroastrian.[1]

1 The paramount importance of a Moslem being attended only by a Moslem doctor and the whole question of medical etiquette is treated at length in *Al-Madk͟hal*, vol. IV, p. 133 of Ibn ul-Ḥaj (Misr Press, Cairo, 1943). See also *Ma'álim al-Qurba*, ch. 45.

There was no objection in either sex to the taking of the pulse. It was always the right wrist that was presented to the physician, for the right hand was used for all honourable purposes, the left for all actions which, though necessary, are unclean. The physician attending Sa'd-ul-Doula refused to take his pulse from the left wrist even though his patient being paralysed down the right side was unable to offer him the correct hand. After the pulse the urine was inspected or instructions were given to send a specimen to the physician's house so that he might be acquainted with its contents before the next visit. He then made his diagnosis and wrote out a prescription. A copy of this prescription he was compelled by law to leave with the near relatives of the patient.

It was customary for a doctor to receive his fee in advance if called to a patient at night. Muḥammad ibn Dániyál, an oculist of Mosul and later of Cairo who died in 1311, describing in a shadow-play a night-call, makes the doctor say:

> I appeal to God against the stoned Satan. Who is it wandering round in the dark night? Who is it that startles me from my bed in the sheltering night? Who calls me from my slumber, when the food has scarcely been digested from my stomach, so that my strength has disappeared and I am nearly dead of palpitations? For it is not customary to call a doctor by night unless one brings him a money cheque and harnesses mules and horses for him.

In a case which was chronic and required many visits it would appear that the physician received his fee only on the conclusion of the case. If the patient recovered, there was in most cases no question of refusal to pay. But if the case ended fatally, the relatives could, if they chose, present themselves before the chief physician of the city and show him the copy of all the prescriptions which had been ordered for the sick man. If in his opinion they were proper and suitable for the case and the physician had shown no negligence or fault, he would declare that the man's life had reached its allotted span and that the fees must be paid. If on the other hand he found evidence of neglect, he could say to the relatives: 'Exact the blood money for your kinsman from the physician, for it is he who slew him by his poor skill and negligence.'[1]

Similarly barbers could be sued if a circumcision went wrong.[2] Sa'dí tells the story of a patient with some disease of the eyes, who instead of going to an ophthalmologist consulted a farrier.[3] The treatment was unavailing and the condition grew worse. The patient then brought an action for damages and had him summoned before a judge. But he lost his case on the grounds that he was a fool, for only a fool would expect a farrier to treat successfully a disease of the human eye. Bar Hebraeus, too, records an amusing defence set up by a doctor when summoned for his unsuccessful treatment. The doctor agreed to cure a patient of tertian fever for a certain sum. His efforts only succeeded in converting the tertian into a semi-tertian fever. The doctor, however, demanded half his fee, as he claimed that the disease had been reduced by half.

Shaykh Muḥammad al-Mahdí al-Hafnaví mentions a similar case in which the patient complained that through the culpable ignorance of a physician his wife suffered from an imperfectly set fracture of the shoulder. The case was settled in favour of the doctor and not only had the patient's husband to pay full fees, but he was also fined for impertinence.[4]

Of even greater interest is the mention by Bahá'-ul-Doula of the case of an Indian in Ray, who was treated for a considerable time for some disease of the kidney. The disease appeared to have been cured when quite suddenly the patient had a relapse. He then brought a suit against his doctor for deficient prescribing and excessive charging. Bahá'-ul-Doula together with some others was asked to act as arbitrator. The result was highly satisfactory to all parties. For the court ordered the patient to pay further fees, the doctor to give more medicine, and the patient to leave Ray and go to the hills for a short rest. In 40 days he returned completely cured.[5]

1 *Ma'álim al-Qurba*, ch. 45. 2 Ibid. ch. 44. 3 *Gulistán*, vol. VII, p. 14.
4 *Contes du Cheykh el-Mohdy*, vol. I, p. 255. 5 *Khulásat-ul-Tajárib*, f. 64b.

An interesting problem is the size of the fee, about which there is a good deal of information hidden in various medical anecdotes. A midwife after the delivery of a female child according to a story in the *Arabian Nights* received a robe of honour and a thousand gold pieces.[1] But this was in the household of a king. The fee of a master physician in the house of a merchant was only one dirham for a visit according to another tale.[2]

As to-day, the fee varied according to the status of the physician and the status of the patient. Másawayh, when still unknown and a 'road-side' physician in Baghdad, received from a servant whom he had successfully treated for ophthalmia, a daily allowance of bread and meat and sweets and a promise of a monthly salary of a few silver and copper coins. This must have been on the low side, for Másawayh's expression of thanks was mistaken for a complaint, and he was at once assured that the allowance would be increased. When the *wazír* fell ill and Másawayh was equally successful with him, the salary rose to 600 silver dirhams a month, food for two mules and the services of five slaves. When finally he reached the rank of ophthalmologist to the caliph, his salary was fixed at 2000 dirhams a month and presents worth 20,000 dirhams every year, together with fodder for his mules and the services of a number of slaves. Jibrá'íl, the ophthalmologist to al-Ma'mún, only received half this fee and, when he was deprived of his office for an indiscreet remark, his salary was reduced to 150 dirhams a month.[3]

These fees paid to the ophthalmologists are a trifle compared with the gigantic fees which the physicians were wont to receive. Al-Jurjání[4] immediately on his arrival at the court of the Khwárazmsháh was allowed a salary of 1000 gold dinars a month. Rhazes for the successful treatment of Manṣúr, the *amír* of Bukhara, received a horse with its harness, a cloak, a turban, a set of arms, a slave boy and a slave girl. Besides these he was assigned in Ray estates which brought him in every year 2000

1 *Arabian Nights* (Suppl.), Night 662.
2 Ibid. (Suppl.), 'Tale of Attaf'.
3 *I.A.U.* vol. I, p. 171.
4 Ibid. vol. II, p. 31.

golden dinars and 200 ass-loads of corn. At the time when Másawayh was receiving 2000 dirhams a month as ophthalmologist-in-chief to Hárún-ul-Rashíd, Jibrá'íl, the physician, was receiving 10,000 dirhams a month. Thus, says the biographer, Másawayh became socially the equal of his teacher, but financially he was still far behind him.[1]

The biggest fixed income of them all was that of Bukht Yishú' bin Jurjís. His salary from Hárún-ul-Rashíd was 10,000 dirhams a month. In addition to this he received presents whenever the caliph was bled, whenever he administered a purge, and on all the great feasts, both Christian and Mohammedan. The value of these was estimated to be over 300,000 dirhams a year. From the household of the caliph he received a retaining fee of 400,000 dirhams. He was also physician to the Barmecides who paid him a yearly 2,500,000 dirhams for his services. In addition to all these he received from his private practice about 500,000 dirhams a year. This gives a total income not far short of 4,000,000 dirhams a year, or reckoning the dirham to be a little less than a shilling, about £175,000 per annum.[2]

Abú ul-Fazá'il Muhazzib ibn ul-Náqid took over 300 dirhams a day in consulting fees,[3] though this was in Cairo, not in Baghdad. The fees were handed to him, wrapped up in paper. He used to place these in empty eye-salve jars, without undoing the wrappings and declared at the end of the day that he did not know which of his patients had paid him with silver and which with gold coins. A similar disregard for fees was found in medieval Persia. When Tavernier visited Ispahan in 1670, no consulting physician handled money, but it was remarked that his apothecary always found 'a way to have the doctor satisfied for his pains'. The custom survived until the present century. When I first went to Persia it was still usual for a physician attending a high-class patient to receive his fee in a sealed envelope. It was considered highly unbecoming to the dignity of a physician to discuss a fee.

1 *Chahár Maqála*, p. 85; *I.A.U.* vol. I, p. 72.

2 *I.A.U.* vol. I, p. 136, and *Maṭraḥ-ul-Anẓár*, p. 118. 3 Ibid. vol. II, p. 115.

Hence it was always an exciting moment to open the packet, when well outside the house, and see whether the fee was larger or smaller than anticipated.

There is no mention of any surgeon being attached to the staff of the caliph, so that it is a matter of conjecture how much a master surgeon could charge royalty. In private practice the surgeons demanded such a fee as they thought their client could pay. Ibn Waṣíf, for instance, much against his will, consented to operate on a case of cataract for 70 dirhams, when the patient protested that he could not pay more. Half-way through the operation a bag of gold slipped from the patient's girdle. Whereupon Ibn Waṣíf returned him his fee and abandoned the operation only half finished.

I have not come across any mention of the fee that was paid for a simple venesection in 'Abbásid times. It is stated in the list of Jibrá'íl's fees that he received 50,000 dirhams each time that he bled the caliph.[1] In the seventeenth century in Ispahan the standard fee was 12 qasbaqs.[2]

Abu Sa'íd Yamání of Basra, who wrote a commentary on the 'Questions' of Ḥunayn and a pamphlet on the 'Examination of Doctors', once took Ibráhím bin Sinán's place for six months as chief of the board of examiners. He received during this time a fee of 1000 tumans a month.[3]

Probably only the senior members of the medical staff of the court received a regular salary. The remainder had to eke out their existence by the numerous presents which the caliphs and shahs distributed with such a generous hand when things were going well. In later days the court physicians were graded and each received more or less the pay of his rank. Authorities differ on the exact salaries that were paid to them. Probably the salaries themselves varied from reign to reign. The chief or *ḥakím-báshí* drew about 1000 tumans a year: the others a smaller sum, corresponding to the favour in which they were held. The sovereign

1 Ibid. vol. 1, p. 136.
2 du Mans, *Éstat de la Perse*, p. 177.
3 *I.A.U.* vol. 1, p. 238.

himself was often quite ignorant of how many medical hangers-on he possessed or how much a fit of generosity might cost him. S͟háh Sulaymán in a fit of pique once made a sudden demand for a statement of how much a year was expended on his court doctors and astrologers. He was told that it amounted to 22,000 tumans.

At times unscrupulous ministers did not hesitate to pay their own medical attendants out of the caliph's purse. Thus, Ḥassan bin Muk͟hallid, *wazír* to al-Mu'tamid, was once under the treatment of a certain physician named Daylam. Happening to be present when the caliph underwent a successful venesection, he was bidden to draw up a list of the physicians attached to the court and to assign to each a reward according to his rank. In his list he included his own physician Daylam, who as a matter of fact was quite unknown to the caliph and who had never set foot within the palace. Al-Mu'tamid signed the order and to his astonishment the physician received the next day a bag containing 1000 dinars, brought by a servant of the royal treasury. The *wazír* laughed heartily when he recounted to Daylam how he had secured this present for him from the unsuspecting caliph.

In many instances no doubt the huge presents which a patron gave to his physician for some particularly pleasing piece of work are exaggerated by the tellers in order to show his generosity. Thus, when Abú Qurays͟h for the second time foretold the birth of a son and in fact Hárún was born, it is said that al-Ma'mún and his courtiers piled up so many trays of gold and silver coins before him that the heap towered above his head.

Even more generous, and for far less reason, was al-Mutawakkil. During the hot weather his doctors forbade him to take mustard with his food. Buk͟ht Yis͟hú' III, however, said that he would prepare for him a special dish containing mustard in abundance, but from which no harm should come to the royal stomach. Al-Mutawakkil ate to repletion that night and awakening in the morning with no pains of indigestion rewarded Buk͟ht Yis͟hú', it is said, with 300,000 dirhams and 30 suits of clothes. To conciliate al-Ṭayfúrí and to retain his services this same caliph made him a yearly allowance of 3000 gold dinars and presents whose value amounted to more than 50,000 dirhams.[1]

On the other hand many of the smaller practitioners must have come near to starvation if a run of ill luck gave them a series of unsuccessful cases. Bad debts are common enough to-day; they must have been even more frequent then, when the caliph was a chronic bankrupt and when the grandees of the court lived in daily fear of a royal levy. A certain Sharaf-ul-Dín of Ispahan, more commonly known as Ḥakím Shifá'í, lamented in a rather coarse verse the refusal of one of his more aristocratic patients to pay for a laxative draught that he had prescribed for him.

Even if you are Sám, the son of Naríman, or great Rustam himself,
You cannot carry off my mixture without paying for it.
Either you must pass over the money for what you have drunk
Or you must drink what you have passed.

Another story is told of Abú Duláma, a wag of the time of the Caliph al-Mahdí, which brings no credit either to the legal or the medical profession. Abú Duláma

once called in a physician to attend to his son who had fallen ill, and agreed to pay a certain sum in the event of the patient's recovery. When his son was restored to health, Abú Duláma said to the physician: 'I call Heaven to witness that we have nothing in the world to pay you with. However, cite the rich Jew so-and-so before the judge and I and my son will go before him and swear that the Jew owes you money.' The physician immediately brought the Jew before the *qází* of Kufa, claiming a certain sum of money. The Jew naturally denied the debt, and the claimant saying that he had witnesses to prove it, went out to bring Abú Duláma and his son into court. The elder of these two scoundrels had anticipated that the judge would make some inquiry about the character of the witnesses, and so in the ante-chamber he recited in a loud voice for the *qází* and all to hear:

'Such men as screen me, find in me a screen;
And if men pay, I run their sins to ground.
Would'st cleanse my well, thine own though far from clean?
Then all shall know what filth in thine I've found.'

1 *I.A.U.* vol. 1, p. 142.

He then entered the court and gave his evidence. The *qázi* listened carefully, and having apparently given it due consideration, said: 'I have accepted your declaration and admit your evidence.' Being convinced, however, that they were false witnesses, he himself paid the money in question out of his own pocket and dismissed the Jew out of fear of Abú Dulâma's tongue.[1]

How the patient received the medicine which was ordered for him opens up another interesting question. The separation of the medical from the pharmaceutical profession, not yet complete even in England, had already begun under the caliphs. The rapid increase in the *materia medica* and the greater skill in compounding which this demanded, must have called for a special body of men. Certainly all the big hospitals had a pharmacist on the staff who had charge of the drugs only and not of patients. In ordinary outside practice the usual method was for the doctor to prescribe and compound his own mixtures. Apparently a doctor on his visits often carried with him certain stock remedies, for Rhazes once apologized for administering simple barley water to a patient with meningitis, saying that that was all that he had with him. In a few cases the patient merely received directions how to find and prepare his remedy for himself. This is the point of an anecdote in the *Laṭá'if-ul-Tawáif*:

One day a certain man went into the desert and buried 1000 gold coins at the root of a tree and went his way. When later he came back to the spot, he found that the root of the tree had been dug up, the soil turned over, and all the gold taken away. He was distracted and hastened to the Judge of the city. In secret he told him what had happened. The Judge then said to him: 'Go away and come back in three days; but during these three days tell no man what has happened.'

Then the Judge sent for a Physician of the town who was a veritable Restorer of Creation, and asked him privately if the root of that particular tree had any special medical properties. The Physician told him that it had. He then asked him if he had recently prescribed that root to any patient. The Physician replied that he had, and that so-and-so had been ill and had now recovered, being treated by this very root.

1 Ibn Khallikán, vol. 1, p. 538. Quoted by Levy in *A Baghdad Chronicle*, p. 39.

'In fact', added the Physician, 'I told him about this very tree. He then went off to get the root, took it and was cured.'

So the Judge farewelled the Physician and sent for this patient. He made him sit before him in a private room and spoke to him with gentleness and cunning. Then he admonished him and quoted many verses and traditions and so softened his heart that he confessed and restored the 1000 gold coins to their owner.

When treating a patient of high rank the doctor was expected to swallow the first draught of the medicine as a guarantee of his good faith. When the Persian ambassador sent by Nádir Sháh to the court of St Petersburgh fell ill at Astrakhan, he was very indignant when Mr Malloch, the English doctor in attendance, refused to conform to this custom, and even desired to have him beaten for this refusal. He ultimately got his revenge by refusing to pay him more than £3 for all his attention.[1]

Often the patient bought his drugs from pedlars, though probably the wandering chemist relied for his sales either upon his own diagnosis and treatment or upon his clients prescribing for themselves. The story in the 779th Night of the *Arabian Nights* shows that it was the custom to purchase all kinds of remedies from these pedlars, for

the lad, donning Jewish garb, shouldered a pair of saddle-bags and went about crying: 'Ho, aloes good for use. Ho, pepper good for use. Ho, collyrium good for use. Ho, tutty good for use.' Now, when the woman saw him, she came forth the house and hailed him: 'Ho, thou Jew', and said he to her: 'Yes, O my lady.' Then said she to him: 'Hast thou with thee aught of poison?' Said he: 'How, O my Lady? Have I not poison with me of the hour? And whoever shall eat thereof in a mess of sweet milk and rice and clarified butter shall die within that time.'

In other cases the relatives went to a druggist direct to get what they required, without any previous consultation with a doctor. The story of Morgiána in the 629th Night shows that the druggist himself was in the habit of dispensing without any examination of the patient.

1 Cook, *Voyages and Travels*, vol. 1, p. 411.

Morgiána went quickly to a druggist's shop and asked of him a drug often administered to men when diseased with a dangerous distemper. He gave it saying: 'Who is there in thy house that lieth so ill as to require this medicine?' And she said: 'My Master, Qásim, is sick well-nigh unto death. For many days he hath not spoken nor tasted ought of food, so that we almost despair of his life.' Next day Morgiána went again and asked the druggist for more medicine and essences such as are adhibited to the sick when at the door of death, that the moribund may haply rally before the last breath. The man gave the potion and she taking it sighed aloud and wept, saying: 'I fear me he may not have strength to drink this draught. Methinks all will be over with him ere I return to the house.'[1]

Certainly the majority of physicians prepared their own compounds. Even the most highly placed did not think it beneath their dignity to do so. Rhazes we know did so, for he wrote: 'I have prepared an extract of turbith and found its action similar to that of scammony. I have also prepared in the same way an extract of colocynth from colocynth pulp. I used to mix it with kernels of almonds and tragacanth and sugar. Thus administered it is less repugnant.'

More rarely the patient went with a prescription to a regular drugstore and there bought what was ordered. It was in Baghdad that the first public pharmacy was opened. By the seventeenth century it had become the usual method, at any rate in the large towns, although it was still customary in the smaller places for the patient to prepare his own infusions and decoctions. Pills, powders and solid drugs were handed to the patient wrapped up in little envelopes.

The owner of such a store was known as *Al-'Aṭṭár* or 'Dealer in Perfumes' or by the Persian term *Dárfarúsh* or 'Seller of Remedies'. The druggist, like the rest of the medical confraternity, came under the watchful eye of the *muḥtasib*. It was his duty to see that only such persons who had a knowledge and experience of drugs dispensed them, and also 'to inspire the makers of syrups

1 *Arabian Nights* (Suppl.), Night 629.

with the fear of God and warn them of divine punishment and immediate penalties'.[1] These 'immediate penalties' were fines, beating of the soles of the feet, and the wooden hat, a sort of ambulant pillory.[2] Before the days of drug standardization the frauds perpetrated by the druggists exceeded even the frauds of the quack practitioners. There was scarcely a drug in common use which was not adulterated by the unscrupulous either by mixing in a cheaper and less potent variety or by the actual admixture of a similar but different drug. An attempt to rectify this was made by the official adoption of the Great Pharmacopoeia of Sábúr bin Sahl and later its supersession by the Pharmacopoeia of Ibn al-Bayán and that of Ibn ul-Tilmíẕ.

Not only did the *muḥtasib* inspect the drugs; he had also the right to inspect the methods of preparation. For this purpose he frequently made his visits at an unexpected hour and could, if he wished, inspect the shop even after it was closed for the night. He was especially enjoined to see that the vessels in which the excipients, such as barley-water and rose-water, were prepared, were kept clean and scoured. During the day the various drugs were exposed on trays, coloured and neatly arranged, in front of the shop.[3] By night shutters of reeds and palm were placed over the shop in order to keep out dogs. By day it was customary only to spread a net across the shop front as a sign that the owner was out or asleep. Old and smelly jars were destroyed by order of the *muḥtasib*. Tinning was to be renewed every three months.

Lax though the rules regarding drugs may have been, as the result of the laws governing ceremonial purity and impurity a considerable body of public health ordinances had come into being before the overthrow of the caliphate. The duty of seeing that such ordinances were carried out belonged not to a physician but to the *muḥtasib*. The regulation of food and drink and the prevention of infectious diseases through the public bath came

1 *Ma'álim al-Qurba*, chs. 24, 25.
2 Chardin, *Travels in Persia*, vol. VI, p. 129.
3 Al-Rúmí, *Masnaví*, bk. ii, v. 280.

within his authority. In the case of the bath it was his duty to see that the water was kept clean and fresh, that the stone floors were scrubbed, and that the washing of felt and leather or anything that caused a bad smell within the bath was not allowed. Sufferers from leprosy and skin diseases were to be rigorously excluded. The possibility of contracting syphilis in the bath was noted by 'Imád-ul-Dín.

The rules about food exposed for sale were particularly severe. All slaughtering was to be done in official slaughter-houses. Goats' flesh was to be kept apart from mutton and marked with saffron. The tails were to be left hanging on the carcasses until the last moment to serve as a further distinguishing mark. The flesh of ewes was to be kept apart from that of rams; the flesh of sick animals was to be kept outside the shop and not mixed with sound carcasses. Such flesh was forbidden to be sold to public cooks.

At the end of the day's work the butcher was supposed to sprinkle his chopping block with salt and to cover it with palm matting to prevent dogs from licking it and to keep vermin away. Similarly, fryers of fish were ordered to wash their baskets each day and to impregnate them with salt. All unsold fish was to be salted in the evening and any that had gone bad was to be conveyed outside the city and thrown upon the public dung-hill. The cleansing and cure of fish was forbidden in any place but the one especially allotted for the purpose.[1]

Public eating-houses were inspected by the *muḥtasib* from time to time. He could order the cooking pans to be changed, if he thought fit. He could even seal up their utensils at night after his inspection in order to make sure that they were clean for the work of the following day. In all cases these vessels were to be kept covered up and protected against flies and insects.

In later 'Abbásid times the *muḥtasib* was known as the *qalandar*. He had the right to punish, even with death, gross neglect of the health of the public. It was not unknown for a

1 Ibn ul-Aṣír, vol. x, p. 173, quoted by Levy in *A Baghdad Chronicle*, p. 204.

baker to be thrown into his own furnace for selling poisonous corn and for a cook to be boiled in his own cauldron for imposing on his customers carrion or putrid meat.

Finally come those most important articles of diet—water and milk—the source of so many diseases in the East. The water supply of Baghdad was of two classes, the best water being derived from wells, the less good being taken from the river. The water was hawked around the city in large jars, which were kept covered by a perforated lid or by palm leaves. Water was sold to the passers-by by means of smaller pots, which were dipped into the large jar. It was strictly forbidden to drink direct from the main jar or to allow the hand to enter the water when filling the drinking pot. It was the duty of the *muḥtasib* to see that the small drinking pots were scoured daily and fumigated. It was strictly forbidden for a seller of well water to augment his stock by mixing it with river water. If such had occurred and it came to the knowledge of the *muḥtasib*, it was his duty to punish the offender by pouring away his water and closing his shop. A similar punishment was meted out if the jars were found uncovered or the drinking pots dirty.

River water was conveyed in a water-skin or open bucket. In order to maintain its purity the Caliph al-Muqtadí forbade the keepers of public baths to void their waste water into the Tigris and had special pits dug for its reception. It was forbidden to sell water for drinking purposes which had been put into new water-skins, for it was held to be affected by the tanning. Such skins were to be used only for the carrying of water to mills or presses or to builders' yards for the making of mortar. Only when the skin was free from tannin was it permissible to use the skin for the sale of drinking water. In the public bath it was compulsory to keep a large porous water-jar and this jar was to be labelled 'Public Drinking Water'.

The rules which governed the selling of milk were even more stringent. All vessels that were to contain milk were to be kept covered and washed daily. All dairies were to be whitewashed and paved and the roofs frequently renovated. The skimming of milk was unlawful; its dilution with water was even more strictly forbidden. It was the duty of the *muḥtasib* and his assistants to guard against such adulteration. Various tests were devised to check it. Among these was the dropping into the milk of a piece of water moss. If adulterated, a line of division became apparent between the water and the milk. Another test was to immerse a hair. If the milk was whole, some beads of milk would adhere to the hair; if it was diluted the hair would be drawn out free from milk.

Leaving public health now and passing to surgery, it may first be remarked that the subject of surgery among the Arabs has been the object of far less research than their medicine, partly because it is far less important and partly because far less was written on the subject by the Arabs and Persians themselves. There are, I believe, no classical monographs on the subject. The Persian medical student had to have recourse to foreign writers. Of these the most famous were Abú ul-Qásim Khalaf al-Zahráwí of Cordova (about A.D. 1000), who wrote a section on surgery in his *Kitáb-ul-Taṣríf*, or 'Book of Explanation', and Ibn ul-Quff, an Egyptian Christian of about A.D. 1250. Even Ḥájjí Khalífa is compelled in his review of works on surgery[1] to quote a translated work of Hippocrates and a Turkish version of a Greek manual as the most typical and authoritative works. In another place he quotes a work which I imagine does not exist to-day and which would be of the greatest interest. This he calls 'A Discourse on the Operations which are performed in Hospital'. Rhazes is said to have written a book on fractures and a monograph on surgery. There are also very good surgical sections in the *al-Manṣúrí* of Rhazes, Book VII, and in the *Liber Regius* of Haly Abbas, Book IX.

In the post-classical period the material for estimating the position of surgery is slightly more. There are the same remarks scattered through the big text-books of medicine. Occasionally, as in the case of the *Khuláṣat-ul-Tajárib* of Bahá'-ul-Doula, an

1 Ḥájjí Khalífa, *Kashaf-ul-Ẓanún*, vol. II, p. 589.

early sixteenth-century writer, a whole section is given over to discussing the principles and practice of the art of surgery. But in general, most writers seem to follow the dictum of Ḥájjí Khalífa that 'the use of Surgery is very great, but the practice and doing of it are more difficult than the acquiring of the theory of it'. In consequence, they leave it at that.

I have, however, discovered in the Bibliothèque Nationale of Paris a manuscript entitled *Zakhíra-i-Kámila* or 'The Perfect Treasury', in which the writer states in his preface that there being no good book on surgery he proposes to devote the whole of the second part of his book to that subject. It is in consequence a work of extreme interest and I am astonished that it has not received any notice whatsoever from medical historians. It is mentioned neither by Leclerc nor by Fonahn. It was written in the middle of the seventeenth century.

The position of a surgeon in the times of the caliphs was one of honour. The surgeons of Islamic times were not looked down upon by the physicians, as they were in medieval Europe. The ultimate position of inferiority which was forced upon surgeons is in part attributable to Avicenna, who taught that surgery was an art which differed from medicine and was an inferior one. The commentators gladly spread this idea, for it fitted so well the theological views of the inherent impurity of the flesh. It also frequently involved a breaking of the ecclesiastical law which demanded that the genital organs should always remain covered. One Moslem writer even deprecated the operation of cutting for stone in the bladder on the grounds that it necessitated an exposure of those parts upon which the eye of a believer could not rest without sin. In spite of this Haly Abbas in the *Liber Regius* appears to consider treatment by drugs and treatment by surgery of equal importance, though it is true that he does not deal with surgery until he reaches the ninth book. The biographers, too, do not write in any disparaging way of those whom they call surgeons. They figure on the lists of the staff of the hospitals of Baghdad as the equals of the physicians.

True to the example of Galen, who was both the leading physician and the leading surgeon of Pergamum, the physicians of Baghdad seem to have engaged also in surgery. Rhazes and Avicenna both made contributions to the art, which cannot have been proposed on purely theoretical grounds. But the cleavage between surgeons and physicians and the development of specialization was already beginning. The lists of the staffs of the various hospitals show a division into a medical and a surgical branch. In the post-Mongol period the cleavage was complete. Bahá'-ul-Doula, for instance, was unwilling to perform any operation except under the greatest necessity. In his great text-book he refuses even to describe the treatment of gangrene, since he is writing for physicians. 'Master Surgeons know it well and there is no need for me to go into detail.' Nor will he attempt to set a broken limb:

> Since bone-setting is a form of surgery and is a dangerous practice, a skilled Master is necessary to watch and to learn from. Hence I have not described these operations in full detail, as is done in works on Surgery and Fractures. But I have written out the general principles, so that if there is no Master at hand and the need is very great, a brief reference may be made to this work.

It is also clear that in Safavid times, as in 'Abbásid times, all surgery was not yet in the hands of the blood-letter, the barber, and the charlatan.

The same factors, of course, which militated against surgery in Europe, were also present in Persia. The knowledge of anatomy and physiology was not greater in the times of Avicenna than in the days of Harvey. The uncertainty of what structures the surgeon would meet and what would be the effect upon the human economy of division or ablation of an organ caused the Persian and Arab surgeon to hold his hand and hence to make no advances in the art of surgery. The edict against post-mortem examinations, common to the medieval Catholic Church and to Islam, took away the easiest method of acquiring surgical knowledge. The great bugbear of ancient surgeons, sepsis, was so common that the same Persian word meant both a wound and pus. The unsatisfactory efficacy of water, oil or wine to prevent contamination made surgery a risky proceeding and led honest and cautious men to look upon it either as a desperate remedy or as a short-cut for those whose lack of skill and knowledge did not allow them to adopt more orthodox methods.

Then, too, there was the question of pain and the amount of suffering which a patient could endure with ultimate advantage. 'In diseases for which operation or cautery is the treatment', wrote Bahá'-ul-Doula, 'take care that the treatment is less dangerous than the disease.' To avoid this dilemma and to render surgery more safe and more possible mankind at all times must have searched for some form of analgesic. Homer says that Helen dropped a drug into the wine, as an antidote to grief and pain. In a later age Galen wrote: 'In cases of severe pain we narcotize with opium, for as Hippocrates teaches, moderate narcotism relieves pain.' This passage cannot have been unknown to the Persians. Closer still to their land were the Scythians, who, Herodotus says, used to inhale the smoke of burning herbs when operations were being performed. And on the other side of them a Chinese surgeon Hoa Tho was wont to use hemp for his operative cases.

In spite of the certainty that the Arabs and Persians used some form of anaesthesia, it is still uncertain exactly what they used and even how they used it. Two degrees of anaesthesia are to be recognized. The first is implied by the Arabic word *mukhadir*, which means an intoxicant or, as we should say, a drug. Of these the most powerful according to Avicenna is opium. Others less powerful are mandragora, poppy, hemlock, hyoscyamus, deadly nightshade (that is, belladonna), lettuce seed, and snow or ice-cold water. Such drugs produce insensibility to pain either by making the part very cold, that is cold both in the thermometric and in the humoral sense, or by exposing it to toxic properties which interfere with its normal sensation.

That Avicenna used these for his operations is quite clear, for in another part of the *Canon* he writes:

'If it is desirable to get a person unconscious quickly without his being harmed, add sweet-smelling moss to the wine or lignum aloes. If it is desirable to procure a deeply unconscious state, so as to enable the pain to be borne which is involved in painful applications to a member, mix darnel water in the wine. Or administer fumitory, opium, hyoscyamus (a half drachm dose of each), nutmeg or crude aloes wood (four grains of each). Add this to the wine and take as much as is necessary for the purpose. Or boil black hyoscyamus in water with mandragora bark, until it becomes red. Add this to the wine.

A similar meaning is to be ascribed to the word *tabannuj*, which occurs in the *Alfáẓ-ul-Adviyah* of 'Ayn-ul-Mulk, a seventeenth-century writer. It can mean nothing more than 'deadening by means of Bang' or hemp. To this use al-Rúmí refers when he writes: 'They give opium to the wounded man that they may extract the point (of a spear) from his body.'[1]

But that this is not the whole story is equally clear. There was another process of anaesthesia which was known by the word *tanwím*, which means to cause or induce sleep and exactly corresponds to narcotize. This is the word which 'Alí bin 'Ísá uses when he describes his more painful ophthalmic operations. Thus, in the *Taẕkirat* occurs the phrase: 'Before putting the patient to sleep raise the lids'; and again in describing the operation for splitting the lid he says: 'You must first put the patient to sleep, then evert the lid.' Similar directions are given in the case of the removal of hydatids, of the removal of pterygium, and for the ablation of pannus. In the ophthalmic work attributed to Ṣábit bin Qurra, the same sort of phrase occurs. 'The operation shall be done at the margin of the iris on the patient after you have put him to sleep.' He too uses the word *tanwím*.

The use of some form of anaesthesia can be traced into the period which followed the fall of the caliphs. 'Do not fail to understand', wrote Bahá'-ul-Doula, 'that every treatment which

1 Al-Rúmí, *Maṡnaví*, bk. ii, v. 1503.

involves severe pain or discomfort requires first the administration of a strong drug to the Faculties. After this has taken effect begin the operation.' I have discovered seven references to anaesthesia in his *Khuláṣat-ul-Tajárib*. In two of them he uses the phrase *bayhúsh kardan*, that is, to render insensible, and in the other cases the Avicennan word *mukhadir*. The word *tanwím* does not occur.

In the *Khirqa-i-Khánum*, a late seventeenth-century work, there is a chapter devoted to anaesthesia. Here the word used is *bayhúshdárú*, or drugs of insensibility. The writer states that he is quoting from a work entitled *Dastúr-ul-'Amal Khúrdan-i-Sharáb* or 'The Uses of Wine Drinking' by Qáẓí bin Káshif-ul-Dín, of which there is a copy in the British Museum (Add. 19619. i). There is also a concluding chapter in the *Zakhíra-i-Kámila*, which is contemporary or slightly earlier than the *Khirqa-i-Khánum*. The chapter is headed 'On Anaesthetic Drugs which are used for Amputations, Incisions, and Bandagings, so that the patient may not be aware of what is being done'.

There can be no doubt what the so-called *mukhadir* drugs were. Avicenna is sufficiently explicit. Their general use is further testified to by Firdausi in the *Sháhnáma*, when he speaks of an anaesthetic being administered to Rudába dissolved in wine. Bahá'-ul-Doula frequently refers to an anaesthetic pill, called the *Ḥabb-ul-Shifá* or 'Healing Pill', which he says may also be administered in the form of an electuary. He says that it is made up of ginger, rhubarb and datura. According to the *Khirqa-i-Khánum* the anaesthetic may take the form of a drink, a snuff or a pill. The directions for the preparation of an anaesthetic snuff repeat the complicated pharmacy which was fashionable in those days. 'Take the flesh of a sheep: free it from fat: cut it up into lumps: and in the centre place some braised henbane seeds. Set this in an earthenware jar beneath a heap of horses' dung until worms are generated. Then place the worms in a glass vessel until they shrivel up. When required, take two parts of these and one part of powdered opium, and instil into the nose of the patient.'

An exactly similar prescription appears in a contemporary work, the *Ṭuḥfat-ul-Mu'manín*, suggesting either that this method of anaesthesia was used by Persian surgeons of those days, or else that both writers were deriving from a more ancient source.

Whether 'Alí bin 'Ísá refers only to such opiates in his accounts of his operations is not known, for he gives no indication whatever what anaesthetic he used. Perhaps the answer, if further answer there be, will come through one of the as yet unexplored books of the alchemists. Abú ul-Qásim al-'Iráqí, a thirteenth-century alchemist, gives several recipes in his *'Uyún-ul-Ḥaqá'iq* or 'Essences of the Truths' for narcotic preparations, and suggests many non-medical uses for them. According to Holmyard one of them runs: 'Take equal parts of henbane, Egyptian opium, euphorbia, and liquorice seeds. Grind each of them separately and mix the whole by pounding. Then place some of the mixture upon any kind of food you like and whosoever eats thereof will sleep immediately.' A second recipe describes an incense which should put to sleep all the members of an assembly, particularly a convivial one. The main constituents are the seeds of mint, anemone and black henbane, euphorbia, Egyptian opium, tamarisk, expressed juice of jasmin and a kind of crocus. The mixture was to be compressed in a copper tube, placed in moist dung to ferment and finally dried. The method of application was to throw some of the dry powder, together with wood of aloes, into a censer burning rose oil. The author guarantees that every individual in the company will fall asleep, 'especially', he adds, 'if there has been wine in the assembly'.[1] The formula is of no interest, but what is of interest is that here again is a suggestion of narcosis by inhalation, a method which Mesue Junior had suggested in the formula which he invented and termed the anaesthetic sponge.

More certain than ever am I that the last word in anaesthesia rests with the alchemists and not with the physicians and surgeons. The author of the *Zakhíra-i-Kámila* describes an anaesthetic that

1 *Proc. Roy. Soc. Med.* vol. XXIX, p. 103.

he himself invented, which produced sleep within a few minutes, and which in one case kept the patient unconscious for seven days. So careful is he of his secret and so fearful of any ignoramus or malefactor using it that he wrote his prescription in the secret language of alchemy.

> Since this drug is to be used in the treatment of fellow men, let a man consider whether he knows any one competent and let him learn from him. Thus shall I be guiltless. And I hope that he who is incapable will learn the method of its use and bear it in mind, that he will abide by the word of God and the commands of the Prophet, and that after instruction by some competent person he will offer up prayers for the success of this humble one.

Then follows the prescription in a cryptic form. Whether any one can read this riddle to-day, I do not know. If not, his useful secret has gone to the grave.

Whatever the method of anaesthesia may have been, the range of operations which the Persian surgeon was willing to undertake was astonishingly wide. Surgery was divided into three branches and hence there was a certain amount of specialized surgery. Some preferred the surgery of the vascular system, which meant that they confined themselves to phlebotomy and its complications. Others preferred what was called tissue surgery; such men engaged in what would now be called general surgery. A third class confined themselves to the surgery of bones and the reduction of fractures and dislocations and were pure orthopaedic surgeons. Ophthalmic surgery was a speciality which was quite distinct both from medicine and from surgery. The caliphs employed their own personal ophthalmologists, just as they had their personal physicians. It is said that Jibrá'íl the ophthalmologist (not a member, be it noted, of the Bukht Yishú' family) was the first every morning to enter the apartment of the Caliph al-Ma'mún. It was his duty daily to wash the eyelids and to anoint the eyes of the caliph when he woke up after the night and afternoon sleep.[1]

1 *Hist. Dynst.* vol. IX, p. 164.

The surgery of the eye was certainly the most advanced, perhaps the only contribution to later ages, of Arab surgery. There is scarcely any operation of to-day which was not attempted, and often carried out with equal success by the Arabs of Baghdad. The specialized instruments used in their operations run into scores. They have been well described by Hirschberg in his *Das Buch der Auswahl*, accompanied by illustrations. Casey Wood has done the same service for English readers in his *Memorandum Book of a Tenth-Century Oculist.* Among these instruments is the forerunner of the injection syringe, a hollow needle, invented by 'Ammár bin 'Alí of Mosul, for the extraction by suction of soft cataracts. This was still in use by eye-surgeons in the seventeenth century in Ispahan. Fr. Raphael du Mans describes it as an instrument with a triangular barrel, open at either end for the plunger and needle and pierced by a hole in the middle for the exit of the evacuated fluid.[1]

The operations upon the head that I have remarked, include amputations of the uvula, this being an ancient Iranian operation, removal of tonsils by means of a two-forked prong, paracentesis of the drum of the ear, the removal of nasal polyps, and the excision of the whole tongue for malignant growths. Amputation of the tongue was also practised as a mode of punishment. So skilfully was it done that in one case at least the victim spoke better after the operation than he had before. Swelling of the inner canthus was treated by an incision down to the bone and the application of a red hot cautery. To Avicenna must be given the credit of introducing the treatment of lacrymal fistula by probing, when he suggested the introduction into the channel of a medicated probe.

The usual dental operations are described in the text-books, but I have never seen any suggestion of artificial dentures, although an Arab in the West suggested the replacing of lost teeth by the teeth of an ox. That the ancient inhabitants of Persia did not escape the almost universal plague of dental caries is

1 du Mans, *Éstat de la Perse*, p. 178.

evident from a passage in the *Zendavesta* which runs: 'There shall be no hump-backed, none bulged forward, no impotent, no lunatic, no poverty, and no lying there; there shall be no meanness, no jealousy, no decayed teeth, no leprous to be confined, nor any of the brands wherewith Angra Mainyu stamps the bodies of mortals.' To Mesue the Younger has been ascribed the first use of gold to stop cavities. He was certainly prolific in his dental prescriptions. He had also remarked upon the phenomenon which we now call sympathetic pain, for he advised that, when a tooth was aching, it should be extracted as speedily as possible to prevent the pain from being communicated to the neighbouring tooth.[1]

As far as operations on the head are concerned, I have not come across in the course of my reading any case of trephining. Branding was common as a treatment for insanity. Among the rarer cases of disease of the head is one of osteomyelitis of the skull. Bahá'-ul-Doula says that a master surgeon removed the diseased bone and replaced it by a piece of bone from the skull of a dog. The missing meninges were replaced by a slice of cucumber. The scalp was sutured over the wound and successfully reunited and the patient is said to have lived for many years more.

It was, of course, in cases of cancer that the most drastic operations were performed. Avicenna's description of the treatment of malignant disease might have been penned to-day. The only hope of cure, he says, is to take the disease in the early stages. The excision must be wide and bold; all veins running to the tumour must be included in the amputation. Even this is not sufficient; the affected area should be cauterized. Even then, Avicenna adds, cure is not certain. He quotes the case of a woman who had one breast removed for cancer. A few years later the growth recurred in the other breast. It is interesting in the light of modern therapy for malignant tumours to note that Bahá'-ul-Doula after stating the orthodox surgical measures adds that in his opinion no treatment is of any value except the application of lead dissolved in aqua fortis.

1 See Lindsay, *History of Dentistry*, pp. 11, 18.

Descending to abdominal operations, the subject becomes even more astonishing, for it is apparent that the surgeons of the so-called decadent period freely opened the abdomen and drained the peritoneal cavity in the approved modern style. When the Turk who murdered Mardávíj returned to his companions saying that he had ripped open his belly, he was bidden to return and cut off his head also. They remembered that they had among them a bedmaker whose belly had recently been cut open by a surgeon and stitched up, and that the bedmaker was now alive and well. Leaving anecdote aside, there is plenty of evidence for this assertion in serious medical writers. Al-Jurjání, describing a peritoneal abscess, writes that the only treatment is to incise the lower abdominal muscles, deepen the incision through the peritoneum, insert the hand and remove as much pus as possible, and then to leave in the wound a drainage tube. Bahá'-ul-Doula adds that the patient should be nursed after the operation in the sitting-up position and that, if necessary, another drainage tube should be inserted in the other flank. In another place he suggests that a special drainage tube might be made with a very fine point at one end and an air-tight bag attached to the other. If a small hole were now to be made in the centre of the tube, the pus might be evacuated by suction and the need for laparotomy be avoided. He thus anticipated Fowler and his position and Potin and his aspirator.

To a young, unnamed surgeon of Shiraz is to be attributed the first colostomy operation. It may well have been a case of malignant growth of the large intestine, for it is said that he tried innumerable purges without effect. At last, in despair, he took a lancet and plunged it boldly into the bowel. The colic was cured and the patient lived for some time after, although, as might be expected, the wound never healed. Possibly he was inspired to take the bold step by an account of a spontaneous enterostomy, which Avicenna had related in the *Canon*.

Liver abscesses were treated by puncture and exploration. A certain surgeon of Qazvin gained great repute by his skill in recognizing the right moment to insert the cannula. Similarly, an Arab, resident in Persia, was famous for his punctures of the spleen. It is recorded that he used a needle, heated to redness in a fire, and that he gave no anaesthetic to his patients.

Presumably it was only their ignorance of anatomy which prevented Persian surgeons treating rupture by operation. For their description of the forces which produce a hernia are excellent and it is difficult to see why they did not attempt to carry out a radical cure. Hydrocoels they classified as a watery species of rupture. Bahá'-ul-Doula describes an amusing case of a spontaneous cure in a man who had a rupture, or more probably a hydrocoel, as big as a melon. When on horseback the tumour rested on the saddle in front of him and he covered it with a special cloth. One day a drunken Turcoman met him on the road and demanded to know what was in his saddle-bag. When told, the Turcoman imagined that he was trying to deceive him and raised his club to hit him over the head. The poor man ducked to avoid the blow and the club hit the hernial sac with such violence that the sac was burst and the man fell from his horse. A surgeon was called who sewed up the wound. On recovering his health the man found to his delight that the rupture was completely cured.

It is in dealing with calculi of the urinary tract that the Persian surgeons are seen at their best. 'When physic avails nothing', wrote Avicenna, 'and you desire operation, it behoves you to choose for the work one who knows the anatomy of the bladder, who is acquainted with the space which lies between the two vasa deferentia, who understands the relative positions of the arteries and the fleshy parts of the bladder, and who will take care of all that needs care. Then there will be no injury to the reproductive system of the patient, no haemorrhage, and no chronic unhealing fistula.' Some of the more bold were prepared to remove stones from the kidneys by an incision in the loins. Avicenna stigmatizes this as a painful proceeding and an unreasonable operation. By the time of al-Jurjání such a method was entirely abandoned.

He writes that he had never heard of a surgeon performing such an operation nor even seen it described.

It was not until the stone was ascertained to be lying in the bladder that operative measures were usually considered. In the days of the Caliph al-Náṣir a surgeon named Ibn 'Akásha had a great reputation for his skill in such operations. In the later times of Shah Isma'íl there was another famous surgeon who had removed by operation hundreds of stones, some as big as a walnut or small apple. It is interesting to learn that the tradition of supra-pubic cystotomy continued among Persian surgeons to our day, for Dr C. J. Willis of the Telegraph Department in Persia, writing in 1879, says that lithotomy was frequently performed above the pubes and was invariably fatal.[1]

A stone impacted in the urethra was made to slip back, if possible, into the bladder. If this failed, it was removed by an incision into the urethra. The same procedure was adopted in a case of retention of urine, if a catheter could not be passed. In cases of obstinate stricture a small tube was inserted into the urethra proximal to the stricture and 'thus the patient is relieved from death, even though life be not very pleasant'. Occasionally the incision for retention was made in the abdominal wall. But the great difficulty in getting the wound to heal made cautious surgeons avoid this route, if possible. 'But even if the wound will not close', said Bahá'-ul-Doula, 'it is better to live with it open than die with it shut.'

Besides passing a catheter there were other, less surgical, methods of dilating the urethra, which were nevertheless recommended by surgeons. Avicenna suggested placing a reed within the channel and blowing down it, a procedure which was also used to cure an imperfectly descended testicle. Ghiyáṣ-ul-Dín suggested the insertion of a twig of saffron or the placing of a live louse within the meatus. A similar remedy was recommended by Ḥamd-Ulláh al-Mustaufí of Qazvin for strangury.[2]

1 *Brit. Med. Jour.* vol. XXVI, p. 4 (1879).

2 *Nuzhat-ul-Qulúb*, p. 45.

Even now the list of operative procedures undertaken by surgeons of those days is by no means complete. The excision of varicose veins and of haemorrhoids was a regular method of cure. Fractures were as satisfactorily treated then as they were in Europe until the discovery of X-rays. Many devices were invented for exerting traction upon the displaced fragments. When replaced, the limb was set in plaster of Paris, a treatment forgotten and not rediscovered until 1852. Abú Manṣúr Muwaffaq had already described it in the tenth century.

Amputations of arms and legs, both for pathological conditions and in cases of accident, were common. Later Persian surgeons lost the art of these operations, for Dr John Cook[1] states that when he visited Persia in the suite of Prince Golitzin in the year 1747 some Persian officers, who saw him amputate a leg, remarked that they believed that no such cure had ever been effected in their country. Whether artificial limbs were ever used is doubtful. Ibn Khallikán says that a certain grammarian, named al-Zamakhshárí, suffered the amputation of a leg after falling from his horse and used to walk about afterwards with a wooden crutch. The Arabic word he employs is not the ordinary word for a crutch and is not to be found in any dictionary. Possibly, therefore, it is a technical word meaning an artificial limb.[2]

Amputation as a punishment survived up to living memory. In such cases the executioner knew nothing of the art of surgery. The limb was struck off by repeated blows of a chopper or short sword and the stump dipped into petrol or oil. Until the accession of the present dynasty it was not an uncommon sight to see a sad procession making its way to the Mission Hospital. In the centre was a man, ghastly white, with one arm covered by a blood-stained cloth. He was on his way for a more elegant re-amputation.

Minor surgery was for the most part left to the barbers, known technically as *dallák*. It was they who opened abscesses, removed

1 Cook, *Voyages and Travels*, vol. II, p. 356.
2 Ibn Khallikán, vol. I, p. 547 and vol. III, p. 322.

the uvula in infants and possibly also their tonsils, and performed the essential operation of circumcision. In some cases this last operation was performed by a regular surgeon. Chardin tells the story of an Armenian provost of Julfa who turned Mohammedan. The ceremonial circumcision was performed by 'one of the Domestick Chirurgions of the Great Pontif'. The operation was very painful and it was two or three weeks before the provost could walk again.[1]

In other cases the operation was performed by a *mullá* or *qází*, that is a priest or a judge. In the case of adults, who would usually be renegade Christians, the *qází* was often satisfied with but little ceremony. In the event of the candidate being the child of a nobleman the operation was accompanied by as much pomp as a wedding.

> Kindred and friends in their best equipage assemble at the parents' house, as a symbol of their joy presenting him with gifts of sundry prices; and after small stay, mount the boy upon a trapped courser, richly vested, holding in his right hand a sword, in his left his bridle; a slave goes on either side, one holding a lance, the other a flambeau, neither of which are without their allegories. Music is not wanting, for it goes first, the father next, and according as they are in blood, the rest; others follow promiscuously. The Hajji attending at the entrance into the mosque, helps him to alight, and hallows him. To work they straightway go: one holds his knee, a second disrobes, a third holds his hands, and others by some trivial conceit strive to win his thoughts to extenuate his ensuing torment. The priest (having muttered his orisons) dilates the prepuce, in a trice with his silver scissors circumcises him, and then applies a healing powder of salt, date-stones, and cotton wool; the standers-by, to joy his initiation into Mahometry, throwing down their *munera natalitia*, salute him by the name of Mussulman.[2]

Among the poorer classes there was no such ceremony. When the operation was finished, the foreskin was thrown into the chicken-pen or eaten by sterile women who yearned for motherhood.

1 Chardin, *Travels in Persia* (Argonaut Press), p. 79.

2 Herbert, *A Relation of some Yeares Travaile* (Broadway ed.), p. 250.

Sháh ʻAbbás the Great was often pleased to dabble in medicine and surgery. He much enjoyed preparing tinctures of fruits and compounding drugs. As a surgeon he was skilful above the average. His favourite operation was the castration of his own slaves. His mortality rate is said to have been very low.

When Sháh Sulaymán wanted two singing boys castrated for his use within the harem, it was a French surgeon who was called in. He was offered a large fee and performed the operation quite successfully upon both. When the Frenchman asked for his money, he was bidden first to turn Mussulman.[1] On his refusal the minister of court 'bid him be gone like a Rascal, telling him withall that he did not think the Religion of the Christians had permitted such acts of villainy'. The operation was, in theory at least, also forbidden to Muslims. There was, however, a large demand for eunuchs which the barbers did their best to meet. The mortality after the operation was enormous and a barber with a low fatality record was more highly valued than the majority of surgeons.

In the realm of gynaecology there is very little to record. Firdausi indeed describes the Caesarian section which produced Rustam. Al-Aḥnaf ibn Kais is also said to have been born *natibus cohaerentibus* which rendered a surgical operation necessary, though more probably the author means that the child had an imperforate anus, not that the mother was incapable of normal parturition.[2] I have never found the method of performing this operation described in any work on medicine, and I am therefore inclined to think that Caesarian section was only a fiction of Persian poets. Even cancer of the womb was usually left untreated. In the classical period all cases of uterine disease were attended to by the mother of the patient or by a friendly midwife or neighbour. Haly Abbas when he speaks of procedures involving the female genital organs, always uses the feminine form of the verb. But in later days the pelvis was not so utterly

1 Tavernier, *Travels in Persia*, vol. v, pp. 8, 219.
2 Ibn Khallikán, vol. I, p. 641.

neglected by male surgeons. Cervical polyps were amputated: sterility was treated by the passage of sounds through the cervical canal: and abortion was produced by the insertion of metal probes, mallow stalks, or paper soaked in ginger. The regular and only treatment of atresia of the vagina was surgical. That this operation was carried out by male surgeons and not by midwives is shown by the statement of Bahá'-ul-Doula, who after discussing the diagnosis and treatment adds: 'Master Surgeons know well the method of the incision.'

Nor was the practice of obstetrics entirely confined to women. This I deduce from the fact that all the large systems of medicine contain a chapter on the management of difficult labour. The midwives were for the most part ignorant women and could scarcely have been expected to possess, far less to read with understanding, such works of learning as the *Canon* of Avicenna or the *Thesaurus* of al-Jurjání. Yet the former devotes a long chapter to the treatment of pregnancy, including a passage on dystocia, and the latter a similar chapter with a section on the induction of labour both by means of drugs and by instruments.

The subject of sex, the satisfaction of the sexual appetite, birth control and all that these subjects imply, was treated with considerably more freedom of expression than is usual even to-day. Sex entered so much into the daily life of the oriental that in this sense all the physicians of those days were gynaecologists. Avicenna seems to have felt that the subject was perhaps beneath the dignity of a physician, for having discussed the matter in the usual manner, he adds: 'It is by no means disgraceful for a physician to speak of the enlargement of the male organ and of the narrowing of the female who receives it and of her pleasure. Nay rather it is eminently proper, for it is by these means that the act of birth follows.'

In the latter days the congress of the sexes was magnified into a distinct science, known as the *'Ilm-ul-Báh*, and was looked upon as a branch of medicine just like anatomy. 'This Science', says Ḥájjí Khalífa, 'is part of Medicine or rather the chief part of all books on Medicine.'[1] Like the other sciences it became the subject of specialized study, and monographs, which the majority of persons to-day would call purely pornographic, came to be composed.

Books on this subject there must have been from the earliest time. It was to India that the first exponents of the *'Ilm-ul-Báh* turned. Among the works which they borrowed was one which still circulates in Persia to-day. This is the *Alfiyya Shalfiyya*, a work frequently illustrated with the lewdest of miniatures, which are themselves extremely interesting because, like the illustrations in the manuals of anatomy, they seem to be a traditional type. The same poses and figures are repeated in manuscripts of widely differing dates. They must represent the survival of a very early traditional painting.

The meaning of the title is lost. Late Persian writers interpret it to mean 'The Story of the Woman who had a Thousand Lovers' and it was therefore called *Alfiyya*, from the Arabic word *alif* meaning 'a thousand'. The *Fihrist* mentions two recensions, a greater and a less. Abú ul-Faẓl-i-Bayhaqí speaks of a summer house where a certain prince Mas'úd had the walls adorned with pictures illustrating this work. Abú Isḥáq At'ima (*floruit* A.D. 1410) attributes the work to a physician who wrote it as an aphrodisiac for a distinguished patron. Popular tradition ascribes it to al-Warráq, a fourteenth-century poet. But probably the work is much older than either of these. The prose version is the usual one to find in Persia to-day.

Possibly the first Persian to produce one of these pseudo-scientific works was Samú'l bin Yaḥyá al-Maghribí. Born about the beginning of the twelfth century in Spain or Morocco he fled to Baghdad, probably on account of religious persecution, and finally settled in Meragha. Here he wrote a medical work called *Kitáb-ul-Mufíd* or 'The Useful Book' and later his *Nuẓhat-ul-Aṣḥáb fí M'áshurat-il-Aḥabáb* or 'Delight of Comrades in the Conversation of Friends'. The first part of this second work according to modern views would be written off as pornographic

1 Ḥájjí Khalífa, *Kashaf-ul-Ẓanún*, vol. II, p. 8.

and not medical at all; the second part is strictly gynaecological. A medieval commentator has written inside the cover of the copy preserved in the Escurial in Rome the following note which sums up the contents:

> Tractatus...medico-anatomicus de mulieribus, ubi scelestissimus ac impudentissimus author agit de mulierum conversatione, de earum venustate, de mediis illas lucrandi eisque placendi, de requisitis illarum, quae sunt appetendae, reprobandaeve, de earum ornatu, vestitu, de modo componendi fucos, de medicamentis, cibo, potu ad venerem ciendam, de modo impediendi conceptionem procurandive abortum, atque de aliis impudentissimis rebus ad coitum pertinentibus, quas ego ob verecundiam praetermitto.

Contemporary with al-Maghribí and one to be included with more justification in a work that purports to deal only with Persian medicine was Shaykh 'Abd-ul-Raḥm ibn Naṣr of Shiraz, who died in Aleppo in 1169 and wrote the *Al-Íẓáḥ fí Asrár-il-Nikáḥ* or 'The Revelation of the Secrets of Marriage'. The original is in Arabic, but very early a Persian translation was made under the title of *Kanz-ul-Asrár* or 'The Treasury of Secrets'.

In the fifteenth century flourished al-Suyúṭí, that prolific writer whose literary output covered the whole area of Moslem science from commentaries on the Qur'án to unblushing pornography. I have already spoken of his 'Medicine of the Prophet'. His *Al-Báh fí Ḥukm-il-Nabbí* or 'Sexual Relations as ordered by the Prophet' is the work of a theologian who has studied all the precepts of the Prophet with regard to the gratification of the sexual desires. Though his bias was always towards theology, yet al-Suyúṭí wrote a few purely medical works. Among them was his 'Tract on the Cure of Children' and a discourse on the use of the depilatory.

The only examples of works on the *'Ilm-ul-Báh*, which are available in translation so far as I know, are the *Ananga Ranga* and the *Kama Sutra*, which are of course Indian, and the *Rauẓat-ul-'Aṭṭar fí Nuzhat-il-Kháṭir* or 'Garden Perfumed for the Relaxation of the Spirit', a sixteenth-century work in Arabic by Shaykh

Nafzawí. A translation of this last has been made into French by an anonymous writer. An English translation was made, I believe, by Sir Richard Burton, but remained in manuscript at the time of his death. It was found by Lady Burton and, together with his notes of extreme value on the subject, was destroyed by his wife in a frenzy of holy indignation. Shaykh Nafzawí was an inhabitant of Tunis, but he quotes al-Ṭabarí by name, tells several anecdotes about Baghdad, and admits in his preface that the work is largely founded upon Persian and Indian sources. Although the strictly medical part is less than in most of such books, it can be taken, I think, as a fair example of the medico-pornographic works which did duty for gynaecology in Persia from the twelfth to the seventeenth century.

Another very interesting and late work on the same subject is the *Khirqa-i-Khánum dar 'Ilm-i-Ṭibb* or 'Woman's Patches in the Science of Medicine'. This work is from the pen of Murtaẓá Qulí Khán Shámlú, the son of a governor of Khorasan and a favourite of Sháh Sulaymán. The work is therefore dated to the latter half of the seventeenth century. The first chapter of his book deals with the causes of sterility. To test whether the condition is the fault of the man or the woman the author suggests that the woman apply an onion to her private parts. If a second party can appreciate the smell of the onion in her breath, then the cause of the sterility does not lie with the woman. Another test is for both parties to pass water on to some barley seed. If in both cases the barley turns green and neither of the heap of seeds dries up, the fault lies with the woman. This is a variation of a much more ancient Egyptian test by which the woman passed water on to spelt and on to wheat. If the wheat grew, she was pregnant of a male child, if the spelt grew she was not pregnant at all.

Of the remaining chapters of this very interesting and hitherto unknown work, several are devoted to the technicalities of sexual intercourse, but others are of greater general interest. The chapter on anaesthesia I have already mentioned. There is another chapter on tobacco smoking and the effect that it produces on sore throats. There is a chapter on the treatment of syphilis with a quotation from an unnamed European writer. The whole book is, in fact, of great interest.

Reverting to more strictly medical subjects, a word may be said in conclusion on the technique of surgical operations and of blood-letting. On the day before a major operation the patient's system was cleansed by laxatives and phlebotomy. On the day of the operation he abstained from all food. If he felt sick, he was allowed to take a little lemonade or infusion of grapes or tamarinds. In the case of an operation performed with no anaesthetic, the knees were tied one to the other; the hands were also tied together or to the thighs. When an anaesthetic was administered the patient was prepared beforehand by a pill of opium, given three to four hours before the operation, or, if he was an habitué of opium, by a preparation of datura.

The site of the incision was washed in water and was often further sterilized by an embrocation of astringent wine.

When the operation was completed, in the case of a laparotomy the bowel was sponged with warm water and then with warmed wine or vinegar. Many kinds of suture were in use for the closing of the incision. In the case of a resection of the bowel the two ends were sewn together with fine gold thread. Another method was to hold them together with ants. The largest species of these insects that could be found was selected. They were made to bite the two separated ends of the gut while the surgeon held them together in close apposition. The insect was then decapitated, the body thrown away and the head left *in situ*. After the completion of the suturing the gut was washed with hot vinegar and returned to the peritoneal cavity. The wound was then closed, particular care being taken to sew up the peritoneum separately from the muscles.

The commonest sutures used for the closure of the skin wounds were thread or cotton or silk. Mesue Senior recommends strong silk for the suturing of arteries. Rhazes is said to have been dissatisfied with sutures of this nature and to have introduced sheep-gut sutures, which he obtained from harp players. Avicenna suggested pigs' bristles as less likely to cause infection of the wound, though their use was condemned on religious grounds by the Sháfi'ite school. The followers of Málik and Abú Ḥanífa, two other orthodox schools of thought, allowed them. When the very finest suturing was required, as in the case of operations on the eye, the hair of a woman was used.

The making of needles was entrusted to a special guild, the members of which took an oath not to mix soft iron needles with steel needles. The best needles were known as *al-musawwada*, had round eyes, and were sharpened three times and then polished. Sometimes special needles were prepared to meet the requirements of operating surgeons. Thus, 'Ammár bin 'Alí directed that his needles should be a hand's breadth in length without counting the point. The length of the point was to be equal to that of the top-joint of the thumb. A small button was to be attached to the needle to separate the point from the shaft. The point was to be triangular, as he held that an angular wound healed more quickly than a round one. It was the duty of the *muḥtasib* to see that no needle fell below specification.[1]

The operation of phlebotomy was performed with as much care, at least in theory, as was a major operation. When engaged in opening a vein the phlebotomist was bidden to hold the lancet between the thumb and middle finger; the index finger was left unoccupied in order to discover and hold steady the desired vein. Of the veins in the arm the cephalic vein was considered the healthiest and most desirable for the operation. Bleeding from the basilic vein was held to be dangerous on account of the subjacent brachial artery. In the case of the vena salvatella the incision was made lengthwise: in most veins it was oblique. In the leg the veins usually used were the interdigital veins and the long and short saphenous veins. Occasionally blood was let from the vein in the fraenum of the tongue and on rare occasions from the temporal vein.

1 *Ma'álim al-Qurba*, ch. 57.

Among the lower classes bleeding was usually performed in a garden or court-yard, though bleeding in public was forbidden. The patient squatted on the ground and a small hole was dug in the earth beside him. The operator put a ligature around the arm, massaged the desired vein, and finally plunged in the tip of the lancet. The filling of the hole in the ground showed when enough blood had been let. When this moment arrived or when the patient fainted, the barber took a little soil, rubbed it on the vein, and applied some strands of cotton, and to keep them in place tied up the arm with the patient's own handkerchief.

The indications for the operation of phlebotomy were many. There were held to be three main reasons. The first was for the evacuation of a phlethora of blood. This was the justification for the regular venesection of every adult in the spring. The second great indication was when it was desired to turn aside the blood flowing to a disordered part. If the object was to relieve pain, it was usual to bleed from a vein as near as possible to the site of the pain. If it was desired to prevent pain, it was usual to bleed from the most distant vessel. In both cases the vein opened was on the same side as the lesion. The third indication for phlebotomy was when it was desired to allow free movement of the blood and vital spirits.

The proper time for performing venesection was before midday, after the digestion of the morning meal and after the bowels had moved. Each organ of the body was believed to be connected with one of the signs of the zodiac. To let blood from a member during the sign of the moon governing that part was a perilous procedure.

If it was desirable to remove blood, but for some reason venesection was contra-indicated, the use of wet or dry cups was preferred. Cupping serves the same purpose as venesection, but removes the rarefied rather than the more viscid blood. The best time for cupping is the middle of the month, when the humours are in a state of agitation, and during the time when the moonlight is increasing. During that period the brain was held to be increasing in size, just as the river water rises in tidal rivers.

Finally, it was sometimes desirable to remove blood by means of a leech. In their choice of a suitable leech the Persians followed Indian opinion. The type considered most suitable was of the colour of duck-weed and had two longitudinal lines running down the back.

CHAPTER XI

THE MONGOL DOMINATION

WITH the destruction of the caliphate the supreme power in the Middle East—it would almost be true to say in the world—passed into the hands of the victorious Mongols. The dying Chinghíz Khán had divided up his empire between his four principal sons. The third, Ogotáy, was named Kháqán or supreme *khán*. In 1251 his brother, Mangú, succeeded him as Kháqán and promptly gave orders for two new expeditions to set forth—one against China under Qubiláy, the other against Baghdad under Húlágú. With the first there is no need to deal: the result of the second has already been described.

Thus once again Persia suffered a successful invasion; and once again, as in the days of the Arab conqueror, the invading forces brought no contribution with them to native Persian medicine. Yet the Mongols were not altogether destitute of appreciation of the benefits of science. It is true that in their rude way they ranked astrology and medicine of equal value in the prevention and treatment of disease. But possibly their astrologers were as proficient in medicine as were their doctors. Certain it is that as soon as they met scientists of culture and deep learning, when they first came into touch with the Persians, this attitude of theirs was considerably modified. Chinghíz Khán, for instance, attached to himself a physician who was captured at the sack of Samarqand. For Chinghíz Khán suffered from some chronic disease of the eyes. It is related that this physician was particularly hideous and had a most unpleasant manner. Nevertheless, so invaluable were his services to Chinghíz Khán that he worked his way more and more into his favour. After the capture of the city of Urganj the physician was emboldened to ask for a certain beautiful slave girl as his share of the booty, who had been allotted to Chinghíz Khán. The general agreed and the girl was handed over to the doctor.

But the girl was by no means pleased to suffer his hideous embraces and a few days later again the doctor made a petition to Chinghíz Khán. This time it was to ask that the girl might be chastised and compelled to obey her new lord. But now the physician had overstepped his limit. The old Mongol lost his temper, launched into a tirade against men who served the enemy of their country and could not make women obey them, and finally had the physician put to death and took the girl back to himself again.

Whatever good Persia may ultimately have obtained through the conquest of the Mongols, it is clear that the immediate result was one of material and scientific disaster. The Mongols cared nothing for human life nor for aesthetic treasures. The first big city to fall before their onslaught was Merv. This was destroyed by their general Tulúy in 1220. The geographer Yáqút has left a contemporary account of the city as he knew it before the sack and how he found it afterwards. It was once filled, he says, with libraries, men of science and writers. But when he returned he found that 'the people of infidelity and impiety roamed through these abodes: that erring and contumacious race dominated over the inhabitants, so that those palaces were effaced from off the earth as lines of writing are effaced from paper, and those abodes became a dwelling for the owl and the raven; in those places the screech-owls answer each other's cries, and in those halls the winds moan responsive to the simoon'.

From Merv Tulúy marched upon Nishapur, which after 8 days of siege met with the same fate. Here perished Quṭb-ul-Dín al-Misrí, the greatest of the pupils of Fakhr-ul-Dín al-Rází. An African by birth, a student in Egypt, he had come to Persia attracted by the fame of the teaching in Ray. He wrote much, both on philosophical and medical subjects. Nor were his opinions always quite orthodox, for in his commentary on the *Canon* he ventured to say that al-Masíḥí and Fakhr-ul-Dín were both superior to Avicenna in clarity and accuracy.

Two years later Chinghíz Khán dispatched another force to

destroy Herat and in the sack of that city the great Najíb-ul-Dín al-Samarqandí perished. Although he wrote several other books, mainly upon pharmacological questions, his reputation throughout the Islamic world rests upon his book called *Al-Asbáb wa al-'Alámat*, that is, 'Aetiology and Signs'. This book was the subject of an Arabic commentary by Nafís bin 'Iwaz of Kerman 200 years later, which he called the *Sharḥ-ul-Asbáb* or *Mújiz-ul-Asbáb*, that is 'A Commentary on the Aetiology', and which he dedicated to Ulugh Beg. This became in turn subject of another commentary and translation into Persian, the first two works being written in Arabic. This last version was called the *Ṭibb-i-Akbarí* and was written by Muḥammad Akbar Arzání in 1701 and dedicated to the Moghul Emperor 'Álamgír. To this I shall have to refer again later.

It is said that 1,500,000 persons were massacred in Herat and that a short time afterwards a body of troops sent back to search for survivors killed another 2000. The only bright spot in this terrible tale of destruction is the story that the children of Fakhr-ul-Dín al-Rází were spared on account of the greatness of their late father. The truth of this story is certainly open to doubt.

Ray, Qum, and Qazvin met with a similar fate, and though the difficult passes which lie between Hamadan and the Mesopotamian plains saved the caliphate for the moment, the delay was only of a few years. By the fall of Baghdad the loss to science was even greater than was caused by the destruction of the ancient cities and universities of Persia. Arab culture suffered a blow from which it has never recovered. Yet the very completeness of the destruction formed the means of fresh learning. The invincibility and the cruelty of the Mongols was sufficient to ensure a period of peace following the destruction of the caliphate. Their ruthless transport of captives from one side of Asia to the other meant that Chinese learning was now brought into direct touch with Arab culture. The wideness of the empire led at once to a decentralizing of learning and the absence of fresh fields to conquer induced the later Íl-Khháns to devote their energies to science and the arts. As for medicine, their ignorance compelled them to encourage those captives who could enable the maimed and wounded to take the field again as soon as possible. Hence, it is found that soon orders were given that smiths, artisans and physicians were to be saved from the general massacres and sent to wherever there might be need of them. Physicians, moreover, were exempt from taxation. Within a few years of Mongol occupation physicians of the conquered race were to be found occupying the very highest positions of State.

Húlágú reigned as Persian Īl-Khán for seven years after he had captured Baghdad. He fixed his capital at Maragha, a town in the north-west corner of modern Persia, and here with the help of a Persian he built his famous observatory of which the ruins are still to be seen to-day. The Persian who was his right-hand man in this matter was Naṣr-ul-Dín al-Ṭúsí, surnamed al-Muḥaqqiq or 'The Investigator'. This man, born in the year 1200, was brought up at Tus, and found his way to the court of the Caliph al-Musta'ṣim. Though a man of science, his interest in medicine was not great and there is no reason to believe that he was employed there as a court physician. His downfall was due to some verses of which the caliph disapproved. He was thrown into prison and escaping turned to Húlágú shortly before he set out on his expedition against Baghdad. Another story makes out that he was captured and carried to Húlágú by force. It is also said that the information which he gave to the Mongol leader made easier his successful attack upon Baghdad.

In the court of Húlágú he was more successful than he had been at Baghdad. He rapidly rose to power and was soon placed in charge of the revenues of all the schools of the Mongol Empire. Anecdote relates that he once saved the life of Húlágú when an unskilful phlebotomist had opened an artery by mistake for a vein. A negro in the company at once applied a bow string as a tourniquet and kept it applied to the arm until the bleeding ceased. The wound in due course suppurated and to Naṣr-ul-Dín was given the duty of deciding whether to open the abscess or not. He was fortunate in his decision and Hulágú recovered without further haemorrhage.

As soon as Baghdad fell, Húlágú gave orders for all astronomical books to be collected, for the wisest Baghdadi astrologers to be summoned, and for an observatory to be constructed on a mountain near Meragha. Naṣr-ul-Dín was placed in charge of the work and in a dozen years accomplished what was expected to take thirty. He died full of honour in 1274, being the first scientist to flourish under Mongol rule. His work did not endure for long, for in the time of Sh̲áh Isma'íl the observatory had fallen into decay and required extensive repairs. This work was entrusted to a certain Gh̲iyáṣ-ul-Dín of Shiraz, an astronomer simple and not also a physician. His methods were very different from those of Naṣr-ul-Dín. He incurred the shah's displeasure by the inordinately long time that he took to complete the work, 'for three years were spent before the cycle of Saturn was finished'.[1]

A few years later, also at Meragha, there died a rather different character, also a physician and also only secondarily interested in medicine. This was the great Christian Abú ul-Faraj Gregory, son of Aaron, usually known as Ibn ul-'Ibrí or Bar Hebraeus. His father was also a physician and was his first teacher. He was born at Melitene in 1226 and left his home to complete his medical studies at Damascus. Here he stayed to do post-graduate work, for he states that he was set in charge of patients at the al-Núrí Hospital. But he played truant to medicine. In his hours off duty he studied Greek and Arabic and already knowing Syriac betook himself to a study of history, philosophy and theology. Later he took orders and becoming a bishop was elevated to sees of increasing importance until at last he was nominated Metropolitan of the Jacobites.

His importance to later generations lies in the great work *Muk̲h̲taṣar-ul-Duwal* or 'History of the Dynasties', which he left behind him. This, although a general history, also contains many

1 *Aḥsan-ul-Tawárík̲h̲*, p. 137.

medical biographies. It is strange that the four great medical biographers of Islam lived, wrote and died within a few years of one another. Al-Qifṭí, who wrote the *Ta'ríkh-ul-Ḥukamá*, died in Egypt in 1248. Ibn abí Uṣaybi'a, whom I have had to quote so frequently, flourished in Damascus about 1250. Ibn Khallikán flourished in Egypt about 1270. And Bar Hebraeus died in Persia in 1286. On these four writers is built up the greater part of what is known about medicine during the time of the caliphs of Baghdad. All information given by later writers is either borrowed from them or, if not borrowed from them, is scanty and inaccurate.

Among the more strictly medical works of Bar Hebraeus is a general compilation similar to the *Continens* of Rhazes. He also wrote an abridgement of Dioscorides and of Ḥunayn; he commented on Hippocrates, Galen and Avicenna; and he is said to have prepared, but never completed, a translation into Syriac of the *Canon*. His 'History of the Dynasties' was written both in Arabic and in Syriac. The two versions are not quite the same. Probably he modified his Syriac version to suit the tastes of Islamic readers. The Arabic version was translated into Latin by Pocock in 1663 and in this version is readily accessible to European readers.

Húlágú died in A.D. 1265 and was succeeded by his son Abáqá Khán, who in turn was succeeded by his younger brother Takúdar Oghlú. Takúdar had been baptized into Christianity under the name of Nicholas. But on his accession he proclaimed himself a Moslem and took the name of Aḥmad. At this time the Mongols were at war with the sultan of Egypt. His conversion to the faith of the sultan seemed to Aḥmad a suitable moment to suggest an armistice. He therefore collected a special embassy, which should carry to the sultan a letter announcing his profession of faith and offering him terms of peace. Included in this embassy were two Persian physicians Kamál-ul-Dín and Quṭb-ul-Dín. Their letter of credence has survived. From the fact that Kamál-ul-Dín is given the title of Shaykh-ul-Islám and 'Model of the

Learned', and Quṭb-ul-Dín is called 'He whose word is sure', it would seem that both were not only doctors of medicine but also of law. The letter was found acceptable to the sultan and peace was concluded in 1282.

Of Quṭb-ul-Dín's early history and of his medical attainments it is possible to form a just judgement. For in the following reign of Arghún, who ruled as Íl-Khán from 1284 to 1291, a Jewish doctor, Sa'd-ul-Doula, was created *wazír*. This *wazír* showed great favour to Quṭb-ul-Dín and in return Quṭb-ul-Dín dedicated to him a work which he entitled *Tuḥfat-ul-Sa'diyya* or 'The Present to Sa'd'. This book, written in Arabic, is another of the many commentaries on the *Canon* of Avicenna and is of interest only because in the introductory chapter the author describes his own life and early struggles. He was born in Shiraz in 1236, he says, being the son of Ẓiyá'-ul-Dín Mas'úd al-Kázarúní, the ophthalmologist, and a nephew of the physician Kamál-ul-Dín abú ul-Khayr al-Kázarúní. From his early youth he had the desire to become a doctor. Under his father he began to study diseases of the eye as a speciality. His abilities and his father's influence secured for him a post in the Muẓaffarí Hospital in his native town at the age of fourteen. This post he held for ten years.

But the practice of medicine had not for him the attraction of philosophy. Avicenna, the prince of philosophers, became his hero. With avidity he began to read the *Canon*. For help with the difficult passages he turned first to his uncle and then to Muḥammad ibn Aḥmad al-Kayshí, and finally to Sharaf-ul-Dín Zakkí al-Búshkání, who was reputed to be the greatest authority on Avicenna of those times. None of these, however, nor the commentaries which were procurable, satisfied him. He therefore started to travel, always on the look-out for any work on Avicennan philosophy of which he was unacquainted. He journeyed through Khorasan, through the two 'Iraqs, through Baghdad, and then on to Byzantium. While still dissatisfied with his own knowledge, he was invited to accompany his uncle on the special embassy to Egypt. He eagerly seized the opportunity to visit a land which till now had been closed to him. In Cairo he found the perfect commentary for which he had searched so long. Three, in fact, he found which resolved all his difficulties. One was by Ibn ul-Nafís and was no doubt the *Mújiz-ul-Qánún*. The second was by Muwaffaq-ul-Dín Ya'qúb ul-Sámarrí. This was a gigantic work entitled *Sharḥ-ul-Kuliyát min Kitáb-il-Qánún* and attempted to solve all the difficulties that previous writers had found in Avicenna's masterpiece. The third commentary which he found was the *Kitáb-ul-Sháfí fí Ṭibb* of Abú ul-Faraj ibn ul-Quff, a pupil of Ya'qúb ul-Sámarrí. These, together with some other works which he found in Egypt, enabled him to grasp the full meaning of the whole of the *Canon* with such clearness that he determined to write a commentary himself. In the very year of his return from Egypt he set himself to the task. The *Tuḥfat-ul-Sa'diyya* is the result.

In addition to this work on general medicine Quṭb-ul-Dín wrote a treatise on his own speciality—treatment of diseases of the eye, a commentary on the *Canticum* of Avicenna, and books on jurisprudence, philosophy and astronomy. He died in A.D. 1311.

The apostate Aḥmad did not live long to enjoy his new faith, for his nephew Arghún, the son of Abáqá, persuaded the soldiery that the Moslems were receiving an unjust preferential treatment. The army therefore revolted and, capturing Aḥmad, put him to death by breaking his back and set Arghún on the throne. Arghún chose as his personal physicians Sa'd-ul-Doula, the Jew, of Baghdad, and Amín-ul-Doula, whose nickname was Khwájá or 'The Eunuch'. The former soon abandoned medicine for politics and Amín-ul-Doula was left alone with the responsibility for the Íl-Khán's health. In spite of the wisdom with which the early Mongols selected their advisers, they were as a whole a superstitious and absurdly credulous race. His credulity cost Arghún his life. There came to his court one day an Indian jogi who claimed to possess the secret of an elixir of everlasting youth. Arghún at once took the jogi to himself and bade him prepare his elixir. In vain did Amín-ul-Doula and other orthodox physicians beg the Íl-Khán to put such foolish notions out of his head. Arghún would have none of them and, when the preparation of the elixir was completed, began a course of treatment.

Fortunately for the world the constituents of this elixir are preserved in the Persian chronicles. One historian says that it contained olives and sulphur; another adds liquid gold, silk and henbane seeds. For eight months the Íl-Khán received this magical preparation and then after the fashion of Brahmins entered upon a 40 days' fast. On the conclusion of the fast, so far from feeling younger, he felt considerably worse. In his despair he turned back to Amín-ul-Doula for advice, who recommended a change of air. Arghún left Tabriz and was soon well again.

With his restoration to health his unreasoning belief in quack medicine returned and he again took counsel with the jogi. Again the jogi prepared for him a draught, which he gladly swallowed and again he fell ill. This time he appears to have had some cerebral trouble and his state got daily worse and worse. Alms were distributed to the poor throughout the land, but still his condition did not improve. At last the jogi announced that one of his women, named Túqjáq, had bewitched him. When accused of this by the nobles of the court, the wretched woman admitted that, like other women, she had had an amulet prepared in order to conserve his affection. But it was now too late to save him. Arghún sank and died, a martyr to his superstition, a triumph for orthodox medicine. A few days before his death Sa'd-ul-Doula, who was accused by his adversaries of hating Islam and of giving lucrative posts to his co-religionists, was imprisoned and put to death. A pogrom of the Jews of Baghdad followed.

There were now three claimants to the Íl-Khánship. All three gained the supreme power in turn, but it was only the third, Gházán, a son of Arghún, who is of any importance. Gházán succeeded to the throne in 1295 and promptly proclaimed himself a Moslem. At the same time he repudiated the supremacy of the

Kháqán and thus became the founder of a new and independent dynasty in Persia. In token of this he transferred his seat of government to the ancient city of Tabriz. Tabriz, or Tauris, has played an interesting part throughout Persian history. Whether the city existed in Sassanian days is uncertain. Persian tradition ascribes its foundation to Zubdat-ul-Khátún or 'The Flower of Ladies', who was a wife of Hárún-ul-Rashíd. They say that she fell sick and was cured by a Persian physician. When she asked him what reward she could give to him, he replied that what he most desired was that she should build a city to the honour of his memory. The city was built and was called Tabriz, for *ṭibb* means 'medicine' and *riẓ* is the root of the verb which means 'to pour forth' or 'scatter'. Others, who find a difficulty in explaining why the *i* of *ṭibb* has been changed to an *a*, claim that not the wife of Hárún-ul-Rashíd but one of his generals was cured of an ague there. For *tab* means 'fever' and *raft* means 'gone'. All traditions agree that the refounding of the city was somehow connected with medicine.

Among his courtiers in his new city Gházán found a Persian from Hamadan whose name was Faẓl Ulláh bin abi il-Khayr bin 'Alí, usually known by his title Rashíd-ul-Dín, who had been a court physician to Abáqá. So high an opinion did he form of him that he immediately appointed him his *waẓír*. For 22 years Rashíd-ul-Dín held this post and was a loyal servant to the Íl-Khán. The credit for the construction of the fine buildings at Tabriz is usually given to Gházán; it might more justly be given to Rashíd. He founded colleges, hospitals, and libraries. One whole quarter of the city was named after him. This quarter is said to have contained 24 caravanserais, 1500 workshops and 3000 private houses, besides gardens, shops, mills, weaving and dyeing establishments, paper factories and a mint. There were 200 professional readers of the Qur'án with fixed salaries. A special street, in which dwelt the divines, juris consults and traditionalists, was situated near a quarter for students. Here he also had constructed a new hospital, which he placed under the direction of a certain Muḥammad ibn ul-Nílí. Letters are extant from Ra<u>sh</u>íd-ul-Dín addressed to his son and other people ordering them to furnish large quantities of drugs for the use of this hospital. The hospital must have been a very large one, for he demands as much as 300 maunds (about 15,000 pounds) of some of the oils and a yearly supply of nearly 100 maunds of each of aniseed, agaric, mastic, lavender, dodder and wormwood. In one of these letters, summarized by Professor Browne in his *Arabian Medicine*, he states that 50 physicians were attached to the hospital, who had been attracted to Tabriz from India, China, Egypt and Syria. Each physician was responsible for the training of ten students. In addition to the physicians on the staff of the hospital were surgeons, oculists and bone-setters, each of whom was in charge of five students. All these resided in a special street at the back of the hospital and had a regular allowance paid to them in money and kind.[1]

Ra<u>sh</u>íd-ul-Dín did not, however, confine his attention to the capital. The hospital of Hamadan, the city where he was born in 1247, had fallen into an unsatisfactory state through the misappropriation of its revenues. He appointed a new physician Ibn Mahdí to take charge and bade him pay more regard to the welfare of the patients and the proper supply of drugs than his predecessors had done. He also made arrangements for the auditing of the accounts for the future.

Even further afield a hospital at Shiraz came under his regard. For here, too, the old Atábegí Hospital had fallen into decay. He had it rebuilt and re-endowed and a new physician named Maḥmúd ibn Ilyás al-<u>Sh</u>írází was appointed to its charge. Ra<u>sh</u>íd seems to have had a great regard for this physician, for in another letter he ordered the governor of Baghdad to make a present to him of 100 dinars in cash, a cloak of grey squirrel, and a horse or mule with its saddle. Among the works of Ibn Ilyás are the *Laṭá'if-ul-Ra<u>sh</u>ídiyya* or 'Pleasures of Ra<u>sh</u>íd', a work evidently composed in honour of his patron but which is unknown to-day,

1 Browne, *Arabian Medicine*, pp. 103–9.

the *Tuḥfat-ul-Ḥukamá*, represented by a single manuscript now in Constantinople, and a short treatise on 'Treatment and Food', mostly in verse, of which I possess a copy. Rashíd also enlarged and enriched the Persian city of Sultaniya where he constructed a whole new quarter which was called after him the Rub'i-i-Rashídiyya. It contained a new mosque, a new school and a new hospital.

At some period of his wazirate Rashíd was compelled by Arghún to journey through India in order to impress the minor Indian monarchs and princes with the greatness of the Mongol power. Rashíd seized the opportunity to collect there certain useful drugs which could not be found in Persia. Among the rulers with whom he stayed was a certain Malik 'Alá'-ul-Dín. This monarch was much inclined to excess at the table; but so skilfully did Rashíd rebuke him that the royal host instead of being enraged, rewarded him with a handsome pension and on his return to Tabriz sent him a present of some clothes, precious stones, perfumes and carved ivories. Knowing his interest in medicine he included among the gifts some simples, some aromatic drugs and a special lotion for removing freckles.

In spite of all these activities Rashíd found time to carry out the orders of his patron who had bidden him write a history which should show the glories of the Mongol rule. This he accomplished, giving the finished work the title of *Jámi'-ul-Tawáríkh*, or 'Collection of Dates'. It has been partly translated into French by Quatremère. Hence there is no need to say more than that it forms one of the chief sources of our knowledge of the Mongol Íl-Khháns.

Among his written works are a few volumes on medical subjects which are so completely overshadowed by his great history that up till now they have received no notice. That they may contain some notable and original contribution to medicine is suggested by a chance remark in his history. Here he was discussing the Chinese system of sealing contracts by finger-prints and wrote: 'It is usual in Cathay, when any contract is entered into, for the outline of the fingers of the parties to be traced upon the document.' In stating that it was the outline of the fingers that was traced upon the parchment, he is probably wrong. In any case he is not the first to describe this method, for an Arab merchant, named Sulaymán, had mentioned the practice as early as A.D. 851. What is of importance is the remark which follows. 'For experience shows that no two individuals have fingers precisely alike.' If he only meant that their shapes were always dissimilar, the statement is of no interest. If he meant that the impressions of the fingers of no two persons were alike, then surely he is the first scientist to record the value of finger-prints as a method of personal identification.

With a view to preserving his works for later generations he bequeathed money for the purpose of making many copies. His works written in Persian he had translated into Arabic; those in Arabic he had translated into Persian. He even ordered versions to be prepared in Chinese. In spite of all these pains nearly all that he wrote has perished. No complete single copy of any work has come down to us.

Feeling that death was now near Rashíd bade his secretary draw up a list of his property and state his wishes for its disposal. This list shows that he possessed a library of 60,000 manuscripts, many of which were brought from China and India. He also possessed 1000 Chinese syrup jars of great artistic merit and Chinese boxes for electuaries. He was not, however, destined to die just then, for he recovered from his sickness and outlived his master Gházán.

The great Íl-Khán died in A.D. 1304, and was succeeded by his brother Uljaytú, who retained Rashíd-ul-Dín in office. Uljaytú died in 1316 of some abdominal disease and was succeeded by his son Abu Sa'íd, then only a boy of twelve. The lad could have no say in the appointment of his ministers, and the younger men of the court, envious of the long success of the *wazír*, determined to overthrow him. Rashíd was accordingly accused of having caused the death of Uljaytú and was impeached on this charge. The personal physician of Uljaytú, one Jamál-ul-Dín, was summoned to give evidence. Being asked to describe the circumstances of the death of the Íl-<u>Kh</u>án he said:

The King was taken with a violent indigestion, accompanied by an extraordinary diarrhoea with frequent vomiting. Being called and consulted about the treatment, I agreed with the other physicians present that astringents ought to be administered, that the stomach and intestines might be strengthened. Ra<u>sh</u>íd-ul-Dín alone was opposed to this treatment. He maintained that the illness was due to a repletion and that evacuants ought to be administered. We harkened to him and gave to the King a purgative. This increased the diarrhoea and brought him to the grave.

Ra<u>sh</u>íd was accordingly found guilty and was sentenced to death. He was executed together with one of his sons in the year 1318, being then aged seventy-one.

It would be difficult to over-estimate the value of Ra<u>sh</u>íd-ul-Dín's services to the Mongol cause. Born at a time when the unifying influence of the caliph of Baghdad was waning and finally overthrown, he made of Tabriz a new centre. He gave fresh impetus to science and scholarship and fortunately for Persia he threw in his lot with the conquerors instead of flying to an established Islamic power. By adopting Persian as his medium he set the fashion for science to make that language rather than Arabic the language of culture. By his catholic tastes he made the Mongol court of Persia the centre of learning throughout the world of Islam. His reputation as a patron extended from the far east to the west. Nor is this by any means an over-statement; for to one of his agents in Asia Minor he entrusted the duty of rewarding ten learned men who had written books in his honour. Of these, six were resident in Cordova, Seville, and other parts of Andalusia, and four in Tunis, Tripoli and Qayruwan.

Among the protégés of Ra<u>sh</u>íd-ul-Dín was a certain young tax-collector, Ḥamd-Ulláh bin abí Bakr bin Ḥamd al-Mustaufí al-Qazvíní, who was born in the year 1281 and became a revenue officer under the regime of the Íl-<u>Kh</u>án Abú Saʿíd. From his patron he acquired an interest in literature and, though his first book was finished too late to be dedicated to him, it was dedicated to Ghiyáṣ-ul-Dín Muḥammad, the son and successor of Rashíd-ul-Dín. Five years later he produced a vast rhymed chronicle in continuation of the *Sháhnáma* of Firdausi; and five years later still he published his *Nuzhat-ul-Qulúb*, a work which gives to him an honoured place in the history of Persian medicine.

The *Nuzhat-ul-Qulúb* or 'Hearts' Delight' is a scientific encyclopedia. It is divided into three portions. The first deals with the mineral, animal and vegetable kingdoms, chiefly from a pharmacological standpoint. The second portion deals with the structure of man and with his faculties and moral qualities. The third portion is purely geographical. An epilogue is devoted to curiosities which have found no place in the three portions which have gone before. The third portion and epilogue have been translated into English by G. Le Strange; some of the first portion is available in the English translation by Stephenson. The rest is virtually unknown to Europe.

The science of zoology and the veterinary art lagged considerably behind that of medicine. The Avestan text of the early Iranians contains two systems of classification of animals, one religious, one more or less scientific. According to the first classification the animal world could be divided into the good animals that Ahura Mazda created for the benefit of the world, and the noxious animals that Angra Mainyu created for its destruction. Of the good animals, the dog, the horse, the cow, the camel and the cock were the most important; of the noxious animals, the chief were wolves, snakes and flies. In the less theological portion of the *Avesta* is found the second classification. In this the animal world is divided into five kinds. These are those that live in waters, those that live upon the land, those that fly, those that are wild and those that have the cloven hoof.

In the case of sickness of any of the 'good animals', above all in the case of sickness of a domestic dog, it was the duty of the owner to call in a veterinary surgeon. The veterinary service of Sassanian days must have been well organized, for the sacred text states that animals were treated both by drugs and by surgery and that the fees of veterinary surgeons were regulated just as strictly as were those of physicians who treated human beings. In this case the amount of the fee depended upon the value of the animal treated. It is obvious upon reflection that any people who depend entirely upon animals for transport, must very soon evolve some system of treatment of their sick animals in order to prevent economic waste. It is not surprising therefore that dispensaries for sick animals figure in these primitive codes. It is much more surprising that there are not more surviving books upon veterinary medicine and more traces of the early methods of treatment.

Kindness to animals, though by no means a distinguishing mark of Mussulmans, survived after the fall of the Sassanian ideals. Niẓám-ul-Mulk tells the story of a certain pious merchant of Merv, who nursed back to health a dog afflicted with the mange. In a vision God declared to him that this act of his was more pleasing to Him than all his prayers, fastings and pilgrimages.[1] Sinán bin Ṣábit is another example of the care for animals in those days. He founded in A.D. 910 in Baghdad a dispensary for sick animals. He it was that sent out travelling doctors with the orders to attend 'first to men, then to animals'.[2] Herbert, writing in the seventeenth century, remarked on the continuance of this trait of sympathy for animals which he found among the Persians. For 'they not only erect hospitals for lame men and diseased, but sometimes for aged, starved, or hurt birds, beasts, and such creatures'.[3] In the 'Abbásid days it was one of the duties of the *muḥtasib* to see that heavy loads were removed from the backs of pack-animals when they were standing about while their masters rested.[4]

1 *Siyásat-náma* (Schefer's edition), p. 191. 2 *I.A.U.* vol. 1, p. 221.
3 Herbert, *A Relation of Some Yeares Travaile*, p. 332.
4 *Ma'álim al-Qurba*, ch. 8.

In Islamic times the veterinary surgeon was also the blacksmith. A somewhat greater knowledge than the mere ability to pare a hoof and put on a shoe correctly was expected of him and any loss of property, which he might cause, by inexperienced cutting, bleeding or branding was punishable by the *muḥtasib.*[1] The number of diseases which attacked animals was reputed to be 320. The methods of treatment of the various diseases of the various animals brought to the dispensaries were no doubt largely traditional and empirical. A large amount of Greek veterinary knowledge was also circulating in Baghdad. I have in my private collection of medical manuscripts a pseudo-Aristotelian fragment, written in Persian. The preface states that it is a translation. It is clear that the translation is not a very early one; but it may well be that although the original version was not Greek, it was a Pahlaví collection of Greek veterinary lore.

The manuscript is short and is entitled 'The Book of the Horse, a Pamphlet of Aristotle the Sage or Farasnáma'. The last translator has added an interesting preface:

> This book has been collected from the sayings of Aristotle the Sage in praise of horses, the good and the bad, their faults and virtues of breeds and uses, and their proper colour. It was composed for the Two-horned One, as men called Alexander the Great. It was translated by the Imám of These Times, the Sun of the People and the Faith, Moulána Muḥammad bin Ḥusayn (may God have mercy upon his soul) out of the language of the Turks into the language of the Persians, so that any one who might have difficulty with the Turkish tongue, should be able to dip into this book whenever he had need and might learn all that is connected with a horse.

There was a Muḥammad bin al-Ḥusayn al-Ṭúsí to whom is ascribed a work on metals now in the St Sophia Library in Constantinople. This work is called *Tansúkh-Náma-i-Ilkhání fí 'Ilm-il-Ma'daniyát*. The Turkish-sounding title suggests the possibility that the translator of the *Farasnáma* and the writer of this book are the same.

1 *Ma'álim al-Qurba*, ch. 40.

The Persian version of this Aristotelian work is divided up into thirty chapters. The first chapter is a description of a horse in general and claims to be the beginning of the original work. 'Thus spoke Aristotle: If you wish to recognize a good horse from a bad, see that it is tall, of good proportions, with a lower lip larger than the upper' and so on. All the chapters up to the ninth deal with the various tests which should be applied to see if a horse is sound. With the ninth the writer begins his descriptions of the diseases to which a horse may fall sick. In the twenty-sixth chapter he deals with wilful poisoning. It is amusingly worded:

A good horse should not be entrusted to any and everybody. For should such a person be hostile to the owner, he may mix in the horse's food some mullein or hellebore. Both these are poisonous to horses. The signs of poisoning by mullein are that the horse throws itself on to the ground and quivers all over. The right treatment for this is to give a maund of hot ghee which should be poured down the animal's throat.

Another veterinary work which has survived in a translation is the 'Pharmacopoeia of a Horse' or in the Arabic title *Aqrábádẓín fí 'Ilm Ṭibb-il-Khayl*, of which the original author is unknown. It does not claim to date back to the days of Alexander, but the preface shows that even in its present form it is a work of the thirteenth century. The translator's preface runs thus:

'The Pharmacopoeia of a Horse' treats of the recognition of thoroughbreds and the cure of their diseases. The book when discovered was written in Armenian and is now translated into Arabic. It discusses the breeds of horses, the points of a horse, the diseases which attack horses, the causes of such diseases and the methods of combating them whether by medicine, bleeding, amputation, or incision. It also tells how to manage a horse asleep and awake. The Arabic equivalents of the names of the medicines and drugs were unknown. But by chance among the prisoners of war there was discovered an Armenian surgeon who explained these terms in Arabic and gave the technical equivalents. Truly he was a man well versed in his profession.

The author of the work tells us that he has only written down what he has learnt by experience and those things of which he is sure. He adds that the original work was removed by the king of the Armenians from the archives of the caliphs in the school of Baghdad after his expedition with the conquered army. The original was in Arabic; he had it translated into Armenian. So 'Right comes into its own again. May God aid us in our objective and enable us to carry through what we propose.'

The first chapter of the original pharmacopoeia dealt with the treatment of diseases of horses and the distinction between a good and a poor horse. It was the work of the physician Muḥammad ibn ul-Khalífa Ya'qúb, an Arab by extraction, helped by a Persian of learning one Sa'd-ul-Dín bin ul-Ẓáhir. It was translated (that is, the second translation, from Armenian back into Arabic) by Maḥbúb, the Armenian, and his collaborator Abú ul-Faraj, who had a thorough knowledge of Arabic and was well versed in all languages. 'The book was carried off from the school of Baghdad by the king of Armenia in the reign of al-Ẓáhir Rukn-ul-Dín Baybars, King of Egypt (whose tomb may God make bright).'

This last paragraph dates the retranslation. For Abú ul-Faraj is almost certainly the celebrated Bar Hebraeus who died in 1286. The Sultan Rukn-ul-Dín is the sultan who reigned from 1261 to 1277. In the museum at Leiden there are two manuscripts which deal with horses called *Kitáb-i-Furúsiyya* and *Kitáb-ul-Khayl*, or 'The Book of the Horse'. These are written by one Muḥammad ibn Ya'qúb, whom Fonahn also calls Ibn Akhí Khúzám al-Khayli. They are both in Arabic and I imagine that they are the work of the same writer.

The Persians themselves seem to have made very few contributions to veterinary medicine, if the extant works on the subject are any criterion. For the most part they were content with translations. There is a Persian version of a Sanscrit work called the *Risála-i-Ṭibb-i-Aspán*, that is, 'A Pamphlet on Equine Medicine', by Zayn-ul-Amín. There is another translation from the Sanscrit, known as *Qurrat-ul-Malik* or 'Lustre of the

Monarch', of which a manuscript exists in the British Museum. And Muḥammad Qásim bin Sharíf Khán made a translation of an Indian work which he called *Tuḥfat-i-Kán-i-'Iláj* or 'Present of the Quarry of Treatment', which again deals with horses. A more important work is the *Kanz-ul-Hidaya* or 'Treasury of Gifts' by Fakhr-ul-Dín bin Aḥmad al-Rúdbárí from a fourteenth-century manuscript by al-Malik al-Mujáhid 'Alí.

The great Fakhr-ul-Dín al-Rází, whose work I have discussed elsewhere, did not disdain the study of veterinary medicine. In his great *Jámi'-ul-'Ulúm* or 'Collection of Sciences' he has written a chapter on the animals of the chase and on remedies applicable to various animals. It is indeed strange that a race like the Persians who were so athletic and so fond of sport, should devote so little attention to their animals. All the works described above deal with horses. There are also a few that deal with hawks. But I have never discovered a monograph on dogs or camels, although the former were essential for their sport, the latter for their comfort.

Less scientific information on zoological subjects is given by the commentaries on the classical poets. Animals and similes drawn from animal life play a great part both in the early Arab writers of the desert and in the later polished poets of the caliphs' court. Many names and *epitheta ornantia* were introduced. Philologists eagerly seized upon these often obscure words and built up learned discourses upon the themes which they suggested. In these cases the object of the treatises was not primarily scientific, but philological. Amongst such works is a book on animals, described as 'containing every curious sort of information', written by the learned Shaykh al-Jáhiz of Basra. The *shaykh* suffered from an early age from exophthalmos and was therefore also known as al-Ḥadaqí or 'The Goggle-Eyed'. He died in the winter of 868 from a complication of diseases. He himself used to say:

Maladies of a contrary nature have conspired against my body. If I eat anything cold, it seizes on my feet; if I eat anything hot, it seizes on my head. My left side is paralysed to such a degree that if it were torn with pincers, I should not be aware of it; and my right side is so afflicted with gout that if a fly walks on it, it would give me pain. I suffer also with gravel which prevents me from passing my water. But what bears hardest on me is the weight of ninety-six years.[1]

Besides these sources of knowledge there must also have been a certain amount of traditional zoology introduced into Persia by Greek soldiery and Western travellers and kept alive by the translations of the Greek classics. Evidence of such knowledge is to be found in the Greek names for snakes, for instance, and in the statement of al-Mustaufí that if the tongue of a frog be laid upon the heart of a sleeping woman, she will tell whatever she may have done. Stephenson points out that this statement is found in Pliny who quoted it from Democritus.[2]

In addition to all this al-Mustaufí had at hand two quasi-scientific works on natural history. One is entitled *'Ajá'ib-ul-Makhlúqát* or 'Marvels of Creation' and was written by Zakaríyyá bin Muḥammad bin Maḥmúd al-Qazvíní in Arabic in the year 1263. He rewrote and enlarged it in 1275 and died in 1283. To him has been given the title of 'The Pliny of the Arabs.' But the title is ill placed, for he has not the merits of Pliny nor was he an Arab. The other zoological work is the *Jámi'-ul-Ḥikáyat* or 'Collected Stories' of Núr-ul-Dín Muḥammad 'Aufí. This work, too, was written in Arabic and consists of a large collection of anecdotes, detached narratives and miscellaneous notices. To al-Mustaufí belongs the credit of having composed the first zoological treatise in Persian.

Nevertheless, al-Mustaufí can scarcely be called a first-hand observer, even though he remarks that the proboscis of a mosquito is hollow and that parthenogenesis is common among bees. He was a compiler, a collector, even a plagiarist. There is little or nothing original in the *Nuzhat-ul-Qulúb*. Yet for the first time the interest appears to be scientific rather than literary or

1 Ibn Khallikán, vol. II, p. 408.
2 Stephenson, *Trans. of Nuzhat-ul-Qulúb*, p. xiii.

curious. It is true that he frequently gives Mongol, Turkish and Arabic equivalents for his Persian names. But such philological notices are brief, and he rapidly passes on to a description of the animal and to its use in medicine. Hence comes the value of the work; for it is an excellent commentary on the animal preparations which were used by Persian physicians of his day.

The classification of animals used by al-Mustaufí is of the simplest. He divides the whole animal world into three classes, those that inhabit the land, those that inhabit the sea, and those that inhabit the air. Yet a more subtle classification is suggested in the introduction when he says: 'Every animal that goes on two legs, takes a single mate, and while mated is jealous. All those that go on four legs become enamoured of numerous mates. Those whose ears project from their heads bring forth their young; and those whose ears do not project lay eggs. And every animal that has horns, is without upper front teeth.'

Other zoologists followed. There is the famous bestiary in the Pierpont Morgan Library in New York, famous for its illuminations, called the *Manáfi'-ul-Ḥayáwán*, or 'The Uses of Animals', transcribed at Meragha about A.D. 1300. There is a work in the National Library in Paris, also called the 'Marvels of Creation', but not the work of al-Qazvíní. This was written in 1388 by a certain Aḥmad Marví for the library of the Sulṭán Aḥmad Khán in Baghdad and is illustrated. Another imitator, and the only other Mohammedan zoologist of importance, is the Egyptian Kamál-ul-Dín Muḥammad bin Músá al-Damírí, who finished his *Ḥayát-ul-Ḥayáwán* or 'Lives of Animals' in 1371. Here again is to be seen the strange phenomenon which I pointed out in the case of the medical biographers. All the first-class zoologists lived and wrote within a few years of one another.

CHAPTER XII

THE EMPIRE OF TAMERLANE

WITH Uljaytú and Rashíd-ul-Dín no longer on the stage the empire of the Íl-Khâns crumbled away. Abú Sa'íd indeed reigned for 20 years, but dying childless left the kingdom a prey to disorder. The rule of the puppet Íl-Khâns succeeded and Persia was in practice divided into two parts. The northern portion, ruled over by the Jalayr family, of whom Shaykh Ḥasan Buzurg is the most important name, made Baghdad their capital. The southern portion, held by the Muẓaffarids, was ruled from Shiraz and Kerman. Continuous fighting between these two families and between members of the same family left Persia an easy victim to any outside invader. Once again the invasion came from central Asia; this time it was Tamerlane, a Barlas Turk, who set up a new empire with Samarqand as his capital.

Tamerlane is perhaps the greatest conqueror Asia has ever produced. The name Tamerlane, by which he is known to Europe, is derived from his nickname Tímúr-i-Lang or 'The Lame Tímúr', for he was wounded in the foot in a minor encounter in Afghanistan. He was born in 1335, the son of a chief of a Turkish tribe. The lawlessness and divided loyalties of Transoxiana suggested to him that to capture that tract of country would be easy. In this he was successful. The first ten years of his life as a soldier were spent in consolidating his position and in conquering the neighbouring states of Mongolia on the east and Khiva on the west. It was not until 1380 that he began his career as a world conqueror by attacking Herat. Again he was successful and again there came a pause while he made sure of his position, and it was not until four more years had passed that he entered Persia. Ray fell in 1384, Ispahan in 1386, and Shiraz and Baghdad in 1392.

With all Persia now under his rule Tamerlane looked further afield and planned expeditions against India, Russia and Syria.

By virtue of these last two campaigns he came into touch with European powers. From Henry III of Castile he received an embassy who sought his friendship, for Henry believed that anyone who fought against the Syrian Turks must be a friend to the Christians. A letter sent back by the ambassador describes the passage of the embassy through Tabriz. Though no longer the capital, the city still contained about a million souls. When the Spaniards reached Samarqand, where Tamerlane had established his court, they were enchanted with the city. They described it as being 'a little larger than the city of Seville, being surrounded with gardens and vineyards'. The inhabitants were mainly captives brought from every part of the empire.

Tamerlane was already an old man when he met the Spanish embassy; yet he rallied sufficiently after their departure to set out in the winter of 1404 on a big expedition to subdue China. This winter was exceptionally severe and the army suffered much from the cold. In February of the following year Tamerlane himself caught a chill and though attended by a Persian physician named Maulána Faẓl Ulláh Tabrízí died in a few days, being then aged 71. He left his kingdom to his grandson Pír Muḥammad, the son of his eldest son Jahángír. Him he made his sole heir. But unfortunately Pír Muḥammad at the time of his grandfather's death was only 22 years of age and besides was absent in Kandahar, of which city he was governor. Advantage of this was taken by Khalíl Sulṭán, another grandson. Winning to his side the army and the grandees, he took possession of Samarqand and ruled there for seven years, until he was deposed for sheer incapacity by his uncle Sháh Rukh, who then ruled until his death in 1447. Pír Muḥammad thus never obtained the throne to which he was by law entitled. But a more lasting honour was his, for to him was dedicated the only Persian monograph on anatomy which has survived. This work does not contain much more detail than is to be found in the anatomical sections of the great compendia of medicine. But thanks to Dr Karl Sudhoff, who has published the anatomical designs which decorate the India Office copy of this work, it enjoys a reputation considerably beyond its merits.

It is convenient at this stage to consider the place that the study of anatomy held in the medical studies of the Persian. It is easier for historians to form a correct judgement about the progress in this branch of medicine than for them to judge of any other speciality. For Dr Max Simon in his *Sieben Bücher Anatomie des Galen* (Leipzig, 1906) has published the text of the Arabic translation of the seven books of Galen which no longer exist in the original Greek and has added an Arabic-Greek-German vocabulary of technical terms. The same service has been rendered to French readers by Dr P. de Koning in his *Trois Traités d'Anatomie arabes* (Leyden, 1903), which are a translation of the anatomical portions of the *Liber Regius*.

With the decay of the Alexandrine school of medicine and the death of Galen the study of anatomy declined. Marinus about A.D. 100 had discovered and described the inferior laryngeal nerves, the mesenteric glands and possibly the vagus. Galen a few years later contributed yet more to the world's knowledge and in his various books standardized anatomical teaching for many centuries. It is strange that there followed this lull and lack of progress. Academic lethargy is comprehensible even when the cause is not apparent. Wars and unsettled conditions, so far from being unfavourable to the study of anatomy, might well be expected to contribute something to it. Surgery, which is but applied anatomy, makes rapid strides when the world is full of wars and civil disturbances. But, though the civilization of Rome in those early centuries was being constantly threatened by the barbarians and war was continuous, no contribution of importance was made to the basic study of anatomy and surgery.

It is impossible to acquit the Church of her share in the retarding of this knowledge. Jundí Shápúr, the glory of the Sassanian Empire and the leading medical faculty of the world, produced nothing. There is not even a mention in history of any anatomist coming from that school. If Jundí Shápúr was indeed a Christian foundation and under Christian discipline, it is not necessary to look further or ask again why the great hospital failed to produce an anatomist.

Islam adopted the same attitude towards dissection that the Christian Church had done. Ibn ul-Nafís apologizes in his commentary on the 'Anatomy' of Avicenna that he is not able to supply first-hand information. But 'the veto of the religious law and the sentiments of charity innate in ourselves alike prevent us from practising dissection. That is why we are willing to be limited to basing our knowledge of the internal organs on the sayings of those who have gone before us.' Post-mortem examination in order to discover the cause of death was strictly forbidden. The most that was allowed was to see whether a death was a violent or a natural one. It is related that the body of a prisoner, who died in the Palace of Baghdad from what was clearly pulmonary tuberculosis, was submitted to the examination of a jurist and others. They contented themselves with pulling out the hairs of the beard and reported that the prisoner had died a natural death.

A minimum of practical anatomy had been learnt in the Sassanian days when it was the custom to preserve for scientific purposes the bodies of criminals condemned to death. A little more must have been acquired by the embalmers, who were frequently people of intelligence and high rank. It was their custom to remove the brain and intestines of a dead person and for the extraction of the brain a special silver instrument was invented. The heads of famous prisoners, too, were 'dressed' after execution before they were shown to the populace. Thus, Sulaymán Túlúní, the chamberlain, 'dressed' the head of Mú'nis after his murder by the Caliph al-Qáhir and had the curiosity to weigh the brain. He recorded that it weighed six *ratls*, that is about 70 oz., considerably above the average.

In the early days of al-Manṣúr the college of translators did not neglect anatomical texts. But these were not sufficient for Yúḥanná ibn Másawayh (or Mesue). His work as a physician has already been discussed, but his place in the history of anatomy is important because he seems to have been the only one who attempted in that ultramontane age to test for himself the facts of his predecessors. His reputation on this point rests upon a single text, but that authority is the great Ibn abí Uṣaybiʻa.

In the month of Ramaẓán in the year 221 (=A.D. 836) there came to Sámarrá the Ruler of Nubia who brought to al-Muʻtaṣim presents among which were some monkeys. I was with Yúḥanná on the second day of the month of Shawwál in that year. I was reproaching him because he had not been to my house, although Salmawaíh, Bukht-Yishúʻ, and al-Jarísh, all being physicians, had come and visited me, when lo and behold there came to us one of the household pages. He carried with him a monkey which the Ruler of Nubia had brought to Baghdad. And never have I seen a finer specimen.

Quoth the page: 'The Commander of the Faithful sayeth: "Marry this monkey to one of thy All-Blacks." For Yúḥanná kept monkeys and called them All-Blacks and he watched over them day and night. But this command displeased Yúḥanná and he replied to the messenger: 'Tell the Commander of the Faithful that I keep monkeys for a very different purpose from what he thinks. For I am planning to dissect them and to compose a book on the same subject as Galen. And should I succeed, this will be for the glory of the Commander of the Faithful. But in their bodies the arteries, veins, and nerves are too fine. I do not pretend that I can be as lucid on the subject as was Galen with his larger bodies. So I have abandoned my intention through pride. But the body of this monkey is big and, if it proves suitable, then the Commander of the Faithful shall know that I will write for him a book, the like of which has never been written in Islam.'

And he carried out his plan upon this monkey, and there was composed a work which even his enemies found fit to praise, let alone his friends.[1]

It is said that Yúḥanná ibn Másawayh has two works on anatomy to his credit, one called 'The Book of Anatomy' and the other 'The Book on the Formation of Man and his various Parts, on the number of the Muscles, Joints, Bones, and Blood Vessels,

1 *I.A.U.* vol. 1, p. 178.

and on the Causes of Pain'. I do not know if either of these exists to-day.

Contemporary with Mesue and famous both for his conversation and for his abstruse knowledge lived 'Abd-ul-Malik bin Qurayb al-Aṣmá'í, who among his writings on linguistic and antiquarian themes, wrote a treatise entitled *Kitáb-ul-Khalq-il-Insán* or 'The Book of the Making of Man'. Professor Nicholson discussing the position of al-Aṣmá'í in the literary history of the Arabs says that 'he was a favourite guest and that the Caliph would send for him to decide any abstruse question connected with literature which no one present was able to answer' and that his treatise on anatomy 'shows that the Arabs of the desert had acquired a considerable knowledge of human anatomy'.[1]

There were but few subsequent writers who did not borrow from the translations of Galen and possibly from Mesue's book. All the large text-books of medicine included a section on anatomy. Of these the most important were the *al-Malikí* (or *Liber Regius*) of Haly Abbas and the *Canon* of Avicenna. The latter is of importance only because of its length and detail and because it was extensively used by later writers on account of Avicenna's fame in other branches of medicine. But the anatomical sections of the *Liber Regius* are more deserving of notice, for they influenced a considerably wider set of readers than the medical students of the eastern caliphate.

About the time when Mesue was engaged in writing his 'Anatomy', the physicians of the little Italian town of Salerno, whether Jew, Arab or Christian, decided to meet together in order to advance their own knowledge and to train their successors. Thus was founded a school of medicine, known to us as the Salernitan school. The zenith of its glory was reached during the eleventh and twelfth centuries. Among those who frequented the school was one Constantine the African, who died in 1087, just a century after Haly Abbas. He was born in Carthage in 1010, but made his medical studies in Baghdad. Later he became

1 Nicholson, *Lit. Hist. Arabs*, p. 345.

a Christian and a Benedictine monk. Living partly at Monte Cassino and partly at Salerno he employed the knowledge that he had gained in the East to introduce Arab medical works into Europe. Hippocrates and Galen, of course, he selected first to retranslate. But it was the work of Haly Abbas that he chose to give to the world after the translations of the early Greek writers. Constantine's translations were an influence which affected all those trained in the school of Salerno. Thus, indirectly, through the hand of Constantine and the Salernitan pupils as they spread through Europe, a Persian physician became the source of European scientific knowledge.

Of Constantine's translations the anatomical portions of the *al-Maliki*, or *Liber Regius*, which he introduced to the Latin world as *Pantegni*, are of importance in the history of the growth of anatomy. His work was carried on by his pupil Joannes Afflacius, who died in 1103. These works were extremely popular and much copied and gave an impetus to a fresh study of anatomical detail. Like Mesue, the men of Salerno prove or disprove what the ancients had said by animal dissection. Whereas Mesue used monkeys, they used pigs.

Of their works on dissection there were two types, being known as the First and the Second Demonstration. The first demonstration only enumerated the parts of the body, stated where they were to be found, but did not attempt to describe them. The second demonstration is characterized by descriptions which were taken in many cases direct from the *Pantegni*. They were not always accurate, but they were brief and frequently practical. The Persians themselves always claimed that Haly Abbas was to be preferred to Avicenna on the practical side.

Thus, discussing the liver, the Salernitans wrote:

> It is situated in the right hypochondrium and is shaped like a Greek sigma. On the upper side, where with its five lobes, it is joined to the diaphragm, it is convex. If matter gathers here it causes dyspnoea and cough....On that side on which it is attached to the stomach, it is concave, and, as we have said, its five lobes surround the stomach.

Although the number of lobes varies in different animals, there are five in the pig, as I have recently shown you, and certainly the same number occur in man. Upon one of the larger lobes is the gall bladder....

None of the subsequent Persian writers deserves particular mention for his anatomical work. The fashion set by Haly Abbas and earlier writers continued. Al-Jurjání in the twelfth century fills up many pages of his 'Thesaurus' with anatomical descriptions which are in no respect better than those of Avicenna of a century before, which repeat his errors, and show no sign of discontent with his presentation of facts and theories. Even the not strictly medical writers like to include a chapter on human anatomy in their works. Thus al-Qazvíní, the naturalist, when writing about the wonders of the world has a long dissertation upon that greatest of wonders—the human body. The Imám Fakhr-ul-Dín, the theologian, disserts at length upon the mechanism and intricacy of the human constitution as another proof of the excellence and supreme wisdom of God. In fact, about this time an ignorance of human anatomy—at least, of what was incorrectly taught as human anatomy—was the sign of an incomplete education. This motif occurs in more than one place in the *Arabian Nights*, the most striking example being the Story of the Slave Girl Tawaddud, which is so long that it fills from the 449th to the 454th Night. This story, although omitted in many translations of the *Arabian Nights*, is of great interest to one studying the stage which anatomical knowledge had reached in medieval Baghdad. For the writer is presenting in Tawaddud a person who is fully versed in the sciences of her day but yet is not a trained physician. Her answers represent the popular but educated views and scientific beliefs of the majority of the learned classes.

Anatomy was not in those days looked upon as a subject fit only for medical students, but was considered also to be a branch of theology. It would not be incorrect to say that in anatomy theologians and doctors met. Ibn Ṣadr-ul-Dín defines anatomy as the science of the individual parts of the body of animals, of the reason for their composition, and of the miracles of creation and monuments of divine power stored within them. Hence he says that a man ignorant of astronomy and anatomy is a host incapable of receiving the knowledge of God. Even medical writers for the most part adopt this standpoint and, as Ḥájjí Khalífa points out, it was not until the days of the illustrated anatomical monographs that any attempt was made to make anatomy serve as a base for practical medicine.[1]

A notable exception to the generations of mere copyists was ʻAbd-ul-Laṭíf, physician, grammarian, and historian of Egypt, who was born in Baghdad in 1162. At the age of twenty-eight he wrote his book on the human body in which he demonstrated that Galen was in error when he stated that the lower jaw consisted of more than one piece. He even had the temerity to assert that the body was better understood by examination of a living subject than by the reading of the authoritative works of Galen and the Greeks.[2]

The great advance came in the year 1396 when Manṣúr bin Muḥammad bin Aḥmad bin Yúsuf bin Faqíh Ilyás composed his Persian monograph on anatomy, which he dedicated to Amírzáda Pír Muḥammad Bahádur Khán. In the original this work is unnamed. Subsequent generations have agreed in calling it the *Tashríḥ bi al-Taṣwír* or 'The Illustrated Anatomy'. I suppose the fact that anatomical illustrations do not appear in any earlier works is due to another prohibition of Islam—that of the making of reproductions of the human figure. In Mongol days there would be less dislike to such disobedience to the laws of orthodoxy.

Whether this is the earliest anatomical monograph, I am uncertain. There is, or was, in St Petersburg a manuscript entitled *Kitáb dar ʻIlm-i-Tashríḥ* or 'Book of Anatomy' by Ismaʻíl bin Ḥusayn al-Jurjání. I suspect that this is only an extract from the *Thesaurus* of Sayyid Ismaʻíl al-Jurjání. There is also a work in the British Museum entitled *Mukhtaṣar dar ʻIlm-i-Tashríḥ* or

1 Ḥájjí Khalífa, vol. II, p. 297.

2 *I.A.U.* vol. II, p. 201.

'Compendium of Anatomy' by Abú ul-Majd al-Bayzávi. This, which is the only known copy of the work, is incomplete and the date of its composition remains doubtful. All that is certain is that it was written later than 1288, for the author frequently quotes Ibn ul-Nafís. The book is written in Persian and is somewhat fuller than the *Tashríḥ-i-Manṣúrí*. There are no illustrations.[1]

Manṣúr's book is divided up into a dedication, an introduction, five chapters and a conclusion. The dedication and introduction are long and wearisome. There is the usual pious discussion of the wisdom of God in His creation of the human race and the usual fruitless argument about which organ is the first to be differentiated *in utero*. With the first chapter the more scientific portion of the book starts. The bones are here discussed at considerable length. The total number, exclusive of the sesamoid and the hyoid bones, is said to be 248. This is the figure that Tawaddud also gave and it was the generally accepted number by the traditional Islamic anatomists. Later this number was called into question and Ghiyáṣ-ul-Dín of Ispahan in his *Mirát-ul-Saḥḥat* pointed out that it is uncertain how many bones go to form the skull and into how many bones the pelvis should be divided and that the number 248 is therefore only traditional and not scientifically accurate. Shaykh Sa'dí, the poet, gives the number as 200, but I do not think that his figure is to be taken literally. He is only, I imagine, stating a large number which fits his verse.

In the next chapter Manṣúr deals with the nervous system. The nerves were to the anatomists of those days a structure comparable to the arteries and veins. They were the only three structures which were found distributed throughout the whole body. It followed therefore that their functions were similar. Now, arteries and veins are hollow and convey the spirit, the natural spirit from the liver in the case of the veins, the vital spirit from the heart in the case of the arteries. By analogy the nerves must be hollow and convey a spirit. As the nerves issue from the brain, of necessity it is the psychic spirit which they

1 British Museum Or. MSS. no. Add. 26307.

convey from there to the rest of the body. Some nerves, says Manṣúr, are mere tubes, such as the nerves which form the optic commissure within the brain and whose function is to convey the spirit of vision. Other nerves are not so obviously hollow; but even through these the spirit will make its way as 'water through mud or oil through an almond'.

The gross anatomy of the nervous system is well described. There are indeed faults, but these only later generations of anatomists were able to put right. Thus, Manṣúr held that there were only seven cranial nerves, that is, nerves whose origin was from the brain itself. Later anatomists have increased this number to twelve. He further considered the filum terminale to be a single nerve, so that he stated that there were thirty-one pairs of spinal nerves and one odd one.

In the third chapter he deals with muscles, a chapter which is the least satisfactory in the whole book. Muscles were still unnamed in his day. Manṣúr is content to describe the gross structure of a muscle, the varieties of muscle as they appear to the naked eye, and the number of the muscles. This last was always a difficult point with Arab anatomists, for unfortunately Galen, upon whose descriptions they so much relied, contradicted himself in his various works. The *Liber Regius* put the total at 554; Avicenna claimed that there were 570. Ibn abí Ṣádiq in his famous commentary on Galen frankly abandoned the difficulty and wrote: 'Personally I cannot reconcile the statements that Galen makes in each of his books on the subject of the number of the muscles.'

The fourth chapter deals with the veins. When reading this chapter it is needful to divest oneself of all ideas of circulation. Blood flowed centrifugally in the veins according to the Arabian School, just as it does in the arteries. Being a food it was gradually used up and hence the distant veins were smaller than those at the centre. Venous blood started its journey from the liver, just as arterial blood started its course from the heart. The superficial veins had been much studied from the point of view of phlebotomy; about the internal system their knowledge was not so accurate. All veins both superficial and deep originate in the liver and carry hepatic blood together with the natural spirit. There was one vein which was an exception which the Arab anatomists called the arterial vein and which we call the pulmonary vein. This must have been a difficulty from the beginning of time. For in the first place the structure was double; there are two pulmonary veins on each side. And in the second place it was generally acknowledged that all blood had to pass from the heart to the lungs and that some had to get from the right side of the heart to the left side. Avicenna, followed by Manṣúr, held that the pulmonary vessels were double because they had a double function to fulfil. Their first function was to carry blood to the heart and lungs for their nourishment. Their second function was to convey blood to the lungs for aeration. A double function required a double passage. The other difficulty was that blood entered the heart from the liver on the right side but was also found on the left side. Avicenna supposed that there was a visible passage connecting the right and left ventricles of the heart. Galen, who presumably had looked at many human hearts, knew that there was no such passage and supposed that there were invisible channels between the two ventricles. It was an Arab commentator on the *Canon* of Avicenna who refuted both these fallacies and, 300 years before Europe recognized it, described in his work the lesser or pulmonary circulation.

'Alá'-ul-Dín 'Alí ibn abí il-Ḥazm al-Qurshí, known as Ibn ul-Nafís, was born near Damascus, and not being a Persian lies in reality outside the scope of this work. But his masters were probably professors attracted away from the moribund school of medicine of Baghdad by the glories of the new foundations at Cairo and Damascus. Thus, though only indirectly, can Baghdad claim to have produced the discoverer of the lesser circulation. Among the many intellectual activities of Ibn ul-Nafís was a special study of the anatomical works of Galen and Avicenna. These studies he published under the title of *Mújiz-ul-Qánún* or

'Epitome of the *Canon*'. It was a practical work and soon became popular throughout the medical world. It was translated into Persian (though never into Latin, I believe) and was printed at Calcutta in 1828 and again in Teheran at the end of the century.

Ibn ul-Nafís died in Cairo in the year 1288. He is to be distinguished from Nafís bin 'Iwaẕ al-Kirmání, who besides writing his famous commentary on the *Al-Asbáb wa al-'Alámat* of Najíb-ul-Dín al-Samarqandí, also wrote a commentary on al-Nafís' epitome. This work he called *Sharḥ-i-Mújiz-il-Qánún*.

The earlier Ibn ul-Nafís, then, in opposition to Galen and Avicenna, wrote:

When the blood has been refined in the Right Ventricle, it needs be that it pass to the Left Ventricle where the Vital Spirit is generated. But between these two there exists no passage. For the substance of the heart there is solid and there exists neither a visible passage, as some writers have thought, nor an invisible passage which will permit the flow of blood, as Galen believed. But on the contrary the pores of the heart are shut and its substance there is thick. But this blood after being refined, must of necessity pass along the Pulmonary Artery into the lungs to spread itself out there and to mix with the air until the last drop be purified. It then passes along the Pulmonary Veins to reach the Left Ventricle of the Heart after mixing with the air in order to become fit to generate the Vital Spirit. The remainder of the blood, less refined, is used in the nutrition of the lungs. That is why there are between these two vessels (i.e. the Pulmonary Arteries and Veins) perceptible passages.

With these words Ibn ul-Nafís combated correctly, as we now realize, the views of Galen, Haly Abbas and Avicenna.

But to return to Manṣúr. He followed Avicenna in his incorrect theory about the flow of the venous blood within the heart. He also followed him in his statement that the human heart had three ventricles. To the small central ventricle (which actually is non-existent) he gave the name *dehlíz*. He also stated that the apex of the heart was strengthened by a special bone.

The fifth chapter of his 'Anatomy' deals with the arteries and their branches. It was generally taught in the Baghdad School that although the arteries contained some blood, their main function was the transmission of air and the vital spirit. The pulsation of the arteries was recognized as dependent upon the pulsation of the heart. It was also recognized that the isolated heart was able to beat with a rhythm of its own. Al-Jurjání long before had described how the heart of an animal, removed immediately after death, will continue to contract and dilate for some time outside the chest. From this experimental fact he deduced that there was a separate faculty of life inherent in the heart. The same faculty he postulated of the arteries.

Be it known that the movement of all the arteries equals the movement of the heart. Comparing the movement of the heart with those of the arteries there is found neither advance nor retardation; but they are equal. For the arteries are branches which spring from the heart. But, whenever an organ on account of a wound or boil or such-like contains pus, the arteries in the neighbourhood of the wound or boil beat earlier and quicker than the movement of the heart and the other arteries. This is due to the condition present; for arteries in the other organs whose condition is the same as that of the heart, have a movement corresponding to that of the heart to which they are subservient. If arteries could not initiate their own movement, then the pulsation of the arteries of an infected organ would not differ from that of the rest of the arteries. But, since the pulsation of these arteries is quicker and more frequent, we are sure that the movement of these arteries is autogenous.

Taking up this line of argument al-Jurjání was opposed to those who claimed that there was an ebb and flow of blood within the arterial tree. The contraction of the heart and arteries, which was appreciable to the examining finger, was not according to him due to the passage of blood within, as some asserted, but to a bellows-like action of the heart which drew in air from the lungs during cardiac diastole and expelled it into the body during systole. It was this doctrine, that the primary function of the arteries was to carry air around the body, that held back the discovery of the major circulation of the blood.

How they failed to discover it, it is hard to understand, seeing that they believed that at certain points the arteries and the veins communicated. Thus Haly Abbas wrote:

And you must know that during diastole such of the pulsating vessels (i.e. arteries) as are near the heart draw in air and sublimated blood from the heart by compulsion of vacuum, because during the systole they are emptied of blood and air, but during the diastole the blood and air return and fill them. Such of them as are near the skin draw air from the outer atmosphere; while such as are intermediate in position between the heart and the skin have the property of drawing from the non-pulsating vessels (i.e. veins) the finest and most subtle of the blood. This is because in the non-pulsating vessels are pores communicating with the pulsating vessels. The proof of this is that when an artery is cut, all the blood which is in the veins also is evacuated.

And Ghiyáṣ-ul-Dín could write:

The terminal branches of this vessel (i.e. the intra-cranial portion of the Internal Carotid artery) anastomose with those of the vein which has penetrated the brain and the mouths of the two become continuous.

The last chapter is devoted to what Manṣúr calls compound organs. Simple organs he has defined as organs of which the smallest part exactly resembles the whole. Thus, a tiny bone is still a bone and a branch of an artery has still to be called an artery. A compound organ is one which cannot be subdivided. Thus, the heart can be divided up into ventricles and auricles, but none of these alone can still be called a heart. In this chapter, therefore, Manṣúr deals with what we would call organs as opposed to the systems. Such a distinction is not quite accurate, for Manṣúr classes as compound organs the various constituent parts of the renal and generative systems.

The book is further enlarged by a terminal chapter upon pregnancy and embryology. The subject of embryology was an extremely complicated one for physicians of those days. On the one hand they had inherited the traditions and writings of the Greeks, based very largely upon actual experiments. On the other hand, as nominal Mohammedans, they were tied down to the Qur'anic doctrines of intra-uterine life which were a mixture of Jewish beliefs and primitive Arab superstitions. All the writers of the Arabian School were conscious of these difficulties. Add to this the fact that the discovery of the spermatozoon and the ovum was still to be made, and it is evident that to frame a theory of gestation and foetal development which would fit all the facts and all the theories was one of very great difficulty. It is not surprising that all their accounts are rather confused.

The teaching of Muḥammad upon the subject is very rudimentary. There is a curious foreshadowing of the doctrine of spermatogenesis in the verse of the Qur'án, which runs: 'The Lord brought forth from the children of Adam from their backs their descendants and made them bear witness against their own souls.'[1] Native commentators on this verse say that Allah stroked Adam's back and extracted from his loins all his posterity which shall ever be, in the shape of small ants. These admitted their dependance upon God and were dismissed to return whence they came. On the strength of this text theologians taught that the male semen is located in the back bone. It is to this belief that Sa'dí refers in that strange poem of his wherein he describes the excellence of gratitude and draws a parallel between the relation of foetus to mother and man to God.

> From the back of thy father till the end of old age
> Look what honours he hath given thee invisibly.[2]

It was generally held that there was both a male and a female semen, although the sexual cycle in woman was a doctrine still unborn. Others denied that the vaginal fluid was a true semen and claimed that woman made no contribution at the moment of conception. Manṣúr rebuts this latter school by pointing out that a woman is just as much under an obligation to perform the major ablution after a nocturnal emission as is a man and that the major ablution would not be ordered unless there was an exit of semen.

1 Qur'án, part IX, ch. vii. v. 172.

2 Sa'dí, *Búständ*, ch. viii. See also al-Rúmí, *Maṣnaví*, vol. I, v. 1636.

And he quotes the words of the Prophet Muḥammad, who once replied to an inquirer: 'The semen of man is white and the semen of woman is yellow. These join together. When the semen of the male is predominant over the semen of the female, a boy is procreated: and vice versa.'

The formation of semen was very elaborate in popular fancy, if the replies of Tawaddud, as related in the 453rd Night, are to be accepted as the beliefs of the desert Arabs. When asked how the seed of man is secreted, she replied: 'There is in man a vein which feedeth all the other veins. Now, water is collected from the three hundred and sixty veins and in the form of red blood entereth the left testicle, where it is decocted by the heat of the temperament, inherent in the sons of Adam, into a thick white liquid, whose odour is as that of the palm spathe.'

A further contribution to these embryological theories was made by those who had studied Indian text-books. Al-Ṭabarí in his *Firdaus-ul-Ḥikmat* includes an embryological section which is a mixture of Greek and ancient Indian knowledge. The ancient Greek metaphor of the resemblance of the foetus within the uterus to a cheese within a press is no part of Qur'anic tradition, but was introduced into Persia from India by Perzoes. In the introduction to the *Kalíla wa Dimna* (a book brought back to Persia by Perzoes after his Indian journey) occurs this passage: 'Man's seed falling into the woman's womb is mixed with her seed and her blood; when it thickens and curdles, the Spirit moves it and it turns about like liquid cheese; then it solidifies, its arteries are formed, its limbs constructed, and its joints distinguished.' The cheese analogy is not found in any of Avicenna's works, but reappears in the *Liber Regius* of Haly Abbas and in a philosophical work by the Ikhwán-ul-Ṣafá' or Brethren of Purity.

As far as foetal sex is concerned, Avicenna held that sex-predominance was to be found not only in the semen, but in the general constitution of both parents. Some people are boy-makers, others are girl-makers. A boy-making man has muscles not over-developed and yet is not flabby. His veins stand out;

his temperament is hot. The boy-making woman is similar. She is of a happy nature. Her eyes are brown. A male foetus is formed from semen derived from the right testicle. This biological fact is proved, says Avicenna, by the fact that Persian farmers can always breed bullocks by occluding the left testicle of the bull.

The first stage of foetal life, being invisible to the naked eye, the Qur'anic account is accepted without question. 'O People, if you are in doubt about the raising, then surely We created you from dust, then from a small life-germ, then from a clot, then from a lump of flesh, complete in make and incomplete, that We may make clear to you; and We cause what We please to stay in the wombs till an appointed time.'[1] The truth of this statement was held to be proved by the story of the evisceration of Shabíb al-Khárijí. Attacked by the orthodox forces under al-Hajjáj ibn Yúsuf he was defeated and fled to Ahwaz. Crossing the river his horse stumbled and threw him in. Weighed down by the heavy armour that he was wearing, he was drowned. His lifeless body was conveyed to al-Hajjáj, who ordered it to be ripped open. The command was obeyed. The heart was found to be as hard as stone, rebounding when struck against the ground. Within it was discovered another heart, about the size of a small ball. This contained the Qur'anic clot.[2]

Avicenna, neglecting the creation from dust, which signifies the original creation of Adam, re-echoes these words.

> When the womb shuts over the semen, then has arrived the First Stage.... A swelling is present, which is cast into the midst of an humidity, that the site of the heart may be formed. Then to the right and above are formed two other swellings, ramifications as it were, which touch for a while. These next become separate and distinct. The first is the clot for the heart, the second the clot for the liver.... The appearance of this clot is the Second Stage.... And the Third Stage is its conversion into the chief organs; and the generation of the heart and the principal organs is completed.

1 Qur'án, ch. xxii, v. 5.

2 Ibn Khallikán, vol. 1, p. 617.

Manṣúr indeed states that in an abortion on the sixth day the heart, liver and brain were already identifiable. But Avicenna and most writers give 30 days for the development through the Qur'anic foetal stages. After this point embryologists were uncertain what happened. Manṣúr and the Imám Fakhr-ul-Dín held that the heart was the first organ to be differentiated, although the umbilicus was the first to be completed. Rhazes held that the liver appeared first. Avicenna himself was doubtful and in consequence his account is somewhat confused.

The first thing formed which shows distinctly is the umbilicus, but the swelling of the heart, liver, and brain precede the formation of the umbilical cord, although the complete formation of these organs takes place after the complete formation of the substance of the umbilical cord.... The truth is that the first organ to form is the heart.

The complete formation of a male child takes from 30 to 40 days, that of a female 40 to 50. The foetus then rests quiescent for six months, although the mother will feel foetal movement after double the number of days that have passed in the formation of the child, that is to say, from 60 to 80 days in the case of a male child and from 80 to 100 days in the case of a female child. This feeling of foetal movement is also diagnostic of the date of going into labour; for the birth of the child will take place after three times the number of days, that is to say, a maximum of 240 for a male and 300 for a female.

The actual cause of the onset of labour, still a mystery to-day, was held to be foetal hunger. The foetus growing tired of the food roamed about the uterus seeking for something fresh. In so doing it breaks the placental vessels and at once seeks an exit. That is al-Jurjání's view. Manṣúr is content to say that when the foetus is strong enough, it forces its way out which may be at any time after the seventh month.

It is still a popular belief, even among educated people of Europe, that an eight-month foetus will not live. In India to-day the eighth month of pregnancy is referred to as 'the unnumbered month'. Manṣúr will not lend his authority to this view. 'If an eight-month foetus is healthy and strong, he ruptures the membranes and makes his way out and by the permission of Almighty God he survives. If he is extremely weak, he either dies within the abdomen or being born dies because the external air is unsuitable for him.' The real explanation of this belief is given by the astrologers and is quoted with approval by Ghiyáṣ-ul-Dín. 'The first month of intra-uterine life is dedicated to Saturn, the seventh to the Moon. If a child is born in the seventh month, when the Seven Planets have completed their ascendancy, he is destined to live. For the Moon is good fortune. But, if the child is born in the eighth month, Saturn is again in the ascendancy. And Saturn is a star of ill-omen and stands for death. It is therefore highly improbable that an eight-month foetus will live.'

The normal lie of a foetus was held to be in the breech position, that is to say, head uppermost. It was popularly believed that the lie differed according to the sex, a male child facing the maternal back and a female child looking forward. In the case of twin pregnancy one child presented by the breech and one by the vertex. Avicenna reports a case of quintuplets and another case in which a woman had four sets of quadruplets. Contrary to modern experience a case of twins in which the sexes differ has a bad prognosis: for twins of a similar sex the prognosis is good. Manṣúr states that twelve is the maximum number of pregnancies which a woman can endure, that the eating of salt during pregnancy will produce a child without nails, and that a woman and a mare react to pregnancy in a very similar manner.

Manṣúr's 'Anatomy' may be taken as typical of all the anatomical treatises which were produced by writers of the Arabian School. They are all characterized by a blind submission to the writers of the Greek age. Descriptions of bone and organs have become traditional; in many cases whole phrases and sentences are borrowed from an earlier text-book and interpolated in the new. Only very occasionally is the authority of Aristotle and Galen called in question.

Anatomy is not viewed as an exact science, but rather in a scriptural light, from a teleological point of view. It was far more fitting for the Persian to demonstrate the wisdom of God in the creation of man than to find out whether really his body was as he was describing it. It was much more important to explain *why* an organ functioned than to show *how* it carried out this function. The humoral theory with its trinity of spirits lay uppermost in the anatomist's mind. He must make his facts fit that theory.

To a certain extent these were the main causes of anatomical errors which once having crept in remained in the text-books for many generations. But it was also the use of animals for their experimental work and the argument from animal to man that bolstered up many false details. Even Hippocrates, experimenting with the chick, had built up his theories of human embryology from what he had seen in the egg. Yet medieval Persians were not blind to the fallibility of this line of argument and Ghiyáṣ-ul-Dín remarked that 'the proof from this is weak, for the argument from birds to man is not very weighty'.

It is often said that over-classification was another fault of the Arabian scientist. In some cases this is justified, but in the case of Manṣúr it is certainly not. His 'Anatomy', in fact, corresponds for clarity very favourably with any modern text-book. In the realm of theory and hypothesis, in physiology and pathology, it is true that their text-books become involved and difficult to follow. But the closer that they approach facts and practice, the less evident does their love of division and subdivision appear. And in Manṣúr's case any such criticism is quite unjustifiable.

The alternative name, 'Anatomy Illustrated', requires a word of explanation. Simple designs are often found in Arab anatomical writers. The two favourite diagrams are that of the skull and that of the eye. The former is usually included in order to explain the sutures and shows how the lambdoid suture or occipito-parietal suture resembles the Greek lambda, or even closer the Arabic letter *dal*, as Manṣúr points out. The diagram of the eye is purely schematic and is intended to demonstrate that the structure of the eye is divisible into seven layers and three fluids. The lens is looked upon as a fluid, congealed like ice. Meyerhof in his *Ten Treatises on the Eye of Ḥunayn ibn Isḥaq* reproduces three such diagrams. In Manṣúr's 'Anatomy' a new type of picture appears, which is of great interest in the history of anatomy. This is a series of diagrams, each showing one of the great systems of the body. These were not an original work of the Persians. Aristotle in his *De Generatione Animalium* states that he used 'paradigms, schemata and diagraphs' in teaching human anatomy. Colonel Garrison suggests that it was these Greek diagrams which found their way into Persia via the Alexandrian School. For it is generally believed that Herophilus and Erasistratus taught their anatomy by the aid of pictures. Sudhoff considers that the origin of these pictures was either the Nile Valley or the plains of Mesopotamia. Under no circumstances can they be attributed to Persia. The inclusion of details of Greek, Egyptian, and even Hindu origin and the absence of any distinctive Arabian influence make it fairly certain that these illustrations are the residue of classical anatomy.

Typically these anatomical illustrations consist of five plates. So constant is this number that Sudhoff refers to them as the *Funfbilderserie*. The first represents the skeleton, viewed from behind. The head is hyper-extended so that the face looks upwards and backwards. The palms of the hands face backwards. There is no attempt at anatomical correctness. In the diagram shown by Sudhoff thirteen ribs are represented; in my manuscript there are fifteen. The next picture represents the nervous system, the drawing also being made from behind with the head hyper-extended. Frequently the nerves are represented in different colours, the main trunk which runs to the extremities being in black and the smaller nerves in red. An occasional bone as a background is added in green. The cranial nerves are represented by one pair running to the nose, one pair shaped like a question mark representing the optic nerves, one pair running to the ears, and the remaining four pairs of nerves wave helplessly in space outside the skull.

The third and fourth pictures represent the arterial system and the venous system. In these the figure is represented from the front and the head assumes the correct position. The opportunity is taken in these diagrams to represent also the alimentary system. In these two illustrations the various manuscripts show considerable variation of detail. In one of my manuscripts (undated, because the final pages are missing) the centre of the illustration is occupied by a green pear-shaped object which clearly is meant to represent the stomach. Two little black patches on either side of the upper end of the pear are labelled 'liver' and all around is a thick broad band labelled 'diaphragm'. There are also two small red balls attached to the duodenum which are labelled 'right' and 'left' and are presumably the kidneys; while the spleen is unlabelled, but is placed in a relatively correct anatomical position.

The fifth picture represents the muscles and is the least decorative, least accurate, and must have been the least useful of the series. The human figure is again represented from the front. There is no attempt to show the borders of any of the muscles or the direction of their fibres. The figure is a mere outline with notes made here and there stating the number of muscles to be found in the vicinity. It is clear that the Arabs knew less about the anatomy of the muscles than they did about any other part of the body.

Some manuscripts have two more pictures besides these five. The first is one of the gravid uterus in which the foetus is represented as a breech or in a transverse lie. The other picture (which I also reproduce here) shows a naked female figure seen from the front. Large red dots mark the points where scarification should be employed. I think this figure may be a true Persian contribution to the series. It is certainly later than the others. The squatting position has been abandoned. The figure no longer looks rigidly forwards which, as Garrison points out,

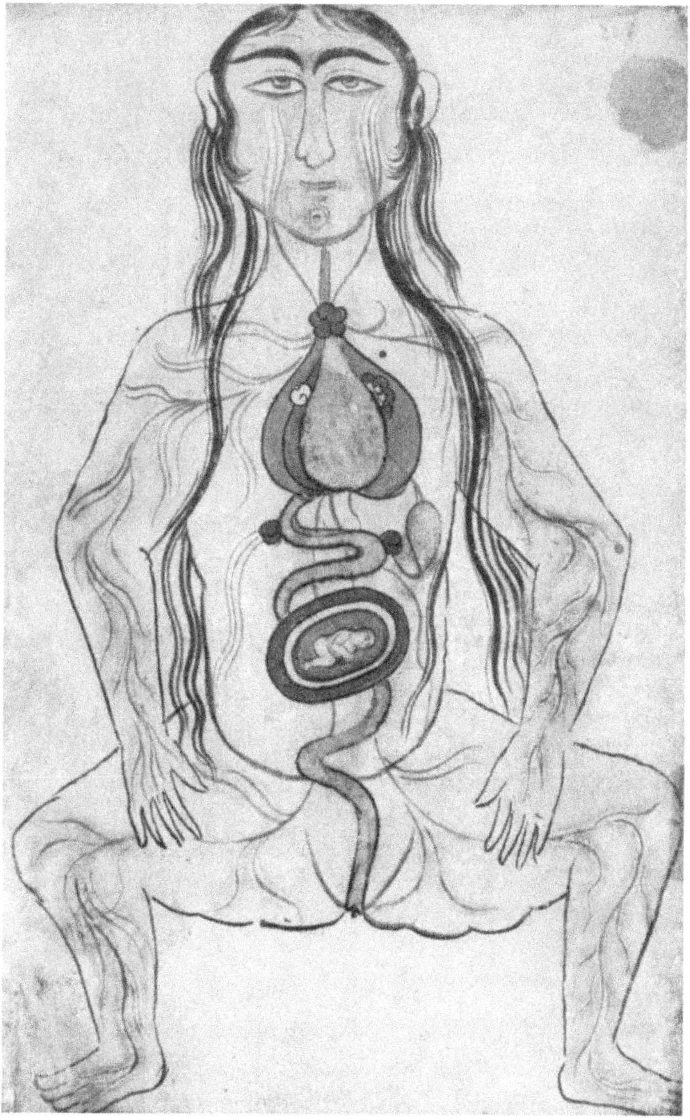

PLATE III. Female figure with gravid uterus

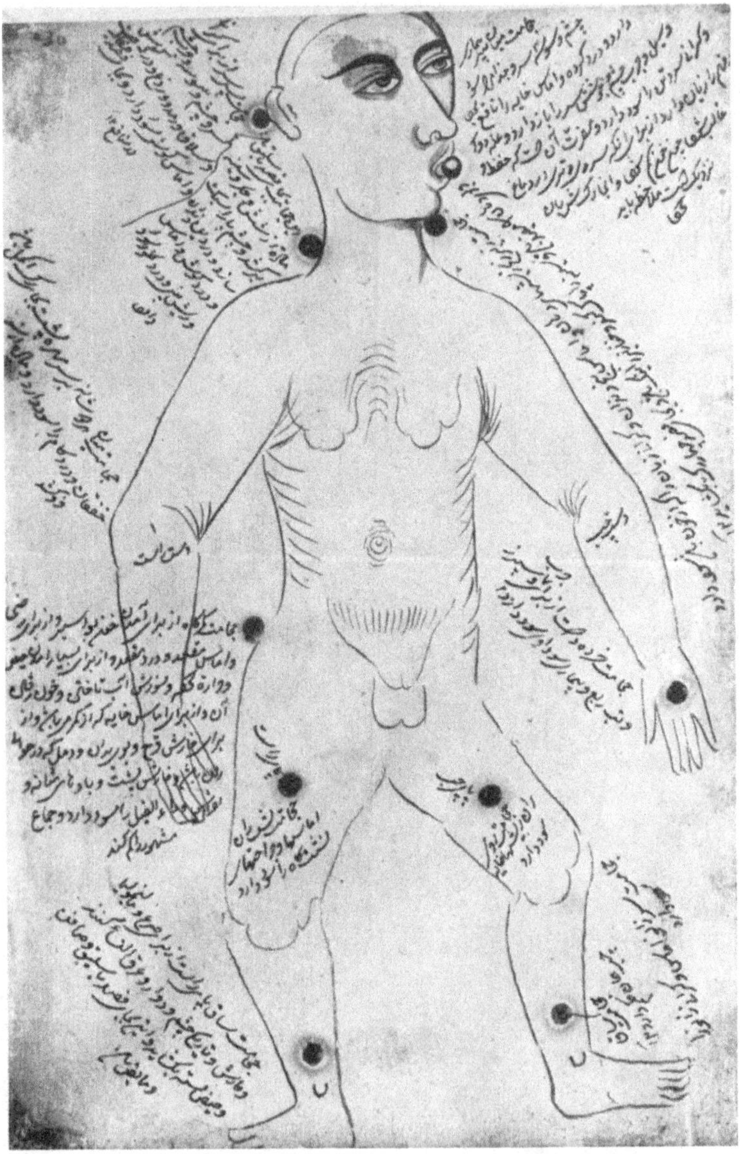

PLATE IV. Female figure showing points where scarification should be made

was typical of the Egyptian and early Greek figures. The breasts are depicted and for the first time an umbilicus is shown. This has affinity to the zodiac-mannikins of the purgative and blood-letting calendars of medieval Europe rather than to the anatomical illustrations of the Alexandrines.

Reproductions of the complete *Funfbilderserie* are to be found in works by Sudhoff, Choulant, Garrison, and in my small *History of Medicine in Persia*. Naficy, in his *La Médecine en Perse* also reproduces a diagram of the skeleton from a manuscript in Paris and a diagram of the eye to illustrate a manuscript of Ḥunayn's work on the eye.

Manṣúr's fame in the west rests solely upon his 'Anatomy'. But in Persia he is also known as the author of two other works. One, which I have not seen, is represented by a solitary manuscript in Calcutta and is called the *Ghiyáṣia* or 'The Aid'; the other is his large *Kifáya-i-Mujáhidiyya*, also known as the *Kifáya-i-Manṣúrí* or 'Sufficiency of Manṣúr', as opposed to the better-known work of the same name by Rhazes. The first title is of the nature of a pun; for it may mean the 'Sufficiency for Strife' (for knowledge or health, presumably) or the 'Sufficiency of Mujáhid'. For Mujáhid-ul-Dín was one of his patrons. The work is dedicated to Sulṭán Zayn-ul-'Ábidín of Cashmir and is dated 1423. It was lithographed in Lucknow in 1873 and is therefore easily accessible. As the contents have been analysed by Fonahn in his *Quellenkunde der Persischen Medizin* there is no need to say more about it.

THE ṢAFAVIDS

A SON of Tamerlane, Sháh Ruḵẖ, succeeded Ḵẖalíl Sulṭán. It is said that he was born while his father was playing chess, who when asked what name should be given to his son, replied 'King and Castle', and the name was given. He had been virtually ruler since his father's death, but it was not until 1409 that the court, sick of the scandals and extravagances of Ḵẖalíl Sulṭán, deposed him and made Sháh Ruḵẖ *de jure* ruler of the whole empire.

Sháh Ruḵẖ now left his son Uluḡẖ Beg to rule in Samarqand and made Herat his capital. His reign challenges comparison with that of Ḡẖázán. His followed the successful, though bloody, campaigns of Tamerlane: the other those of Chinghíz Ḵẖán. Both men were devoted to the arts of peace. Science was encouraged: men of learning were attracted to the court. Both reigns were distinguished for their architects: Ḡẖázán enriched Tabriz, Sháh Ruḵẖ Herat, Merv and Meshed. Long before his time the tomb chamber, believed to be the actual mausoleum built by al-Ma'mún over the remains of Hárún-ul-Raṣẖíd, had been the pride of Meshed. Later it was the burial place of the Imám Riżá. Many generations added to the buildings; even Maḥmúd Ḡẖaznaví added to the shrine and built a wall around it. It was left to a woman Gauhar Ṣẖád, the wife of Sháh Ruḵẖ, to add the mosque which is not only the finest building in Meshed, but also the best example of Mongol architecture. To the shrine of the Imám was added a hospital, at what date I am not sure, and in this there was a regular medical service for the pilgrims and others. The shrine appears to have been used as a kind of Chiltern Hundreds, for the Sayyid Mú'izz-ul-Dín Muḥammad Ispahání after he fell from the favour of Sháh Ṭahmásp retired and died there, and 'Imád-ul-Dín, the physician of Shiraz, after his dismissal from the service of Istajlú, was appointed by the Shah physician to the shrine.[1]

Unfortunately for Sháh Rukh he possessed no adviser comparable to Rashíd-ul-Dín. In consequence there is nothing of medical interest to record among the public works of the Tímúrids. Such scientific fame as they gained is due to the learning of Ulugh Bég during his governorship of Samarqand. He was, like so many of the Mongols, intensely interested in astronomy and he has left behind him some astronomical tables which the Savilian Professor of Astronomy in Oxford in 1650 thought fit to be translated into Latin and published. His two years of reign after the death of his father were not happy for him. For his nephew seized Herat, the Uzbegs plundered Samarqand, and his own son turned his arms against him, captured him, and finally murdered him in 1449.

The state of Persia now becomes one of confusion and perpetual war until the rising of the Ṣafavid family and the consolidation of the empire under Sháh 'Abbás the Great. Chief among the contestants for the supreme power were the two Turcoman tribes known from the device which they bore upon their standards as the Black Sheep and the White Sheep. The Black Sheep allied themselves with the Jalayr family, who ruled in the south. The White Sheep, founded by a grant of lands by Tamerlane, were in constant opposition to them. The greatest of the White Sheep chiefs was Ūzún Ḥasan, who first overthrew the reigning Tímúrid prince, thus making way for the accession of Sulṭán Ḥusayn, and then by defeating the chief of the Black Sheep made his tribe supreme over the western part of Persia.

To a certain Shaykh Junayd of Ardebil Ūzún Ḥasan gave the hand of his sister in marriage. The Shaykh was the direct descendant of the saint Ṣafiy-ul-Dín, whose tomb is to be seen in the mosque of Ardebil to-day, though it is the carpet which Sháh Ṭahmásp presented to the mosque in 1539, which has made the town famous. A son of Shaykh Junayd was presented by Ūzún

1 *Aḥsan-ul-Tawáríkh*, p. 141; *'Alam Árái*, f. 43.

Ḥasan with one of his daughters, who had been born to him by a Greek slave girl. From this union came three sons—Sulṭán 'Alí, Ibráhím, and Isma'íl. The two first died young; the third became Shah of a reunited Persia and the first of the so-called Ṣafavid line. The new dynasty thus had Greek blood in its veins.

Ūzún Ḥasan, having defeated his various rivals in the north and west, abandoned his provincial capital, Amid, and made Ispahan the seat of his government. Here, as ruler of Persia, he received the Venetian ambassadors who came to urge him to unite with the forces of Europe in the extermination of the Ottoman Turk. The mission from Italy was successful and Ūzún Ḥasan declared war upon the Turks. Thus there enters a new influence into the policy of Persia. In 1453 the Turks captured Constantinople and the Ottoman Empire was definitely established. During all this period the Persians wooed or quarrelled with the Turks as it suited their purpose. For the most part the claimant to the supreme power in Persia defied the Ottoman sultan, while his dispossessed rivals sought refuge in the Ottoman court where they attempted to persuade the Sultan to make their cause his.

There were at this period three foreign powers with whom the Persians had relations: the rulers of China, India and Turkey. The last was by far the most important, because she alone represented a potential conqueror. Consequently any Persian ruler who aimed at an independent empire, such as Tímúr had ruled over, was compelled to wage a more or less continuous warfare with the Turks.

Ūzún Ḥasan's relations with them ended with disaster. Though winning his first battle, he was severely defeated in the second and was compelled to abandon Ispahan and to retire to Tabriz, which he now made his capital. Here he died in 1477. His empire was broken up by various claimants to supreme power. The central government was carried on by his son Khalíl, but the outlying districts either struck out for themselves or attempted to unite with the Turkish Empire. Khalíl, after reigning only six months, was attacked and killed by his brother Ya'qúb.

During these last few years the city of Ispahan had become restless under the yoke of the profligate court of Tabriz and pro-Turkish views were predominant. In 1492 the city revolted against Rustam, who was now on the throne of Úzún Ḥasan, but on the appearance of the loyal troops, the governor of the city fled to Qum, where he was captured and killed. The city was again reduced to its White Sheep obedience.

This affection for things Turkish in central and southern Persia was carefully fostered by the Ottoman sultans. Jalál-ul-Dín, the famous mystic poet, received shelter in Asiatic Turkey and lived there all his life, so that he became known to his fellow-Persians as al-Rúmí or the Turk. Two other Persian scholars, less famous than al-Rúmí, were similarly honoured—one Jalál-ul-Dín Dawání of Shiraz, the other the theologian Faríd-ul-Dín Aḥmad-i-Taftazání, who received honorific letters from Sulṭán Báyazíd II.

Ūzún Ḥasan had died while Isma'íl was still a tiny child. His successor promptly sent him and his two young brothers to a castle, where they were kept for four years. They were released to serve a political end and only narrowly escaped a violent death when that end was accomplished. The death of the two elder brothers left Isma'íl the sole heir to the prestige of the Shaykh and his saintly ancestor. When he was old enough to look round, he found all the north-west parts of Persia under the rule of the chief of the White Sheep Turcomans. Khuzistan, Gilan and Mazanderan were independent and under their own chiefs. Yezd and Kerman were semi-independent under a Turcoman governor. Fars was governed by a ruler appointed by the chief of the White Sheep; and Khurasan was the territory of Sulṭán Ḥusayn, the last of the Tímúrids.

The strength of the Ṣafavid family lay in Gilan. Their descent from a saint made the family a rallying point for all the discontented members of the Shí'a faith. Just now these were many, for during the more or less continuous war with the Sunní Ottoman sultans, for the most part the Turks had been successful.

The conquered S̲h̲í'a minority looked for a deliverer of the Faith. In Isma'íl they recognized their champion. The new dynasty was thus reared upon theology and oppression, and it is not surprising that the sovereigns made dogma the test of merit and that in consequence scientific ability was no longer a key to high office. This tendency to intolerance had been growing ever since the days of the Seljúqs, when al-G̲h̲azálí, the famous *Ḥujjat-ul-Islám* or 'Proof of Islam', taught that the study of science was to be shunned 'because it leads to a loss of belief in the origin of the world and in the Creator'.

Within a few years S̲h̲áh Isma'íl acquired by conquest a kingdom which extended from Mosul on the west to Merv in the east, from Baku on the north to Shuster in the south, and so refounded Persia as a separate state. The dynasty which he thus set up is also described as the first national Persian line since the days of the Sassanians. The S̲h̲ay̲k̲h̲s of Ardebil were indeed Persians, but they claimed Arab descent and they spoke Turkish. In consequence, Turkish, Arabic and Persian were all current languages in those days. Persian, however, was the language of choice: even works dedicated to Turkish rulers were often written in Persian. Arabic was now only used as a sop to conservatism or, one often feels, as a *tour de force*.

These events coincide with the renaissance of art and learning, which is found fully developed in the court of S̲h̲áh 'Abbás the Great. It was an age characterized by great writers, such as al-Rúmí, Jámí and Mírk̲h̲wánd, and by great painters, such as Behzád. Though medicine flourished, its glories are far less. Ignorant of a similar rebirth which was sweeping over Europe, Persian physicians wrote, thought and talked as though they were the intellectual successors of Avicenna, as though the scientific world were still looking to them for guidance, as though the primacy of medicine had not passed to another land. Among this vociferous and imitative crowd there is one great exception, who, though almost unknown in Europe, was in my opinion the greatest physician who ever lived in Persia after the passing of the golden age of the caliphs of Baghdad. This was Muḥammad Ḥusayní Núrbakhshí Bahá'-ul-Doula.

The date of his birth is unknown. His father was Mír Qawám-ul-Dín and was a citizen of Ray. I am inclined to think that he also was a doctor, both because it was extremely common in those days for a son to follow his father's footsteps and also because there is found in the text of his only surviving work an unnamed person, whose doings and sayings Bahá'-ul-Doula frequently quotes with an intimate knowledge and reverence which suggests more than the relationship between teacher and pupil. More certain is it that his brother was a doctor, for he mentions him by name, calling him Sháh Shams-ul-Dín, and recounting his successful cure of an impotent man, who was enabled through his treatment to take two wives and to have a son by each.

Bahá'-ul-Doula studied medicine both in Ray and in Herat under Persian and Indian teachers and imbibed a great sympathy for and knowledge of Indian medicine. During part of his life he was attached to the suite of Sulṭán Ḥusayn Mírzá. It was no doubt at his death that he returned to Ray and became the leading physician of his native city. Here he very nearly died of an attack of dysentery, and here in the year 1501 he composed the only book which he is known to have written. Ḥájjí Khalífa says that he died in Ray in 1507.

His book, the *Khuláṣat-ul-Tajárib* or 'The Quintessence of Experience', is exactly what the title implies. It is the quintessence of a life of clinical experience, a summary of the observations of a man trained in the wide school of medicine which only Islam could produce. His quotations show the breadth of his reading. The name of Hippocrates appears twelve times, of Galen thirty-seven times, of Avicenna twenty-seven times, and of Rhazes ten times. Besides these he quotes Ṣábit bin Qurra, Sayyid Isma'íl of Jurjan, Ibn Bayṭár of Damascus, and others too numerous to mention. Only of writers of the western caliphate does he seem to be ignorant.

This work combines the clinical acumen and personal touches

of the *Continens* with the orderly presentation of the *Canon*. It is essentially practical, yet full of original observations and aphorisms. It is, I venture to think, the finest text-book of medicine in the Persian language to be composed after the Mongol invasion. Nor am I alone in my views. For 'Alí Afẓal Qáti' of Qazvin, a physician of the late Ṣafavid period, can recommend to his brother, just starting medicine, only two books in the Persian language, the *Thesaurus* of al-Jurjání and the *Khuláṣat-ul-Tajárib*. The former is, of course, of the pre-Mongol era.

Bahá'-ul-Doula himself must have been a keen observer. Scattered through his works are observations which a physician of to-day can neither accept nor deny. They have never been considered. Thus, Bahá'-ul-Doula asserts that stammerers never become bald, that a black and lustreless pupil in a state of health signifies a short life, that as long as a splenomegalic complains of pain in the left side there is hope of a cure, that a fruit-eater is very prone to catarrh, and that the appearance of pigmentary patches on the face or body of an epileptic heralds the cessation of the fits.

In addition to minor aphorisms, which are scattered throughout the book, there are several original contributions to the clinical study of disease. He was the first to record (as far as I know) the spontaneous cure of cutaneous leishmaniasis after twelve months of ulceration. In his chapter on eruptive fevers he describes three diseases which he says have passed unnoticed up to his time, which, though resembling, are neither small-pox nor measles. He makes one wonder whether he was not describing chicken-pox, german measles, and the Fourth Disease. In his terminal paragraph to the chapter on diseases of the eyes he is undoubtedly describing what is now popularly called hay fever, which was not recognized in Europe until 1819.

I have seen many persons whose brains have become heated in the spring by the smell of red roses. They get a catarrh and a running at the nose. They also had an irritation of the eye-lids, which, when this season passed, subsided together with the catarrh and the nose-running. These people were very little benefited by treatment.

In this connection, however, it is only just to point out that Rhazes had already written a book which he called 'A Dissertation on the Cause of the Coryza which occurs in the Spring when the Roses give forth their Scent'. The resemblance of phraseology is so close that it is almost impossible that Bahá'-ul-Doula should have made an independent observation of this type of hay fever.

His description of an epidemic cough, which occurred at Herat while he was there, can be nothing else but the earliest account of whooping cough. This disease was not recognized in Europe till the end of the sixteenth century and was not described until Willis wrote his monograph in 1674.

Coughs and such diseases as arise from excessive damp air, also sometimes arise from infected air on account of the aversion of the Spirit and the lungs to inhale infected air. I have several times proved this. Twice while I was at Herat, there was a mild infection of the air, which caused a universal cough without catarrh. The cough became so severe that it did not cease until vomiting occurred. Patients grew weak: children lost consciousness. Many people, old and young, fainted from the violence of the cough and in some cases during the first epidemic even died. At last an Indian physician ordered people to eat every day a miscal or more of raw ginger, dissolved in warm water. The second epidemic occurred in the spring and there were fewer fatal cases. The treatment was venesection, laxatives, feeding with powdered ginger, and so forth. I and all my household caught the cough, but by these methods of treatment it subsided in a couple of months. But it did not completely disappear until we had made a change of air.

Contemporary with and in direct contrast to Bahá'-ul-Doula is another physician, who, although as far as I can see wrote nothing original, yet because he represents the opposite school of thought, is worthy of a brief mention. This was G͟hiyáṣ-ul-Dín, a general practitioner of Ispahan. In faith he was a Sunní; in politics he was a pro-Turk. His training and sympathies were all Turkish. His father was a physician named Muḥammad ibn 'Alá'-ul-Dín of Sabzawar, who wrote a book called *Nus͟hka-i-Qawánín-ul-'Iláj* or *Zubdat* or *K͟hulásat*, that is, 'A Note Book', or

'The Cream', or 'The Quintessence of the Rules of Healing'. This was finished in 1466 and was largely based on the *Aghráẓ-ul-Ṭibb* of Sayyid Isma'íl al-Jurjání. The young Ghiyáṣ-ul-Dín was sent to Ispahan, where he made his medical studies under 'Alí al-Ṣadr and Sharaf-ul-Dín Ḥasan Shírází, a skilled physician who 'Imád-ul-Dín says was always drunk with hemp and opium. He then went further south and began to practise in Shiraz. But he did not stay there long and records in his own book that he went to Turkey to make his post-graduate studies. He records cases which he saw at Angora and at Brussa. After working there for an unknown number of years he returned and settled down in Ispahan. Here he wrote his only known work, which in gratitude for the help that he had received from his Turkish colleagues, he dedicated to the Sulṭán Báyazíd II. The book is dated 1490.

The book can be dismissed very briefly. It is entitled the *Mirát-ul-Saḥḥat fí Ṭibb* or the 'Mirror of Health in Medicine'. It is a dull exposition of the Arabian system of medicine, based mainly on the *Thesaurus* of Sayyid Isma'íl al-Jurjání. His source of inspiration is nowhere acknowledged. Many passages from the *Thesaurus* are taken *in extenso* and incorporated as his own. It is redeemed, however, from being an utterly worthless plagiarism by its full and detailed section on drugs, by its exposition of Turkish teaching and Turkish equivalents, and by the concise method in which it reduces the whole subject of physiology, anatomy and general medicine from nine books in the *Thesaurus* to less than 500 folios.

In 1524 Sháh Isma'íl died at Ardebil and there he was buried beside his holy ancestor. He left an orderly and organized kingdom and was succeeded without dispute by Ṭahmásp, who came to the throne as a child of ten and reigned for 52 years, dying in 1576. He made Qazvin his capital. Of his reign a great deal is known both from Persian chronicles and from European writers who accompanied the trade missions which now began to arrive in Persia. Anthony Jenkins came on behalf of Queen Elizabeth. An Italian mission was sent from Venice to persuade Ṭahmásp to wage a more vigorous war upon the Turks. Both missions have left an account of the country as they found it.

A certain amount, too, is known about the social position of the higher members of the medical faculty during this reign, as fortunately two lists of the court officials have been preserved. The Ṣafavid social system changed the feudalism of the old Perso-Mongol regime into a despotism with an absolute shah at the head. The State was made up of three classes—the ruling, the middle, and the working. Of these three classes the first was divided into two groups, the *amírs* and the *tájiks*. The former were mainly Turcomans and comprised the generals, the politicians and the men of action. The latter were made up mainly from the old Persian families, the hereditary repositories of learning, letters and clerical skill. It is into this category that the physicians and better class astrologers and druggists fall.

The chief physician of the royal household now became known as the *ḥakím-báshí*, and being 'the companion of the king's general and private assemblies, he used to enjoy great love and affection'. Feeling the shah's pulse was a prerogative exclusively his. He was responsible for the salary, grants and employment of all the doctors throughout the kingdom. He had the nomination of all physicians to the staff of provincial governors and in all medical matters the prime minister acted as he directed. Subordinate to him was the *'Aṭṭár-báshí* or chief druggist.[1]

In the early part of his reign Sháh Ṭahmásp attempted to put into force, at least in public, the strict moral code of Islam. Wine and music were forbidden; taverns, gambling dens and brothels were closed. In this he was supported by his *wazír* Amír Mu'izz-ul-Dín Muḥammad Ispahání, who unfortunately fell a victim to the plots of the *ḥakím-báshí*, at that time Rukn-ul-Dín Mas'úd al-Kázarúní. The shah foolishly listened to the slanders which his physician breathed in secret into his ear, and expelled his *wazír* from the court. Mu'izz-ul-Dín fled to Meshed, where he died with a reputation for great holiness. The shah soon

1 *'Alam Árái*, ff. 104 et seq., 761–7; *Khuld-i-Barín*, pp. 251–99.

changed his mind with regard to the value of the services which Rukn-ul-Dín had rendered to the State in securing the dismissal of the *wazír* and he caused the physician to be burnt. Rukn-ul-Dín was held by his contemporaries to be somewhat unorthodox in his methods of medicine, but such changes as he made met with general approval.

Among those who suffered from the wave of temporary Puritanism was another royal doctor named Ḥakím Ḥusayn of Shiraz, who had received the title of Kamál-ul-Dín. Caught after having wined too freely he was expelled from the court without further investigation. He took service under a certain Khán Aḥmad of Gilan, a minor governor, who was interested both in the theory and the practice of medicine. And there he died.

His disgrace did not prevent the shah from honouring his son Mauláná Núr-ul-Dín, who seeing what worldliness had brought to his father, adopted a severe and strictly religious attitude towards life. He was therefore chosen to succeed Rukn-ul-Dín, when he perished at the stake. He successfully combined the love of God with a love of medicine, for his contemporaries accounted him a good clinician and he refused the shah's offer to abandon science for politics. After his death another son of Kamál-ul-Dín of the name of Ghiyáṣ-ul-Dín 'Alí succeeded to the post of physician-in-chief.

Other physicians attached to the court of Sháh Ṭahmásp about this time were Mírzá Abú ul-Fatḥ of Tabriz and Mírzá Abú Naṣr of Gilan. Of the former very little is known; the latter is of some importance. His father was a doctor of law; the son became a doctor of medicine, and at first had a military practice in Qazvin. Being called in one day to treat the shah, he had the good fortune to meet with success. He was appointed to the royal household as his reward. Here he became very friendly with Ḥaydar Mírzá, the heir apparent. His rapid promotion turned his head and he is said to have treated his elders and betters with the utmost haughtiness and incivility, confident in his position in the court.

When S͟háh Ṭahmásp died, it was said that Abú Naṣr had brought about his death by putting poison into a depilatory which the shah was in the habit of using. In this he may well have been acting on behalf of Ḥaydar Mírzá, for S͟háh Ṭahmásp had secretly determined upon his death in order to secure the succession to the throne for his second son Isma'íl. At the time of the shah's death Ḥaydar Mírzá was in prison in Qazvin. A small party of his adherents attempted to make him king. But the loyal captains of the late shah cut short his claims by ordering his immediate decapitation. The governor of Qazvin who had befriended him was forced to flee and disguising himself as a doctor attempted to flee to the Turks. But he was overtaken and recognized and was soon after put to death by Isma'íl, who had now become shah. All the adherents in Qazvin of the late Ḥaydar Mírzá were also murdered. Among them fell Abú Naṣr, the physician. His personal unpopularity combined with his political views made it certain that his life was forfeit. He was caught hiding in a stove and was hacked to pieces or else drowned in the pond in front of the windows of the room where he had hidden.

Yet it is quite possible that S͟háh Ṭahmásp died a natural death; for when he was in the mood, he drank most immoderately and was said to consume enormous quantities of opium. His interests were painting and riding about on gaily apparelled Egyptian donkeys, so that a wit of the day remarked that in S͟háh Ṭahmásp's times there flourished painters, writers, asses and Qazvinis.

Workmen of the royal workshops had the right to free medical attendance from the court physicians and to free medicine from the court druggists. To cater for the unprivileged workmen there was opened in this reign in Teheran a charitable dispensary. This was known as the *S͟harbat-k͟hana-i-K͟hayṛiah-i-Pádis͟háhí* or Royal Dispensary of Good Things, and was placed under the direction of a physician named Mírzá Yár 'Alí, a personal physician of S͟háh Ṭahmásp, who in consequence was given the nickname of Ḥakím K͟hayrí. He was a popular physician and one of some skill, for several poems are attributed to him as well as a book on pharmacy. The work of the dispensary prospered under his direction and he found it necessary to call in his two sons to help him. Both became physicians, the one being named Núr-ul-Dín 'Alí and the other Ḥakím Sharaf. Ḥakím Khayrí at the end of his life assumed the habit of a dervish and retired from active life in the world. His two sons carried on the work of the dispensary, Núr-ul-Dín dying in 1622.[1]

The most striking feature about this period is the return to superstition and the immense hold that astrology gained over the minds of all classes, even the highest and most learned. There never was a time when the astrologer was not looked upon with awe and in many cases his word was final. Niẓámí of Samarqand had long ago remarked that there were four servants essential to kings: a secretary for administration, a poet for immortal fame, an astrologer for the ordering of affairs, and a physician for the health of his body.[2] Persian astrologers and Persian physicians made their appearance in the court of the caliphs of Baghdad at the same time. It was al-Manṣúr, the caliph, who summoned Jurjís I to attend his body and Nóbakht, the astrologer, to direct his fate.[3]

Yet many of the great physicians of that age despised the art of the astrologer. Bukht Yishú' is said to have flaunted them deliberately by administering clysters when the moon was in conjunction with an unfavourable planet and by giving draughts when the moon was in opposition to Venus. Nevertheless his patients lived.[4]

In spite of his popularity the position of an astrologer was a delicate one. The line between lawful astrology and heretical star-worship was a thin one. The more orthodox of the caliphs delighted in persecuting heresy and any suspected astrologer ran the risk of a trial as an atheist. In 1192 by the caliph's orders a very respectable physician 'Abd-ul-Salám al-Baghdádí was

1 *'Alam Árái*, f. 43; *Maṭraḥ-ul-Anẓár*, p. 361.
2 *Chahár Maqála*, p. 12. 3 *Hist. Dynst.* vol. IX, p. 145.
4 *I.A.U.* vol. I, p. 143.

examined on such a charge and found guilty. He himself was sent to prison: his books were publicly burned. The sentence was carried out with great solemnity. The preacher for the occasion was Ibn al-Máristání, the director of the 'Aẓudí Hospital. After mounting the pulpit he discoursed against philosophy in general and cursed 'Abd-ul-Salám in particular. And as he dealt with each book in turn, he denounced it, tore it across, and threw it into the flames.[1]

Later al-Damírí contrasted very unfavourably astrology with medicine and even with oneiromancy. Mongol superstition and the general decline in the standard of medical education led to an enormous growth in the belief in the omnipotence of the stars and in man's control over the fate of another by means of incantation and magical rites. In 1551 a *wazír* of Khorasan and an administrator of the shrine of the Imam at Meshed was sent to prison for many years because he was reported to have gained an influence over the stars and over the sun in order that he might be enabled to control the shah. It was said that he kept a yellow calf in the sunlight and stained his face with saffron and tinted his clothes. By the royal command he was shut up in a box with his hands outside 'so that he might not do those things which depend upon the clasping of the hands'.[2]

A little later Sháh 'Abbás was told that the stars portended the destruction of the ruler of Iran. His astrologer royal advised him to abdicate temporarily and to set upon the throne in his place a criminal whose life was already forfeit. The shah was fully persuaded of the truth of the warning and a luckless Christian, a quiver-stitcher, was selected for the honour of averting the royal destruction. For three days he ruled as a king and then was done to death, acting as a conductor to the malign influence of the stars.[3]

Even a serious and learned writer like Bahá'-ul-Doula apparently fully believed in the place of magic in medicine. To

1 Al-Qifṭí, p. 228.
2 *Aḥsan-ul-Tawáríkh*, p. 160.
3 *Chronicle of the Carmelites in Persia*, vol. 1, p. 405.

wipe with a duster, when the moon is on the wane, the body of a child, who has a disagreeable rash, and to say at the same time 'O Moon, even as thou dost diminish, so make these spots to grow smaller', is his most satisfactory method of treating the rash. He also recommends the treatment of malarial fevers by a magic rite which requires the use of a lamb, a thread, a virgin, and a Wednesday night. The rite is of Indian origin, as the incantation which he prescribes shows. For many of the words are Hindi.

In the realm of drugs magic ran riot. Abú Ayúb was wont to prepare a magical ointment for preserving himself against the wrath of al-Manṣúr. In the work of Ghiyáṣ-ul-Dín of Ispahan the magic property of drugs is very pronounced. What could go further beyond the bounds of imagination than his description of a fluid which he names 'Water of Jamh'?

> This is a dust coloured liquid with a vile smell. When stale it looks like ink. It is obtained from the belly of a fish known as the Jamh, found in the China Seas. The peculiar property of this liquid is that if anyone with a broken limb drink of it, at once the limb will become perfect again. But he must take great care that it does not touch the teeth, for it is very harmful to them. Of course it must be drunk after the limb is set.

A drug with the same remarkable properties was believed to exist in the district of Dedesht in Persia. In this case it was a bitumen which was collected from a rock. So valuable was it that the local governor set a guard over it to prevent pilfering and the loss of income which he acquired by selling it. It was said that a cock was cured of a broken leg in 24 hours by the eating of it. Mr Alves, an English surgeon, was induced to try it in a case under his care who had a fracture of both thigh bones. He reported that his patient suffered no fever during the whole of his convalescence. He did not, however, report that the bones reunited any quicker than normal.[1]

Yet with all this credulity there went much scientific thinking and experiment. Rhazes used apes for his pharmacological

1 Ives, *A Voyage from England to India* (London, 1773), p. 217

experiments; Ghiyáṣ-ul-Dín reports the use of cockerels. Bahá'-ul-Doula, too, describes how dogs or cocks may be used to clinch a diagnosis of rabies, much as guinea-pigs are used nowadays in a doubtful case of tuberculosis.

The days of the Mongol domination and the rule of the Ṣafavids were the golden age of the pharmacologists. The polypharmacy of Mesue gave place to specific therapy, and the study of drugs became a specialization in which the leading physicians of the day were not unwilling to indulge. Historically, the first pharmacological monograph to be written in Persian is the work of Abú Manṣúr Muwaffaq of Herat and was composed about A.D. 975. It is called the *Kitáb-ul-Abniya 'an Haqá'iq-il-Adviya* or the 'Book of the Foundations of the true Properties of Remedies'. It was dedicated to the Sámánid Sulṭán Manṣúr bin Núḥ. In this work are described 585 drugs, about which the author has collected data from Greek, Syriac, Arabic, Persian and Indian sources. Not only is it the earliest known piece of Persian prose, but the unique manuscript of it is also the oldest known Persian manuscript in Europe. This manuscript is preserved in Vienna and is a copy made by the poet Asadí in A.D. 1055.

Nearly 200 years later died the greatest of all the Arab pharmacologists, Ibn ul-Bayṭár, whose work had such an enormous influence upon the Persian writers who followed him. Ibn ul-Bayṭár was a botanist rather than a pharmacologist and contented himself with describing an enormous number of simples. He was not a Persian, and though he travelled from Spain to Syria in search of copy for his great book, he does not appear ever to have visited Persia. But his work formed the foundation of many a Persian *Qarabádín* or *Materia Medica* which came later.

Perhaps the greatest of the pharmacists of the Mongol period is 'Alí bin Ḥusayn al-Anṣárí, known as Ḥájjí Zayn-ul-Dín al-'Aṭṭár, who was born in Shiraz in the year 1329. His father, by name Jamál-ul-Dín Ḥusayn, was originally a physician of Ispahan. He had settled in Shiraz a few years before the birth of his son. Al-Anṣárí stood high in the favour of Sháh Shujá', whose personal physician he was. This Sháh Shujá' was one of the Muẓaffarids, who ruled over south Persia after the death of the last true Íl-Khán, Abú Sa'íd. He is chiefly famous because he was the patron of Ḥáfiẓ the poet, with whom therefore al-Anṣárí must have been well acquainted.

Among the works of al-Anṣárí are the *Tuḥfat-ul-Saláṭín* or 'Present of Emperors', an anatomical pamphlet, and a work called the *Miftáḥ-ul-Khazá'in* or 'Key to the Treasures', a work which he finished in 1366. In the Bodleian Library at Oxford there are two copies of this work, one of which dated 1367 is in the handwriting of al-Anṣárí himself, as another hand has noted at the end. The work is divided into three chapters, the first on simple drugs, the second on their rectification, and the third on compound preparations. Three years later he revised this work, adding considerably to the third chapter. The revised work was called the *Ikhtiyárát-i-Badí'í* or 'A Selection for the use of Badí'', being dedicated to the princess Badí'-ul-Jamál. In the course of this work he quotes an enormous number of authorities, ranging from a Socratic electuary which he says Ḥunayn translated from the Greek for al-Ma'mún to an electuary of newts, which was an aphrodisiac 'composed by the late Mu'ín-ul-Dín the physician'. He also quotes a prescription for an electuary which he ascribes to Rashíd-ul-Dín the *wazír*. He died in 1403.

Although the output of pharmacological treatises by no means ceased, it now became the fashion to search for specific remedies. The introduction of smilax, the eastern substitute for sarsaparilla, was hailed by Persian physicians as the discovery of a perfect antidote. Many other substances had already been described as of universal efficacy, but I think there must have been much doubt in the minds of the writers, for they so frequently add at the end of a more than usually incredible statement 'but God knoweth best'. Smilax or China Root, as they called it, was first made known to the Persian medical faculty by the monograph of 'Imád-ul-Dín, who says in his preface that the root was introduced into Persia 'within our own times'. He maintained that it was a panacea for all diseases due to spleen or yellow bile. For 'just as ice and snow fly before the sun, so do these diseases before the China Root'. It is effective, too, in cases of cancer, though he admits that he knows of failures, and in the overcoming of addiction to opium. Skin diseases, scabies, baldness of the head, and leprosy all yield to the Root. Dropsy, colic and palsies are also within the range of its curative powers.

Above all it was found to be efficacious in the treatment of *átis͟hak* (the Persian variety of syphilis), now a very widely spread disease. According to Qáẓí bin Kás͟hif-ul-Dín Muḥammad Ḥamaví Yezdí, a son of a physician to S͟háh 'Abbás the Great and himself the chief priest of Ispahan, who wrote two handbooks on the subject about the year 1650, China Root was introduced into Persia by European doctors in the year 1494, that is the same year that *átis͟hak* appeared. This I very much doubt, both because sarsaparilla is thought not to have been known in Europe before the middle of the seventeenth century and because Bahá'-ul-Doula, who discussed the treatment of *átis͟hak* very thoroughly in his *K͟huláṣat-ul-Tajárib* does not mention the drug. To 'Imád-ul-Dín, therefore, may be given the credit of being the first to describe it. His pamphlet, called *Risála-i-C͟húb-i-C͟híní K͟hurdan* or 'Pamphlet on the Eating of China Root' must have been written about 1550.

The enthusiasm of the Persian pharmacists for China Root was quite equalled by that of their English colleagues. As late as 1870, 345,000 lb. of sarsaparilla, valued at £26,000 were imported into Great Britain, and it was not until 1914 that the General Medical Council finally decided to exclude it from the pharmacopoeia as being an entirely inert drug. Still in some of the less up-to-date chemists' shops can be seen massive glass-jars in the window, proudly labelled 'Sarsaparilla', in golden lettering.

Contemporary with 'Imád-ul-Dín was another Persian pharmacologist who wrote a treatise on the Root. This was Núr Ulláh 'Alá'-ul-Dín, who quotes 'Imád-ul-Dín as still alive and who is in turn quoted by him. And so the subject and the fame of the merits of the Root spread until no writer failed to recommend it. With the introduction of the true sarsaparilla it was almost abandoned and even the name is not to be found in the twentieth-century writers.

The best known of the pharmacists of the time of S͟háh 'Abbás is probably Muẓaffar bin Muḥammad al-Ḥusayní al-S͟hifá'í, who composed a pharmacopoeia which he called after himself, *Ṭibb-i-S͟hifá'í* or 'S͟hifá'í's Medicine'. This work was written in 1556. The arrangement of the subject-matter closely resembles the works of al-Anṣárí. Drugs are arranged in alphabetical order. The main interest of the book lies not in the book itself, for it differs only slightly from its predecessors, but in the fact that it formed the foundation of the *Pharmacopoeia Persica* of Fr. Angelus, the first European to make a study of Persian medicine.

Joseph Labrosse, born at Toulouse in 1636, entered the Order of the Discalced Carmelites and took the name in religion of Fr. Angelus of St Joseph. In 1662 he left France for Rome, where he stayed for nearly two years, studying Arabic. In the winter of 1664 he reached Ispahan and began to study Persian under a Carmelite father of that city. Spurred on by the success of another father of the Community, Fr. Matthew, who having a considerable knowledge of medicine, used it as a means of propagating Christianity, Fr. Angelus determined to add a knowledge of medicine to the detailed knowledge that he had now acquired of Arabic and Persian.

I used to consort with Fr. Matthew at Shiraz [he wrote] and envied his success, seeing him baptise under the pretence of administering a medicine not only children, but even adults. So I began to study both Medicine and Persian. I translated the Aphorisms of Hippocrates into that language....I read many Arabic and Persian books, above all that System of Medicine called the *Zak͟híra-i-K͟hwárazmshahí*. I visited the houses of the learned people of Ispahan and paid hundreds of visits to the shops of the druggists, the pharmacists, and the chemists.

In 1678, Fr. Angelus left the East for his own country and in 1680 he published in Paris his *Pharmacopoeia Persica*. 'Opus missionariis, mercatoribus, ceterisque regionum orientalium lustratoribus necessarium, nec non Europaeis nationibus perutile' as he says on the first page.

This was not the end of his contributions to our knowledge of Persian medicine of his day. Appointed visitor to the Carmelite Convent in Amsterdam in 1681 he succeeded in buying the oriental type which belonged to the heirs of the Elzevirs. He was thus able to publish his *Gazophylacium linguae Persarum*, a dictionary of Persian words translated into Italian, Latin and French. It appeared in Amsterdam in 1684. Chardin, who at this time was the agent in Holland for the English East India Company, read through some of the proofs before the work appeared and very highly commended it. Hyde of Queen's College, Oxford, the greatest English orientalist of the seventeenth century, on the contrary formed quite a different opinion. 'It is quite obvious from his Persian *Gazophylacium*', he wrote, 'where there is such a harvest of errors that to correct them all would require another volume of equal size. Hardly could a woman have made more mistakes in writing than he.' I have more than a suspicion that Hyde was animated by an anti-Catholic bias, errors though there undoubtedly are, for he had already castigated Fr. Angelus for daring to criticize some passages in a Persian translation of the New Testament by Walton.

Although the *Gazophylacium* is not exclusively scientific, far more attention is paid to medical words than to others. It is moreover enriched with interesting little notes about any word which seemed useful or unknown to European readers, just like Schlimmer's *Terminologie* of 200 years later. Of *átishak*, for example, he writes that the Persian authors call it the French Disease. 'Nay rather it should be called the Persian or Turkish Disease, for there is scarcely one person in a thousand who is unaffected by it.' He also states that the medical works most commonly read in his day were the *Thesaurus* of Isma'íl al-Jurjání, the *Ṭibb-i-Yúsufí*, and the *Kifáya-i-Manṣúrí*.

Catholic missions and medicine were closely associated.

Fr. Matthew practised among the Persians when he was in Shiraz and attended the Dutch traders when he was in Basra. Later in India he gained a reputation as a botanist. Another Carmelite, Fr. Damian of Lyons, was personal physician to Nádir Sháh and to 'Alí Qulí Khán, his cousin, who afterwards ruled under the title of 'Adíl Sháh. The Jesuit lay-brother, Bazin, took Fr. Damian's place after his retirement. Fr. Emmanuel afterwards bishop of Baghdad, and Fr. Leander both served as physicians to the Pasha of Baghdad, and in this capacity the former was able to obtain privileges for his Order which even ambassadors would have had the greatest difficulty in obtaining, 'even for a large bribe of money' he adds.[1] In Tiflis, which then belonged to Persia, all the Capuchin Fathers were given the title of physician. It is notable, too, that in Baghdad at the close of the seventeenth century at the time when the Turkish authorities were giving particular trouble to Catholic missions, all the Capuchins were compelled to go about the streets dressed as doctors of medicine. As late as 1827 the Catholic bishop of Baghdad, relating how he was robbed by some wandering tribesmen, first remarked on their politeness, for they removed his new boots from off his feet without even troubling him to dismount. He then adds that when they were about to seize a small chest which contained all his valuables, it was saved by a bandit calling out that it had best be left alone as it only contained medicines.

At the same time that Fr. Angelus was writing his pharmacopoeia, another famous monograph on drugs was being composed by the two Mu'mans, father and son. Their combined work is known as the *Tuḥfat-ul-Mu'manín* or 'The Gift of the Two Mu'mans'. The work was begun by Mír Muḥammad Zamán Tankábuní; it was completed by his son Muḥammad Mu'man Ḥusayní, usually known as Ṭabíb Mu'mana. The book was finished in the year 1669 and is dedicated to Sháh Sulaymán Ṣafaví. It is a pharmacological treatise based upon earlier works

1 *Chron. Carm. in Persia*, vol. I, p. 620.

of Arabic and Indian authorship. It draws its main inspiration from the *Ikhtiyárát-i-Badí'í*. Leclerc, in his *Histoire de la Médecin Arabe*[1], makes a mistake when he states that the book is dedicated to an Indian prince. It is on the contrary entirely Persian. It is written in Persian, in Persia and for a Persian. Like so many other popular works it was lithographed in India before it was printed in Persia. It is easily obtainable now both in manuscript and in cheap printed editions. It was one of the main sources from which Schlimmer drew the information contained in his *Terminologie*.

A study of medieval pharmacy is generally considered a sterile occupation. It is by no means so. Seeing that the whole Persian pharmacological system was empirical, I am inclined to believe that further study would reveal plants and animal products which have escaped modern investigators. The history of the pharmacy of stones is far the most exciting part of Persian therapeutics. None of the ancient writers could resist the lure of ascribing marvellous properties to the strange coloured stones which were occasionally discovered. It is difficult to know what to select for quotation. There is the stone known as Jamast, found in some mines three days' journey away from Medina. This stone protects the wearer from gout and bad dreams and, if set in a cup, is a preservative against drunkenness. There is a glass-like stone found in the crop of a cock, which will protect the wearer against grief and sorrow. Epilepsy can be cured by the Moon-stone, the Swallow-stone, and a dozen others. The most famous of all and the most universal in its potency is surely the Bezoar-stone, a native Persian stone, whose fame spread to Europe and whose very name is a corruption of the Persian words *bád-zuhr* or antidote.

The history of the stone is long and glorious. That it was used in the East before the preaching of Islam is sure. It is stated that it was known to the Hebrews of ancient times, who termed it *Bel Zaard* or 'The Master'. The impetus to its general use was

1 Leclerc, *Hist. Méd. Arabe*, vol. II, p. 330.

supplied by the physicians of the Arabian School. Rhazes mentions the stone both in his *Continens* and in the *Liber Almansoris*. An old English translation of this latter passage runs:

The evill Venoms that doe offende the heart and woorke their effects, O how little profite doeth any cure prove in them, if the Bezoar be not taken, for that doeth resist it. Moreover I myself saw that it did resist the venome called Napelo, which is the venome that doethe penetrate more than al venomes.[1]

Haly Abbas speaks about the stone in the *Liber Regius* and Avicenna in the *Canon* makes several passing references to its efficacy. The first mention of it in European scientific literature would appear to be in the work of Avenzoar, an Arab physician of Seville, about the year A.D. 1140. Later Nicholas Monardes devoted a long account to the virtues of the stone and recounts that one of the Edwards was cured by the use of the stone.

And a King of England, called Edward, was delivered by means thereof from a poisoned mortall wound that the great Soldane with a venomed glaive gave him in a battaile that they fought beyonde the seas neare to the City of Aaron. When hee was almost dead, there was given to him the Bezaar Stone by one who was the great maister of the Templers, which was an order in those daies of great estimation and verie riche.[2]

In England the stone was so highly prized that Queen Elizabeth carried one set in a ring upon her finger. It figured in the London pharmacopoeias from 1618 to 1746. As late as 1808 Fatḥ 'Alí Sháh sent some prized specimens as a present to the Emperor Napoleon I. But the emperor threw them with scorn into the fire. The stone is still in use in Persia to-day. A fair sized stone was once presented to me by a grateful patient; but the cupidity of my dispensary servant overcame his respect for his master's goods, and the stone, together with a quantity of saffron in which it was carefully preserved, disappeared during one of my temporary absences from Teheran.

1 N. Monardes, *Joyfull Newes* (trans. J. Frampton), p. 76.
2 Ibid. p. 83.

The first Persian monograph to be devoted entirely to the subject was again from the pen of 'Imád-ul-Dín. In his work he collected the opinions of all the earlier writers on the subject, so that the true stone might be distinguished from the false. For so great was the demand and so limited was the supply that a trade in the manufacture and sale of spurious stones had arisen. The true stone was a calculus found in the belly of a wild goat that inhabited the north-east corner of Persia. The belly must be understood to include both stomach and gall bladder; Persian writers are themselves undecided which organ was the true source. They definitely exclude the urinary bladder. Artificial stones were an artefact of wax and herbs. Some held that the true Bezoar-stone was only to be found in Khorasan. Others even limited the area to the district known as Shabánkárah, a part of Fars, erected into a separate province by the Mongols. 'Imád-ul-Dín admits that it can be found in other places than these.

The true Bezoar-stone was black or reddish and weighed anything up to 20 *miṣqáls*. The false stone was manufactured from lac and was often undistinguishable by the eye. The Persian test to distinguish the two was to heat a needle red-hot in a flame and to place it on the stone. If the stone is an artefact, as the needle sinks in, it will give out a black smoke; if it is a genuine stone, the smoke is yellow and the tip of the needle turns yellow too. Schlimmer, a Dutchman, writing in 1874, remarks that the Persians of his day still regard the Bezoar-stone as their greatest antidote and that though 'Imád-ul-Dín's method might still be employed to distinguish the true from the false, most druggists who were in doubt would cut the stone in half. The internal composition easily discovered the fraud.

Another feature which now reappears in medical writers is an extensive borrowing from Indian sources. In general I do not think that sufficient credit has been given either to the part that India played in the moulding of Persian theories of medicine—it has been generally assumed, I mean, that all Persian medicine is Greek—or to the attempts of the early 'Abbásids to mould

Greek, Sassanian and Indian medicine into a single comprehensive system. I have already spoken of the visit of Perzoes to India in Sassanian times. I have also mentioned the names of one or two Indians who were in residence in the court at Baghdad. That these were not rare and occasional adventurers is clear from the remarks which the author of the *Firdaus-ul-Ḥikmat* makes when describing some Indian remedies. For he adds that he had collected such treatment of diseases by Indians as were easy and well known to the people of his part of the world. He was writing in A.D. 850, probably at Merv. Not only their practice but also their theory must have been well known in those times. Manka had translated an Indian book on poisons into Persian: Sanjahl, another Indian, had translated Charaka into Persian which had been retranslated into Arabic.[1]

A few decades later the debt to India seems to have been forgotten. Avicenna quotes Indian opinions only about the toxicity of leeches and only mentions the name of Charaka in connection with therapeutics. Rhazes is equally silent.

The only work that I know of which makes a serious study of Indian medicine is the *Firdaus-ul-Ḥikmat* of 'Alí ibn Rabban al-Ṭabarí, a work on general medicine which he composed for his patron the Caliph al-Mutawakkil. It obtained an immediate success and was widely quoted. The text, but not unfortunately a translation, has been made available lately by its publication by the Sonner Druckerei of Berlin. Of this work the seventh and final part concludes with 36 chapters devoted to Indian medicine. 'Alí bases his comments not only on Charaka, but he knows and uses also the works of Susruta, Nidana and Ashtangahradaya.

In the Ṣafavid days, the period of the so-called Persian renaissance, Indian views and Indian physicians seem to have become popular once more. Bahá'-ul-Doula speaks of Indian physicians practising in Ray and in Herat and quotes the clinical notes of many cases of Indian patients whom he attended in Persia. This rapprochement was partly political. The ruler of

1 *I.A.U.* vol. II, pp. 32, 33.

Farghana had been a certain 'Umar S͟hayk͟h, who, dying in 1495, left a young son Ẓahír-ul-Dín Muḥammad, surnamed Bábur or 'The Tiger'. He, after a series of victories and defeats in central Asia, finally retired to India where he founded the Moghul Dynasty in Delhi. At the capture of Merv, when S͟háh Isma'íl was still at the beginning of his career, the sister of Bábur fell into his hands. He treated her with all honour and restored her to her brother. Thus early the Moghul emperors were placed under an obligation to the Persian shahs. A few years later Humáyún, the successor of Bábur, was driven out of Delhi by an insurrection and took refuge at the court of Ṭahmásp.

This debt India repaid when she gave asylum to the Persian scientists who fled to the Moghul court to avoid the distractions and dangers which perpetual internal strife made the lot of all who had the misfortune to be born in Persia in the seventeenth or eighteenth century. Among the more famous of these refugees is Núr-ul-Dín Muḥammad 'Abd-Ulláh bin Ḥakím 'Ayn-ul-Mulk of Shiraz. His best known work is the *Alfáẓ-ul-Adviyah* or 'The Vocabulary of Drugs', which he composed in 1628–9 for his patron the emperor S͟háh Jahán of Delhi. It has been frequently lithographed and printed and it has the distinction of being, so far as I know, the only Persian work on general therapeutics that has been translated into English. For India maintained the reputation of being the patron of Persian learning by printing in Calcutta in 1793 the text of this work and its translation into English by Gladwin.

A more important work of his is that known as *Ṭibb-i-Dárá S͟hikúhí* or 'The Medicine of Darius S͟hikúh'. This is a gigantic work which rivals in quantity, if not in quality, the *Canon* of Avicenna or the *Thesaurus* of al-Jurjání. Darius S͟hikúh was a son of S͟háh Jahán, who was the heir to the throne until he was murdered by his brother Aurungzeeb. The young man had scientific tastes and a literary turn of mind. A few years ago it was customary to attribute this work to his pen. But apart from the improbability that a royal prince would have sufficient medical knowledge to write such a work, a study of the early chapters shows that it is to 'Ayn-ul-Mulk that the authorship must be assigned.

The *Ṭibb-i-Dárá* is an interesting work because it is the swan song of Persian medicine. It was the last great system of medicine to be written in the Persian language. It deserves further study. But to examine the text is extremely difficult, for according to Fonahn there are only two manuscripts of the work in existence. One is in Paris and one is in Calcutta. Leclerc has summarized the former. But his summaries are not to be trusted, for he read Persian with difficulty and makes many errors. According to him surgery is scarcely discussed in this work; even cataract is here treated with drugs. A long chapter on syphilis is of great interest.[1]

Mention too must be made of another physician who left Shiraz for the court of Aurungzeeb. This was a certain Muḥammad Akbar Sháh Arzání, who began to write about 1700 and produced several works of which the most famous are the *Ṭibb-i-Akbarí* or 'Akbar's Medicine', the *Mízán-i-Ṭibb* or 'The Scales of Medicine', and the *Ṭibb-ul-Nabbí* or 'Medicine of the Prophet', to which I have already referred. Of Mirza Muḥammad 'Alaví Khán, physician to Muḥammad Sháh of Delhi and later to Nádir Sháh, I will speak in greater detail when I deal with the reign of Nádir.

Even when the Qájárs had restored internal peace to Persia, it was left to the printing presses of Calcutta, introduced into India 50 years before they reached Persia, to keep alive the Arab system of medicine when it was dying of inanition in its native land. The fanning of the glowing embers was mainly the work of the Baptist Press and the Education Press, supported and encouraged by the Directors of the East India Company. Among their non-scientific works was Macnaghten's magnificent edition in four volumes of the Arabic text of the *Arabian Nights* which for excellence of print and Arabic lettering is still unsurpassed.

[1] Bibliothèque Nationale (Paris), no. 342, Suppl. The MS. contains 1711 folios. The section on syphilis is found on ff. 521 et seqq. For summary of contents see Leclerc, *Hist. Méd. Arab.* vol. II, pp. 332–4.

Among the medical books, in addition to those composed in the Moghul court which I have already mentioned, nearly all of which were printed in Calcutta, is a very interesting one called the *Anís-ul-Mus͟harraḥín* or 'Anatomists' Vade Mecum'. This is a translation by John Tytler of the Company's Medical Service into Arabic of Robert Hooper's *Anatomy*. It was prepared for the use of the Mohammedan colleges which were situated within the Company's jurisdiction. The work contains moreover a very valuable index of scientific anatomical terms. It was printed in 1836. The pity is that 30 years later, when Dr Schlimmer was attempting to do almost the same thing for Persia, he seems to have been ignorant of the existence of this book.

In his translation Dr Tytler was aided by an Indian doctor named Ḥakím Moulvi 'Abd-ul-Majíd, who was a professor of Arabic and physician to the college of the Company in Calcutta. To him too Persian medicine is indebted, for he edited and saw through the press in 1832 the *Al-S͟harḥ-ul-Mag͟hná* or '*Commentatio Absoluta*' of Moulána Sadíd al-Kázarúní. This commentary, usually known as 'The Sadídí', is another commentary on the *Mújiz-ul-Qánún* of Ibn ul-Nafís and thus carries us back to the days of Avicenna. He also wrote a commentary on a relatively unknown *Qánúnc͟hi* which has the merit of containing an excellent glossary of English equivalents of technical Arabic and Persian medical terms.

About this time there appeared in Europe in epidemic form a disease to which was given the name of the shepherd Syphilis. Whether it existed in Europe before the siege of Naples in 1495 is doubtful. It is certain that the form which syphilis now takes was unknown before the return of Columbus from America. A close study of Persian writings prior to the beginning of the sixteenth century shows that it was equally unknown to those parts. Attempts have been made to prove that the lesions of this disease were described by Avicenna and the writers of classical times. There is also the story which Sa'dí relates of the king who suffered from 'a terrible disease the nature of which it is not proper to mention'.[1] If this is considered to be syphilis, then the disease was known to the Persians before its introduction into Europe. But there is hardly enough evidence in this story to draw such a provocative conclusion. The quotations carry no greater conviction of the existence of the disease in the East than do similar arguments of its existence in the West prior to the discovery of the New World.

Of the lesions described by the Arabs and Persians of classical times, those of the disease, which Galen called *Ignis Persicus* and the Persians *Nár-i-Fársí*, bear the closest resemblance to syphilis. Unfortunately, it is not certain with what the disease called Persian Fire is to be identified. Avicenna describes the disease in the fourth book of the *Canon*, and later writers borrow his account without adding any further useful observations. There it is stated to have been an irritating, pustular or vesicular eruption, which causes a blackening of the tissues around, and which on healing leaves a scar similar to the scar of a burn. It is nowhere suggested that the sexual organs are the site of election or that sexual connection is the normal method of infection. The resemblance must have been very close for many Persian observers of the early sixteenth century regarded syphilis as a new form of *Ignis Persicus*. I think, however, the medieval translators were correct in rendering *Ignis Persicus* as anthrax or carbuncle.

Modern historians of medicine, while recognizing that syphilis is a clinical entity, have tried to show that it existed before Fracastoro and others described it. Persian writers, contemporary with its appearance in those parts, attempt the opposite. They saw a new disease, but refused to admit that it was a new clinical entity and attempted to classify it as a novel form of a disease which they already knew. Some therefore called it Persian Fire. Others identified it with leprosy. Others considered it a form of Armenian Sore, thereby linking the disease to the sore which Avicenna had called the Balkh Sore. This last is certainly identical with cutaneous leishmaniasis. There was also a party which called

1 Sa'dí, *Gulistán*, vol. 1, tale 22.

the new disease the European Small-pox. Finally, that most acute of observers Bahá'-ul-Doula recognized it to be a new and distinct disease, though also using the phrase European Pox and Armenian Sore, gave to it the name of *átis͟hak* or the Little Burning Disease. Perhaps it is too much to say that he invented this name. It would be more correct to say that it is in his book that this term first occurs.

The earliest description of the disease in Europe, which admits of no contradiction, is that of Coradinus Gilinus in 1497. His account was followed by a host of others, including that of Fracastoro in 1530, who gave to it the name of syphilis. The earliest account of this disease in the East is from the pen of Bahá'-ul-Doula in 1501. He states that it first appeared in Azerbaijan in the year 1498. From there it spread to Iraq and Fars, and by the time that he was writing only three years later it was scattered throughout Persia. What he called *átis͟hak* was the secondary syphilitic rash. But he also realized that the sore throat and the chancre were other manifestations of the same disease. He even diagnosed a case of syphilitic diplegia. He recognized that the spread of the disease was chiefly by sexual intercourse, though he admitted the possibility of infection through the body vapours given off in the hot bath. Nor did he fail to associate gummata and ulceration with the vanished rash.

With regard to treatment he was not very hopeful.

> Anyone afflicted with this disease and wrongly treated may remain sick for two, three, four or even more years, though without any sores or very few. But, if the rash does not disappear at the time of the final crisis and when the body is full of peccant humours and the spots are many and the treatment unsatisfactory, then the patient will very soon die.

He considers 17 months the normal time before the disease matures within the body and therefore treatment should be continued for nearly two years. He believes it possible, however, for a cure to be affected in less time and he states that he himself has cured several cases by a prolonged treatment with an electuary of mercury. He does not seem, however, to give to mercury the same importance which later writers do. Sarsaparilla was not yet introduced into Persia; zedoary was at first considered the specific for the disease.

A few years after appeared another work in which there is a discussion of the treatment for chancre. It is notable that the Persian phrase used is now *naftat-i-farangiyya* with the alternative title of *ábileh-i-farang*, that is, European pustule or pox. This work appeared in Herat in the year 1511 and was called the *Jámi'-ul-Fawá'id* or 'Collection of Benefits'. It is easily accessible to those who wish to pursue the question further, for an edition lithographed in recent years in Meshed can be picked up in the bazaars of Persia and certain parts of it have been translated into English by Dr Lichtwardt of the American Mission to Persia and published in the *Annals of Medical History*.

The author was one Yúsuf bin Muḥammad bin Yúsuf, who was born in the reign of Sulṭán Bábur, the first Moghul emperor, and was a secretary to his successor the Sulṭán Humáyún, who reigned from 1530 to 1556. His father also was a distinguished physician of Herat and composed an invaluable work entitled the *Baḥr-ul-Jawáhir* or *Jawáhir-ul-Lughat*, that is, 'Sea of Jewels' or the 'Jewel of Dictionaries', which he dedicated to Sulṭán Jalál-ul-Dín Malik Dínár. It is written partly in Arabic and partly in Persian and is a scientific dictionary in explanation of technical, medical and botanical terms. Several manuscripts of this work exist in European libraries and it has been lithographed in Teheran.

The son was a more prolific author. He wrote several books, most of which have survived. The greater part of these writings is in verse, even though their subject is medical. Of his non-medical works the best known is the *Badáyi'-ul-Insha'* or the 'Glory of Style', written for his son. Of his strictly medical works besides the one I have already mentioned, is the *Fawá'id-ul-Akhyár* or 'Benefits of the Best', which he wrote in 1507. His poem on the preservation of health appeared in 1530, and his *Riyáẓ-ul-Adviya* or 'Gardens of Remedies' in 1539, both being dedicated to his patron. Besides these he wrote an *'Iláj-ul-Amráẓ* or 'The Treatment of Diseases' and the *Ṭibb-i-Yúsufí* or 'Therapeutics of Joseph'.

In his chapter on skin eruptions he deals with syphilis at length. The symptomatology of the disease he discusses very briefly, only saying that the disease shows itself by an eruption on the body and by pain in the limbs. His account of the remedies to be applied is long and varied. Mercury holds the place of honour.

Whether Dervish or Shah of his syphilis complains,
To remove all his sores and cure all his pains
Give mercury powders or mercury pills
Or mercury vapour to relieve all these ills.

By now this new Frank disease was becoming well known. Its infectivity was realized; it was in fact much exaggerated. There was a certain *amír*, Ghiyáṣ-ul-Dín Manṣúr of Shiraz, who so excelled in the science of astrology that Sháh Isma'íl sent him to repair the observatory of Khwájá Naṣr-ul-Dín Ṭúsí at Meragha. He is said to have lived in perpetual fear of a venereal infection and in consequence refused even to shake hands with anyone or, when politeness admitted of no excuse, would only grasp the hand of the other through his sleeve. When he was minister, says the chronicler of the *Aḥsan-ul-Tawáríkh*, he relied very largely upon the services of a certain Qáẓí 'Alí of Baghdad. One day one of his friends told him by way of a joke that the Qáẓí was infected with the new disease. Next day, when Qáẓí 'Alí came to the minister for his seal with which to seal certain papers, the *amír* shrank away from him and the practical jokers were delighted to see the *amír* edging away across the room from his astonished secretary.[1] Ghiyáṣ-ul-Dín died in 1541, but it is not stated whether he ultimately contracted the disease of which he was so fearful.

It was not until 1569 that the first monograph on syphilis appeared in the Persian language. This came from the pen of 'Imád-ul-Dín of Shiraz. My translation of this into English has been published by the editor of the *Annals of Medical History*.[2]

1 *Aḥsan-ul-Tawáríkh*, p. 137.
2 *Annals of Medical History*, pp. 4 et seq. New York, 1931.

A comparison of it with Bahá'-ul-Doula's original account shows that from the clinical standpoint Persian physicians had made very little progress. The methods of treatment have considerably improved by the insistence on the value of mercury, both by internal and external administration. The effect of the treatise on a modern reader is marred by the abuse which 'Imád-ul-Dín showers upon Bahá'-ul-Doula, who, he says, 'neglected the usual custom of scholars by not enumerating or even mentioning signs and symptoms... and wrote contrary to the dignity of an author by holding up to ridicule other physicians'. Yet he himself unblushingly plagiarizes Bahá'-ul-Doula and quotes as his own cases of Bahá'-ul-Doula's without any acknowledgement. Of the aetiology of the disease he writes:

Be it known that this disease occasionally results from an infection. The commonest source of this infection is sexual intercourse. The next commonest is that which results from the hot bath; for in the bath vapours, that may be described as noxious, readily escape from the body of the infected person and through inhalation or entry into the internal or external pores of the body produce a great effect. Should one sit in the very place where an infected person has sat, the effect is even greater.

Occasionally an uncovered razor cut off which the scab has been scratched, comes in contact with the razor of one infected and then this disease results. Although this condition is unlikely, yet it has been seen.

The disease is not hereditary. If it occurs in a child, the infection is accidental and is not to be attributed to a congenital lesion.

Occasionally infection results from dining in company, and it is milk dishes which produce the greatest effect when they are served in dinner parties. The virulence is so great in this respect that infection can be conveyed by a cup or a drinking vessel, the owner of which himself has the disease.

It may be conveyed by clothes, especially trousers and drawers, even after they have been washed. Kissing, too, is a source of infection.

Further on 'Imád-ul-Dín discusses secondary and tertiary symptoms. He states that he himself saw a woman with a syphilitic sore throat and another one 'whose feet were useless, like one paralysed', who was clearly a case of locomotor ataxia. He recognized the chronicity of the disease and stated that 'one overwhelmed by this sickness, even though treated, may remain diseased for three or four years or even more'. All this will be recognized as a plagiarism of the *Khuláṣat-ul-Tajárib*.

Considerably more than half the pamphlet is devoted to the treatment of the disease. In addition to the recognized methods of sweating, bleeding and dieting, mercury and sarsaparilla are recommended as specific for the disease.

The best ointment, nay rather a drug to which there is nothing equal, is mercury, which alone without other medicaments is enough, and, though there should be a thousand other drugs, cannot be replaced. The cause of this I will relate later. But of internal drugs, in addition to those which produce elimination or balance that I have already described, there are two other excellent remedies. One is China Root (that is, Sarsaparilla) in various forms, and the other is a drug which contains mercury.

Manuscripts of this work, from which I have so freely quoted, exist in the British Museum, in the library of the Bengal Asiatic Society in Calcutta, wrongly catalogued as the *Qarabádín-i-Masúmí*, and a third is in my private collection.[1]

'Imád-ul-Dín Maḥmúd ibn Mas'úd ibn Maḥmúd was born about 1515. The dates both of his birth and of his death can only be deduced from the statements in his own works and in those of other writers. Thus, Qáẓí bin Káshif-ul-Dín Ḥamaví in his pamphlet on the Bezoar-stone states that he made his studies under 'Imád-ul-Dín; and Ḥamaví died in 1664. Again, in his monograph on the China Root 'Imád-ul-Dín quotes verbatim the first eighty lines of Núr Ulláh's work on the same subject and Núr Ulláh in his own work on the China Root quotes 'Imád-ul-Dín with approval. They were therefore contemporary writers. Núr Ulláh says that he first took up the question of China Root in 1540. Finally, 'Imád-ul-Dín himself says that he composed

1 British Museum Or. MSS. Add. 19,619; and Asiatic Society of Bengal, no. 1557. See also *Iksír-i-A'ẓam* (Lucknow, 1885), vol. IV, p. 380.

his monograph on *átishak* in 1569. He must therefore have been living during the greater part of the sixteenth century.

'Imád-ul-Dín came of a medical family. His father was Muḥammad Bakr, an oculist, who was attached to the suite of Sháh 'Abbás and composed for that sovereign a work on the treatment of common eye complaints, which the shah is said to have carried with him when he left Ispahan in 1602 to attack Tabriz. 'Imád-ul-Dín, when he had finished his studies, was attached to the suite of 'Abd-Ulláh Khán Istajlú, governor of Shirvan. For some reason he fell out of favour and was exposed for a night on a frozen pond in punishment for some misdemeanour. Here he saved his life by liberally dosing himself with opium, and from this night's adventure he contracted the habit of taking opium regularly. Ultimately he wrote a book on the uses and abuses of opium. Next he is to be found as physician attached to the shrine of the Imám Riẓá at Meshed, and here having, as he says, much leisure although lacking books, he composed his monograph on *átishak*.

The interval between the death of Ṭahmásp in 1576 and the accession of Sháh 'Abbás the Great in 1587 is famous only for disturbance and bloodshed. Ḥaydar, Isma'íl and Muḥammad Khudábanda all in turn occupied the throne for a short time and each endeavoured to make his position more secure by murdering all possible rivals. Ḥaydar reigned only a few hours. Some say that he was drugged and then strangled. Others say that he died from an overdose of opium, for he was in the habit of taking large quantities of this drug to subdue the pain of a chronic colitis from which he suffered.

Isma'íl, after putting to death eight members of his own family and seventeen of the leading aristocrats who had the misfortune to be in Qazvin at the time, died before he could murder the princes who lived in the provinces. Alcohol or opium or excess of both caused his premature death, although stories of assassination were also current.

Muḥammad Khudábanda, the third of Ṭahmásp's sons, next

ascended the throne. He was forty-five or forty-six when he came to the throne and was already quite grey. He had a strange impediment in his sight so that when he looked down he could see nothing, but when he raised his eyes he could see as well as anyone. In spite of these disadvantages his rule was the longest of the three brothers and he died a natural death, probably in 1585. What exactly happened after this is obscure. It is generally said that his son 'Abbás (afterwards to be known as 'Abbás the Great) was the virtual ruler of Persia even before his father's death and that the statement of Olearius that Ḥamza Mírzá, the eldest son of Muḥammad Khudábanda, succeeded to the throne, is an invention. A letter written by Fr. Paul Simon, the first leader of the Carmelites in Persia, sent to Rome in 1608, that is, only 20 years after the events that he is discussing, would seem to show that on the contrary it is Sykes and other modern historians who are at fault.

Olearius, writing in 1638, says that Ḥamza Mírzá succeeded Muḥammad Khudábanda and was very soon assassinated by his brother Isma'íl and that Isma'íl in turn ruled for some months and was then murdered by a barber. Fr. Paul Simon confirms this, for he wrote:

> ...The King of Persia is called Shah 'Abbás. He was the second-born. Out of fear of his brother, when his father was dead, he fled into Khorasan, where he lived incognito and poorly, like a dervish among the Tartars there. Some of the principal lords of Persia, partial to a change, offered him the kingdom. They cause his brother [that is, Ḥamza Mírzá or perhaps Isma'íl Mírzá] to be killed by a barber, who cut his throat while shaving him; and they sent for this king, who with the aid of the Tartars subdued many of the provinces which were willing to recognize him. To those lords, who had made the plot against his brother, he gave the lands and money which he had promised; then at a banquet he asked them whether his brother was a good king. They replied: 'Yes.' At once he had all of them decapitated, and he laid in ruins the district where had been born the barber who murdered him.[1]

1 Letter no. 234b of *Casa Generalizia of Carmelite Order in Rome*, quoted in *Chron. Carm. in Persia*, vol. 1, p. 66.

It is probably more correct therefore to say that ʻAbbás about two years after his father's death, being then aged twenty-one or twenty-two, came to the throne without opposition. He then concluded a series of successful campaigns against the Uzbegs and thus made secure his position in the East. His war with the Turks recovered for him Kurdistan, Baghdad and the Holy Places. His frontiers being made safe Sháh ʻAbbás now turned his attention to the internal affairs of the realm. The capital was removed from Qazvin to Ispahan. The whole country was enriched with numerous caravanserais, bridges and hospitals. Many of these were built to perpetuate the name of his chief wife. It is said that this pious lady herself expended the equivalent of nearly half a million pounds sterling in the construction of such public buildings.

In his later years Sháh ʻAbbás was filled with jealousy of his own children. Of the four who might have succeeded him one was murdered, one died a natural death, and the other two were blinded. Blindness in itself constituted an insuperable bar to succession and was inflicted very commonly as deterrent to rival princes. It was also used as a method of punishing malefactors. In pre-Islamic days the method employed was to heat olive oil and pour it while fiercely boiling into the wide-opened eyes. Or the eyeballs were pricked with a red-hot needle. In the days of the caliphs blindness was caused by passing a red-hot sword blade close to the orbit or by the use of a needle or by instilling some chronic irritating substance. Ṣamṣám-ul-Doula was treated by this last method by a certain Muḥammad the Bedmaker to satisfy the jealousy of one of the Buwayhid *amírs*. After several weeks of such treatment, finding that he was still sensible to light, Muḥammad 'cut away the eyes with a lancet'. In the times of the Ṣafavids the operation was performed with considerable surgical skill. An incision was made down each corner of the eye, the lids were then raised, and the eyeball removed by cutting the optic nerve and the intrinsic muscles. The execution of possible rivals who were still in their infancy, was accomplished by the simple process of forbidding their mothers to give them the breast.

As a result of this inhuman treatment there was no competent heir-apparent to succeed Sháh 'Abbás on his death. The first to take the vacant place was his grandchild Sháh Ṣafí, who lost for Persia Hamadan, Tabriz and Baghdad, which again fell into Turkish hands. He died prematurely, only 32 years old, when he was about to set out to recapture Kandahar which had been traitorously handed over by its governor to the Moghul emperor. The shah was addicted to opium. According to his medical advisers this had set up an excess of cold in his constitution and he was advised to counteract it by the use of a sufficiency of alcohol. He very willingly followed the prescription of his doctors, so that the East India Company Agent reported in his Diary, 17 January 1643:

> We are advised that Shah Suffe, late king of Persia, being in May last advanced as far as Cashone in prosecution of his intendments for reducing Candahar to his obedience dyed there unworthily whilest overmuch drinking and other ryots hastened his end.[1]

He was succeeded by his son 'Abbás who restored to some extent the prestige which Persia had lost in the previous reign. He brought Kandahar back once more to his empire and successfully defended his existing frontiers against the Russians and the Tartars. Under his rule the Christians received peace and justice, and it was a bitter blow for them when he died quite unexpectedly one night in the early autumn of 1667. The cause of his premature death was said at the time to be syphilis or else an inflammation of the throat brought on by excessive drinking. In order to keep the news of the death secret as long as possible, the attendant eunuchs persuaded the women of the household to suppress all outward signs of mourning. At daybreak the two chief ministers of state were informed of what had just happened. Unfortunately

1 Diary of the East India Company. Preserved in the India Office Library. Only fragments of this diary have been published.

at his last gasp 'Abbás had been heard to whisper: 'I know that you have poisoned me, but you shall drink a good share of the poison. For I leave behind me a son who after my death shall devour your very hearts.' The two chief ministers saw from these words ruin for themselves and their families; the two attendant physicians were no less depressed. In any case these last two could expect nothing less than exile and confiscation of their property, for this was the normal reward for unsuccessful court physicians. If these words became known, they could hardly expect to escape with their lives.

The late shah left behind him only two sons. The elder, by name Ṣafí Mírzá, was already twenty-one and would probably find himself in duty bound to avenge his father's death. The younger son, by name Ḥamza Mírzá, was then only eight years old and would be obliged to entrust the rule of the country to a regent. It therefore became to the common interest both of the ministers and the physicians to set aside the claims of the elder son to the throne and to prefer those of the younger. Their lives would thus be safe for a space and by the time the young king reached maturity they could doubtless have made their own position secure.

'Abbás at the time of his death was on a hunting expedition in Ṭabaristan. With him was the young prince; the elder was at Ispahan. The young child was thus at hand to receive the crown which the ministers and physicians wished to settle upon him. Nor was it their fault that he failed to receive it. A full conclave of grandees on the following day was won over to their opinion by a series of specious arguments. And had it not been for the totally unexpected and entirely disinterested speech of a eunuch, the throne would have passed without dispute to the younger prince. The eunuch, who was tutor to the young Ḥamza Mírzá and had therefore much to gain from his accession, yet spoke most eloquently in defence of the lawful claim of Ṣafí Mírzá. The grandees were astonished. Apparently a sense of the injustice which they were purposing touched their hearts. For now with an unanimity similar to that which they had shown at the first voting they cast their votes without exception for the accession of Ṣafí Mírzá. Thus contrary to the desire of the great majority of those present Ṣafí Mírzá was elected to be Shah of Persia.

At once a deputation was named which should proceed to Ispahan with the news of the king's death. The two chief astrologers with nine other lords of state formed the commission. By dint of hard riding they reached Ispahan seven days after the death of S͟háh 'Abbás. At first Ṣafí Mírzá refused to see the commissioners. He feared that they had come to put out his eyes. At last he allowed them to approach him and learnt the astonishing news that his father had died suddenly and that he himself was advanced from the position of a quasi prisoner to be the absolute lord of all Persia.

To prevent disturbances it was decided that the coronation should be pressed on with all haste, and the astrologers, who had accompanied the commission for this very purpose, were now consulted about an auspicious hour. They named twenty minutes past ten of that same night as the most favourable moment and preparations were accordingly made for the immediate coronation of the young sovereign. He thus in due legal form ascended the throne with the title of S͟háh Ṣafí II.

The first orders that the new monarch gave were that he completely approved of all that had been done since his father's death. To his brother's plea that he should be allowed to retain his sight, he gave no answer. He bade the physicians embalm the body of his father and carry it for burial to Qum and that at the same time there should be prepared three similar coffins. These were to be carried to Ardebil, Meshed and Kashan without revealing in which coffin the body lay. Thus he hoped that no magic or enchantment could be practised on the soul of his father. To the physicians who had failed to preserve his life, he gave orders that they should betake themselves to the palace at Qum which adjoins the mosque, and there pray to God the remainder of their days for the prosperity of his throne.

Ṣafí now began that round of robbery, rape and riot which has made his name a by-word even among oriental monarchs. It was not long before his constitution began to show signs of breaking down under the stress of continuous dissipation. Whatever medicine his doctors provided for him, he took; but it was all of no avail. The bolder bade him refrain from wine. Though he followed their advice for a few days, it was not long before he was drinking deeper than ever. He began to grow pale and anaemic; his body imparted its weakness to his mind. It was noted that when he rode abroad he wore a handkerchief tied three or four times around his neck, which in those times was a sign that a person was sick. At last he was unable to ride and was forced to travel, like a woman, in a *kajáva* on a camel.

His chief physician at last grew terrified that the shah would die and that he himself would be forced into exile along with the physicians of S̲h̲áh 'Abbás. The astrologers added to his fears by whispering that they could not find in the king's horoscope that he had more than six years to live from the time of his coronation. Of these two had already passed. The queen mother refused to believe that the fault of the king's indisposition lay in himself. She quarrelled with the physician, accusing him of treason or ignorance. The physician at his wit's end what to do began to lay the fault upon the stars, saying that if the king was in a languishing condition and could not recover his health, it was because he had failed to observe an auspicious hour for his coronation. The friends of the physician seized upon this argument and threw all the blame upon the astrologers.

It now became the general opinion of the court that the chief astrologer was the cause of the whole of the two years of sickness. There was therefore nothing for it but to repeat the ceremony on a more auspicious day. Such a day was presently found and S̲h̲áh Ṣafí repeated the whole of the coronation ceremonies. To make matters more certain and utterly defeat the misfortunes which had dogged him so far, Ṣafí changed his name to Sulaymán and henceforth became known as S̲h̲áh Sulaymán III.

The shah seems indeed to have benefited by the second ceremony. But his restoration to health was anything but a blessing to the country. His mismanagement of public affairs reduced the lot of the common people to misery and extreme want. Bread was scarce and very expensive; yet the shah lavished money on buildings and entertainments. The first to feel the wrath of the mob was the chief eunuch of the royal household, who was accused of debauching the king with wine, women and witchcraft. But the shah espoused his cause and the people had to be content with the execution of half a dozen Jews who were said to be his accessories. A few months later this same eunuch fell from favour. One night he was invited to the house of a former *ḥakím-báshí*. When this entertainment came to the ears of the shah, he at once sent for the imprudent physician. He, supposing himself to be on the point of reinstatement to office, donned his best clothes and made his way cheerfully to the palace. On reaching the gate his liver turned to water, for there before him was a rope to tie him up.

In spite of his ill health and all his excesses Sháh Sulaymán reigned for nearly 30 years and died a natural death. According to Fr. Krusinski, a member of the Society of Jesus at Ispahan for many years, the shah was 'confined to his bed for two whole years by a very painful gout during which being shut up within the walls of his harem, none but eunuchs came near his person'.[1]

Sulaymán left two sons capable of succeeding him. One, named 'Abbás Mírzá, was physically deformed. His legs were enormously bowed and he was flat footed. He was quite without ambition and was known in consequence as 'The Dervish'. He was therefore passed over in favour of the other son, Ḥusayn Mírzá, who ascended the throne in 1694 and became known to posterity as Sháh Sulṭán Ḥusayn. In his days the decadence of the House of Ṣafavid reached its limit. It was rare to find him sober. His *andarún*—his collection of women, eunuchs and slaves—assumed gigantic proportions. For many years after his death it was

1 Krusinski, *Memoirs*. Quoted in *Chron. Carm. in Persia*, vol. 1, p. 469.

sufficient to say Kizlarun Ili or 'The Year of the Girls' for every Persian to think of 1700. His council of eunuchs, composed of blacks and whites, brought a spirit of faction into the very heart of the palace. His extravagance of public funds knew no limit. He pulled down the old palace at Ispahan and built a new one regardless of cost. Finally, the sudden execution of his chief and most faithful minister at the instigation of the *mulla-báshí* and the *ḥakím-báshí* laid the country open to the successful invasion of the Afghans. In 1720 came the first invasion which captured Kerman. Two years later came the second. After a terrible siege Ispahan fell and with it Sháh Sulṭán Ḥusayn, and the Ṣafavid Dynasty virtually came to an end.

For eight years the Afghans remained in Persia. At no time was their rule complete. The capture of Shiraz confirmed their hold on the south. But, though Qum, Kashan and Qazvin fell into their hands, in the north their rule was not undisputed, for Ṭahmásp Mírzá, a son of Sháh Sulṭán Ḥusayn, assumed his father's office and held his court in Mazanderan. Still further north the Russians began to nibble all along the Persian frontier, though the only province they occupied was that of Gilan. In the west the Turks seized Hamadan and Tabriz. There was therefore at this moment no paramount power in Persia.

It was not until 1736, the year in which Ṭahmásp Qulí Afshár was crowned Shah of Persia under the title of Nádir Sháh, that Persia was once more a united empire. Nádir was the last of the great Asiatic conquerors. Rising from the menial task of guarding the flocks, he became successively servant to the local governor, governor in place of his master, robber chief, and then general to Sháh Ṭahmásp. In this capacity he succeeded in driving out the Afghans and beating back the Turks. The return of the Turks and their defeat of the shah gave Nádir an excuse for dethroning him. Three years later, having again defeated the Turks and having driven the Russians out of the Caspian provinces, he assumed the throne for himself.

Nádir Sháh only reigned for 11 years. The first part of his reign was glorious, for it included the capture of Kandahar, the successful campaign in India and overthrow of the Moghul Empire, and the subjugation of Khiva and Bukhara. Twice were the Turks defeated, and now the Persian Empire again stretched from the Oxus in the north to the Indus in the south. But riches and prosperity brought with them no profit for Persia. They did but corrupt Nádir and made him a cruel and profligate tyrant. His health became deranged. His own physician Fr. Damian of Lyons wrote of him: 'Ce Roy estoit incommodé d'une intempérie chaude du foye et des viscères.' And a little later: 'Le Roy m'a retenu auprès de luy et, grâce à Dieu ie l'ay guéri des vapeurs et humeurs melancholiques, dont il estoit attaqué.'[1]

On the other hand, India, although the fortunes of battle went against her, gained very considerably from the Persian invasion. Persian culture, which the Mongols had carried with them 200 years before, received a fresh breath of life. Persian medicine and Persian science were reintroduced. When these were dying in their native land, they flourished in the neighbouring kingdom. The printing presses of a later generation of Indians did more to popularize and make known the scientific achievements of the Ṣafavid Persian writers than would have been possible had not a victorious campaign carried Persian culture into the capital of the Moghul Empire. Through the invasion of Nádir Sháh Lucknow and Delhi became once more the home of a decadent and stifled Arab medicine.

His murder in 1747 again threw the country into confusion. His Afghan bodyguard attempted to avenge his fall, but was defeated by the Persian troops and retired to Afghanistan. Sháh Rukh, a grandson of Nádir Sháh, after some fighting finally ascended the throne. He was but a child and the position was one which even a strong and experienced man might fear to assume. The treasury was empty. The cash removed from Delhi was all spent, and he was compelled, so it was said at the time, to melt down the Peacock Throne to provide metal with which to pay his soldiers.

1 *Chron. Carm. in Persia*, vol. 1, pp. 608, 609.

Sháh Rukh was, of course, not left in undisputed possession. He was soon defeated and deprived of his eyes. He was then allowed to remain a nominal ruler of Khorasan, while Karím Khán-i-Zand, Muḥammad Ḥasan Khán Qájár and Ázád, the Afghan, fought for the possession of the rest of Persia. Ultimately Karím Khán emerged victorious and for 29 years was supreme ruler of Persia. He made Shiraz his capital and adorned the city with many fine buildings.

On his death the usual strife broke out. The Qájár claim to the throne was again raised, Ághá Muḥammad being now the claimant. The final struggle lay between him and Luṭf 'Alí Khán, a grandson of a brother of Karím Khán. Luṭf 'Alí was for the moment successful and reigned, if indeed such an uncertain and disturbed possession of the throne can be called reigning, from 1786 to 1794. Luṭf 'Alí, although brave, good looking and a leader of men, drove many of his supporters away by his overbearing and imperious character. After a series of small victories he was besieged in Kerman by Ághá Muḥammad and yielded only when starvation compelled him. He was blinded, taken to Teheran and murdered. The women of Kerman were handed over to the soldiery. Of the men 600 were murdered and 20,000 were blinded.

Among the few who escaped were a son and daughter of Luṭf 'Alí. The former was named 'Alí Khán Mírzá and was then a child of seven. He was castrated by the orders of Ághá Muḥammad, and was employed when grown up in the seraglio of 'Abbás Mírzá who had married his sister. Keppel, who met him in India, described him as 'tall and emaciated; his eyes are large and black, and his complexion is sallow. Though not more than thirty-eight years old, he appears double that age, and his voice and features so resemble those of a female, that when wrapped up in shawls, he might easily be mistaken for an old woman'.[1]

So was founded the Qájár Dynasty.

1 Keppel. *Personal Narrative of a Journey from India to England* (London, 1827), vol. 1, p. 4.

CHAPTER XIV

THE EAST INDIA COMPANY IN PERSIA

IN the year 1611, being the twenty-fourth year of his reign, Sháh 'Abbás the Great sent to the court of King James I of England, an Englishman as his ambassador. This was the famous Robert Sherley. He was authorized by the shah to offer to the English the free and absolute use of two ports in Persia, in return for their friendship and their trade. Three years later, a Mr Richard Steele succeeded in reaching India by the overland route, and related to the British merchants at Surat the enormous advantages which he foresaw from the opening up of trade with Persia. The offer of Sháh 'Abbás was thus unexpectedly seconded. Two years later, the Persian section of the East India Company was founded by the establishment of factories at Jask and Ispahan.

For the first few years of its existence, the Agency in Persia had no regular medical staff. The factories on the coast were probably looked after by the surgeons who arrived at rare intervals in British ships. To the factory at Ispahan, a Scottish physician was attached. This was a certain George Strachan. His life was a strange one. In 1602 he was in Rome, where he entered the Scots College, but apparently never reached even minor orders. A desire to travel took him a few years later to Constantinople. From there he passed on to Syria, the Lebanon and Aleppo. At this last place, having heard that the *amír* of 'Anayza was in need of a physician, with the ulterior object of perfecting his Arabic, he took service with him, although he was at the moment entirely ignorant of medicine. However, he furnished himself with some prescriptions from a Flemish doctor, bought a book or two and started to practise. He was enormously successful, and only with difficulty some three years later did he escape from his patron, whose sister he had married.

He then made his way via Baghdad to Ispahan, where the English had just established a trading house. They, both because they feared he would join the Spanish embassy and because they needed a medical attendant, engaged him as their linguist and surgeon at a salary of twelve tomans a year.

But he was not happy. He was accused of peculation and even of murder, and in August of 1620, he was dismissed from the Company's service.

And Strachan our Antechristian Phesitian, for his fflattering, lying, dissimulation, inconscionable stores of purloynment, with his tentar-hookes of deere penniworthes of plaisters and purges, sowing dissention in the ffactory, his scandalous reporte of poyzoning the Companys servants as the late Agent and William Rhyns, his discouering all the passages of our busines to the ffryers in Espahan, through his confession and disloyall service to the Company, intercepting of their letters. How can he be otherwise, being marryed to a More in Arabia, from whom he tooke his runnagate raunge, leaving wyfe and family to prosecute the divells commission in doing evill; continewally despizeth his owne country, and yts church, And confesseth to haue the dispensation of the Pope to dissemble his Religion in all his Pilgrymage. Whose plague infection to remove from our ffactory (by irresistible reasons to the Agent besides costeth the Company 100l. per annum) hath wrought him to act the devill, to make a compleate nomber of my cappitall Aduersaries.

Thus wrote Robert Jefferis, a factor of the Company at Ispahan. The authorities at Surat, however, seem to have taken the side of Strachan, and Jefferis was dismissed. Strachan was reinstated in the following year, although only temporarily. In Ispahan he spent his leisure instructing the Carmelite missionaries. 'The Fathers have an Englishman as their teacher of Arabic—a good Catholic who had studied in Rome—reading for two hours daily, and having conversation one hour', wrote Fr. Prosper in August 1621.[1]

In 1622 Strachan was in Gombroon, now known as Bandar Abbas, getting ready a house and establishing a factory and

1 *Chron. Carm. in Persia*, vol. I, p. 236.

waiting to take charge of the silk convoy which was about to arrive. Except for the statement that in November of that year he suffered from a severe attack of fever and returned to Ispahan and that he was then superseded by a regular medical officer of the Company, history is silent about the rest of his life. Possibly he came back to Europe. Certainly he intended to do so, for he commissioned Fr. Vincent, a Carmelite father, to take to Rome sixty-one of his books written in Arabic, Persian, and Turkish, and he promised to pay the cost of their transport as soon as he himself reached Rome. In the archives of the Order is Strachan's will in which he bequeathed these books to the Carmelite Convent in Rome. In the Library at Naples there are (or were) several manuscripts with their titles inscribed in his handwriting. In the British Museum, too, are to be found translations into Latin in the small and neat handwriting of Strachan himself of two Persian philosophical works. On the first page of one of these is written: 'Universum seu ut Persae vocant Poculum Mundi: Opera Georgii Strachani Mernensis Scoti in Latinum idioma traducta 1634.'[1] This book was discovered not in Europe but in Baghdad, and the question of his return to Italy still remains doubtful.

His religion, his irregular qualifications, and the complaints which were lodged against him made it undesirable to retain him on the nominal roll of the Company. The minutes of a meeting in Surat, held in March 1621, record that Thomas Quince, who had been sent out for service in Surat, 'though here bee already a suffitient surgeon', was to be dispatched in the following year to Persia 'for excuseinge the chardge and supplyinge the place of an unnecessaire phisition ther entertayned'.

It is clear that from this time on there was a regular physician attached to the factory at Gombroon, though I think that he was the only British doctor in Persia. The Company's agents inland were not supplied with medical advisers. Neither was one included in the suite of Sir Dodmore Cotton, the first British ambassador to the Persian court, who arrived as the representative

1 British Museum Or. MSS. Add. 7720, ff. 63 et seqq.

of King Charles I in 1626, for Herbert, an attaché, has left an account of the ambassador's death at Qazvin and makes no mention of any British physician being in attendance. Later, when he himself fell ill, he 'wanted not the advice and help of the Archiater, the King's doctor; who albeit he was doubtless a very skilled physician, yet did me little good, so malignant was my distemper; albeit I took what he prescribed (part of which I well remember were pomegranate pills, barberries, sloes in broth, rice and sundry other things) and returned what he expected: so that it was hard to judge whether my spirits or gold decayed faster'.[1] He was ultimately cured by a Tartar woman servant who for her fee robbed him while asleep of his clothes and money.

In 1633 Quince was succeeded at Gombroon by Constantine Young who was hurried out to Persia on account of the excess of sickness in the factory. A few years later the factor at Ispahan, mindful perhaps of the recent death of the British ambassador, appealed for the appointment of a surgeon there too. But the president and council at Swally refused the request, remarking that a surgeon was unnecessary as 'fever and fluxes, both in India and Persia, are most familiarly cured by natives of each or either, to whome nor meanes nor skill is wanting'.

In the autumn of 1660 Young was replaced at Gombroon by Richard Brough, who did not stay very long, for the Diary records that Stephen Flower, the agent in Persia, was accompanied by one Thomas Boyce as surgeon, when he travelled up from Gombroon to Ispahan in 1668. In this same year the minutes of the court of directors record that a Mr Samuel Carlton was entertained as surgeon for Persia at a salary of 45*s.* a month. He was also granted by the same court the sum of £5 to spend upon fresh provisions, presumably for the crew of the ship which was to carry him out. Next year his salary was raised to 50*s.* a month. But he received no benefit from the rise, for his mother complained to the court of directors at home that it was not being

1 Herbert, *A Relation of some Yeares Travaile* 1638 (republished in Broadway Traveller series), pp. 208, 221.

paid to him. A stiff letter was therefore sent in the April of 1674 to the president at Surat, bidding him see that the English authorities in Persia paid their surgeon in full.

In 1676, one of the great physicians, whom the Company was fortunate enough to employ, was sent out to India. This was John Fryer. He was born about 1650, educated at Trinity College, Cambridge, and qualified in 1672. He offered himself almost at once to the East India Company and was accepted. 'We have enterteyned Mr John Fryer as Chirurgeon for Bombay', wrote the directors in London, 'at fifty shillings per month to commence at his arriveall, and have furnished the Chirurgery Chest now sent according to the directions of Mr Ward.'

When Fryer arrived, he found that he was supernumerary, and was not really required. He was thus easily persuaded by the Company's agent of Persia, 'representing how highly conducive to the Company's Interest one of my Profession would be there', to put in the first few months of his service in the factories of Persia instead of in India.[1]

He accordingly sailed on 18 February 1677, in a vessel called the *Scipio African*, in the company of a young Franciscan friar, who had been almost bled to death by the physicians of Goa in their efforts to save his life. On 22 March, the party landed without any misadventures at Gombroon. Here Fryer stayed until the heat of the summer forced the agent to seek the cooler hills of the central Persian plateau. Fryer was invited to accompany him, and the party set out for Ispahan on 28 June. After a short stop at Shiraz, they set out again, and finally reached Ispahan on 7 August, 'having accomplished a tedious Journey in the hottest Season of the Year over desolate parching Sands and naked Rocks... seven hundred miles, which we performed in Thirty two Days, abating the Time for Refreshment, and One Day for our Excursion to Persepolis'.

Without any delay, Fryer set out to explore the city. He was first attracted by the druggists, who lived around the gate which led to the Armenian bazaar. These he found to be 'all Jews, who

1 Fryer, *Voyage*, bk. ii, p. 149 and *New Account*, p. 217 et passim.

are very numerous, and live apart, though their Shops are in common with the Natives in the Bazaars, mixed among a Crowd of other Tradesmen; who sell by Retail, and pass without any Brand, having their Synagogues open every Sabbath-day'. Other writers have remarked upon the great number of pharmacies which abounded in Ispahan in those days. Herbert, who had visited the city a few years before Fryer, wrote that there was no lack of 'the knowledge of herbs, drugs, and gums, the Mydan in Spahawn abounding in singular variety, and than which, no place in the world can more aptly be termed a Panacaea, a Catholicon, of herbs, of drugs: a Magazein 'gainst all diseases'.

Of colleges, mosques and Christian churches Fryer has a lot to say, but of hospitals nothing. It is strange that a medical man should omit any mention of a side of life which he was so particularly well qualified to describe and which he had not failed to visit when in Bombay and Goa. It is not as though the great hospitals of Persia had fallen into disuse and been allowed to tumble down. Fr. Raphael du Mans, who was in Ispahan at the time of Fryer's visit, says that every large town had one or two. He even mentions the hospital at Ispahan, saying that in his day it was a large, square building with a cloister into which all the wards, large and windowless rooms, opened. It was not very much used, for when he visited it he found there only one moribund Indian lying on the floor and in another room a solitary madman chained to the wall. It was so unpopular among the townsmen that it was referred to in conversation as the *Dár-ul-Marg* or House of Death.

More observant than Fryer, Sir John Chardin writes that when he visited Tabriz, he saw three hospitals in the city 'very neat and well in repair'.[1] But they contained no inmates and were only used as a centre of food distribution for the necessitous. Hence they were known by the name of *Ach-tucon* or 'Place where they spend a great deal of Victuals'. Similarly the hospital at Ardebil, which adjoined the Great Mosque, was a place 'where daily they

1 Chardin, *Travels in Persia*, p. 354.

give food to all those who go there and many gather in pilgrimages from various parts'.[1]

Of the hospitals of Shiraz, too, Fryer makes no mention. But he does remark that at a little village 20 miles north of Gombroon, where there were some natural hot water springs, there were two 'handsome hospitals... neat and durable works'. These were not Persian foundations, but were built one by the Dutch and the other by an Indian banker in the service of the Company. In his later book which he called *The New Account*, he enlarges on these hospitals and on the nature and source of the water. The springs were still being used for therapeutic purposes a hundred years later, for Dr John Parker, a surgeon of the Company at Gombroon, was sufficiently interested to use them and to take some of the water back to England. On analysis it was found that sulphur was the active principle.

The president of the Company at Surat having died this midsummer and the agent in Persia having been nominated as his successor, the sub-agent at Ispahan was compelled to go down to Gombroon to take temporary charge of the Agency there. Fryer and he, therefore, left Ispahan in January 1678. In their company was a French surgeon bound for Bandar-i-Rig, and probably for India. At Shiraz the party was joined by a Georgian soldier and a French Carmelite friar, who travelled with them the rest of the way to Gombroon. Possibly this friar was Fr. Angelus, the author of the *Pharmacopoeia Persica*, for it was in this year that he returned to France.

From January to April Fryer remained in Gombroon. In the middle of that month the same ship that carried the new president to India returned with the new agent for Persia. This was one John Petit, who being none too strong, desired to leave the coast and reach Ispahan before the hot weather set in. Within a few days, Fryer and the agent set out for the interior. They reached Lar on 8 May, and there, most of the company fell sick. The Europeans were too prostrate to sit their horses, and were carried

1 *Chron. Carm. in Persia*, vol. I, p. 117.

on in litters or in *kajávas*. These latter are pairs of large panniers slung on either side of a horse or camel. Adam Oelschläger, better known as Olearius, the secretary of the embassy from the Duke of Holstein, had a few years before this the misfortune of being compelled to travel in the same manner. 'The Physician and myself', he bewails, 'were set in ketzaweha upon the same camel, whereby we were put to great inconveniences—one proceeding from the violent motion caused by the going of that Great Beast which at every step gave us a furious jolt; and the other from the insupportable stink of the camels, the infectious smell of whom came full into our noses.'

The party remained in Shiraz until the end of May. The agent then decided to push on to Ispahan, but, at the earnest request of a Spanish Carmelite, resident at Shiraz, who had 'been long grieved with a continued Fever and finding no relief from the Country Physicians', the agent left Fryer behind to attend to him and to the English residents in the city. Scarcely was the Spaniard recovered when Fryer himself fell sick. Even before he was recovered, he was summoned to treat the governor of the city, 'a great Saint, because rich and one of Mahomet's kindred'. To please the Carmelite and the Armenian Christians, whose welfare depended so much upon the favour of the governor, Fryer consented to be carried out to his palace:

> Whereupon my Attendance is engaged, and a Million of Promises, could I restore him to his Health, laid down from his Wives, Children, and Relations, who all (with the Citizens, as I could hear going along, pray to God that the Hackin Fringi, the Frank Doctor, might kill him) play'd the Hypocrites, wishing his Death; the first to compleat the Expectation of what he might leave them, the other for his being a Plague to them; as it proved after his Recovery, for they performed as much as he, dismissing me with a Compliment, and no other Reward.

On 6 July, Fryer was sufficiently recovered to continue his journey, and he set out for Ispahan. Again he did not stay long. The port of Gombroon required the presence of another Englishman during the 'time of shipping', and the agent being obliged to remain in Ispahan, as he had failed as yet to secure an interview with the shah, Fryer returned alone to the coast. The news of his arrival, as he passed through Shiraz, was at once conveyed to the governor, who expressed a desire to have some more of the medicine which had effected his cure in the spring. But Fryer, having received no fee for his former services, was not disposed to attend him again. He delayed presenting himself until the caravan had already left the city, and then made the excuse that his servant and his medicine chest were already out of reach. The Sayyid, undaunted, replied that he would send a couple of trustworthy servants to overtake the caravan at the end of the day's march. With this Fryer took his leave.

On his return to the factory, most of those present congratulated him upon his consultation, and inquired what fee he had received. When he replied that he had received just the same amount for the second consultation that he had for the first, one of those present remarked that he was lucky to have come with his hat, and not to have had that stolen from off his head. The servants of the governor did indeed catch him up that evening, but Fryer refused to see them, and they returned empty-handed to their master.

Apparently on reaching Gombroon Fryer fell ill again, for on the last day of November he returned to India, 'being forced by sickness to leave Persia and thereby becoming destitute of employment'. For a short time he remained in Surat, and then came back to England. Here he became an M.D. of his university, and in 1697 was elected a Fellow of the Royal Society. What is of greater interest is that he published his observations upon the internal state of Persia. He discusses the climate, the court, the people and their customs. He also devotes a few pages to the state of medicine as he found it. Seeing that this is the testimony of an eyewitness of a period of which so little is known, I think that I am justified in quoting *in extenso* Fryer's account:[1]

At length I convert myself to that Noble and Excellent Art, so beneficial to the Life of Man, Physick; which though it be here in good

1 Fryer, *Voyage*, bk. iii, p. 94.

Repute, yet its Sectators are too much wedded to Antiquity, not being at all addicted to find out its Improvement by new Enquiries; wherefore they stick to the Arabian Method as devoutly as to the Sacred Tripod, which they hold as Infallible as of old that Delphic Oracle was accounted.

On which score Chymistry is hardly embraced; nor to the Pathological part do they think the Anatomical Knife can bring much Profit: However, many of them have Wealthy Presents from their Grandees.

Whoever applies himself to this Profession, takes a Master of that Calling, who Instructs him in the Stile and ordinary Characters of Medicine; where being thoroughly versed in the Employment, and able to set up for himself, he consults whereabouts the fewest Physicians are planted in the City, and the likeliest place to draw Customers to him; there he joins an Apothecary to make up his Prescripts, and sells them to his Patients, the half of which Gain comes into his Pocket: Thus by degrees increasing in Fame, he covets many Students to Read to, who are sure to spread abroad his Fame, like so many Speaking trumpets, and are sent about in quest of Prey, to bring in Game like so many Decoys.

But the Bait that takes most, are the Women crying up their Man, when he is found to please them by a fair Carriage and voluble Tongue, who never leave off till they have rendered him gracious to all their Acquaintance; who flock to him in Droves, and are as full of chat as a Magpy when she has found an Owl in the Wood at Noon day; nor wants he his Lime-twigs for such sort of Birds, by whose frequenting he arrives at the top of his hopes, and sucks those Riches Galen is said to offer his Disciples: Dat Galenus opes.

But as all the Eggs laid under one Hen do not always prove, so many of this Tribe miss their aim, and after an expence of Time and endeavour, are forced to fall upon other Trades to get a Livelyhood. Here is no presedent License of Practising, but it is lawful for anyone to exercise this Function who has the impudence to pretend to it.

The Suffee retains several in Ordinary, and others in Extraordinary, without any Salary; the Chief of whom is called Hakaim Bashee, and suffers on his Master's Death, not only Banishment from Court, but Dispoyling of all his Goods, and must acknowledge it a Favour to escape with his Life.

In the matter of their Physick, Extracts, or Essences of Plants, Roots, or Minerals, are beyond their Pharmacy; only they use cooling Seeds, and medicines of that nature; so that in repelling a Fever, they make but one work of that and the Innate Heat, where most an end both become extinguished at once; or at least, the Body is left in that condition, that Obstructions or an Ill Habit succeeds; although I am not ignorant, that sometimes after the greatest Care in Chronical Distempers, such things will happen, according to the Experience of Hippocrates, yet in Acute Distempers so frequently to fall into these Indispositions, I cannot excuse the Indiscretion of these Medicasters, whose Patients in Suffahaun seldom pass out of this Life by any other way to their Graves.

Besides this Abuse, their Prescriptions are Pancrastical, a Salve for every Sore, without respect had to difference of Temperament or Constitution; nay, even to the Distempers themselves; but asking some frivolous Questions, viewing the Veins of the Hands and Feet, inspecting the Tongue, they write at adventure. The Apothecary dispenses the Ingredients into so many Papers, and leaves them to be boiled according to his Directions, and given to the Sick Party at such and such hours of such a day, by any good Woman or heedless Servant; who not attending the Quantities of the Liquor more than the Qualities of the Ingredients, boil more or less, not as the Exigency either of the Medicines or the Patient requires, but as if they were to make Pottage, and give him to drink of this heterogenous Broath, sometimes three or four Pints at a time; so that if it fails moving the Belly by its excitative Faculty, yet by its excessive Dose it makes way for Evacuation: And this they do repeat most an end for a Fortnight or Three Weeks together; which if it succeed not, another Physician is consulted; for among such store they think it hard to miss of a Cure; and in that are so opinionated, that if their own Nation cannot give them a Remedy, they think none other can. (Though as to Chyrurgery they are of another mind, thinking the Europeans better at Manual Operation than themselves.) But to proceed, being severely handled by one, they fly to another; and he from extreme Cold things runs upon the other extreme; so that between these two Rocks its no wonder the Patient so often miscarries, and so many concurring Causes joined with their Distemper, hurry them to another World.

Rhabarb, Turbith, and Scammony are dreadful to them; but Senna, Cassia, Manna, and Turpentine are swallowed without any apprehension of evil. Many of their Physicians insist on diets unusual elsewhere, as Goats-flesh, Horses, Asses, and Camels flesh; for which reason they have distinct Shambles for the same purpose.

Avicen, Averroes, and Rhasis, are known Authors among them; and among the most Learned, Galen and Hippocrates, and some more Modern, who have treated of Botany, and Human parts.

Their Law forbids them to inspect a dead Carkass; they therefore lean implicitly on what they find among Ancient Anatomists, and yet think themselves at no loss in that Science; whence it is their Practice is lame, and their Theory no more than the prating of a Parrot.

Hence it follows they are imperfect in the Chyrurgeons Art; they can tell how to protract slight Wounds into Length of Time, but for things of real danger they are to seek which way to handle; especially where

'Ense recidendum ne pars sincera trahatur.
The knife is used to part the dead, and give
The Vital Part occasion to live.'

Yet they are bold enough with the Blood, where they command Phlebotomy, bleeding like Farriers.

The Endemial Diseases of this Country, are Phrensies, Plurisies, Peripneumonies, Empyemaes, Catarrhs, distempers of the Eyes; Red Gum, which besets our Children in Europe, is pernicious to Old Age here; S. Anthony's Fire, or more properly the Persian Fire, impressing on the adust Blood the nature of Atrabile: But the fashionable Malady of the Country is a Clap, scarce One in Ten being free from it; which the unbounded Liberty of Women, Cheapness of the Commodity, and the encouragement of their filthy Law, are main Incentives to. And to back this Lewdness, they bring the Example of their Prophet Haly, who lying down without a Female Companion, is reported to be the Author of this doughty Dialogue between the Earth and him, wherein the Earth upbraided him by saying, 'Whilst you lye on the Ground an unfruitful Log, a burthen to my sides, I sweat and labour in producing Vegetables, Minerals, and Animals for your use; Why then do you not busy yourself in getting Children, to transmit your Offspring to Posterity?' Which pleasing Reproof of the Venerable Prophet's recommending to his easy Disciples, they embrace with both Arms, while the Poyson creeps into the Marrow of their Bones, so that they are not come to Maturity, before they are rotten; though by reason of the Pureness of the Air, it seldom or never arrives to that height of Cruelty as in Europe; inasmuch as when any are so dealt by it, they reproach it with the Frank Disease, Atecheque Fringi, when it breaks out into Sores and Ulcers, after it has seized the whole Mass of Blood, and eats them up alive; while they wear theirs dormant almost to extreme Old Age, which makes them not much solicitous for Remedy, nor are there any who profess its Cure.

There is another Infirmity as general almost, proceeding from their Ceremonial Washing, when they exonerate, too frequent using of Baths, which causes a Relaxation of the Muscles of the Anus, whereby the great Gut of the Fundament falls down: Most of them by a Fulness of Body are subject to Hemorrhoids; but what chiefly vexes them, walking or riding, (putting them into miserable Pain, and contorted Postures of the Back, and whole Trunk of the Body), is a Fistula in Ano, which they contract from their Athletick Temper, and constant being on Horseback; as has been observed not only by Sennertus, but Platerus, Fernelius, and others: Nor does it seldom fall out, from their aptness to Venery, and proneness to make use of Boys, that they are afflicted with terrible Mariscae, or swoln Piles of several forms, by them called Obne; wherein Worms, as they perswade themselves, are bred, that excruciate them with such an Itch as they cannot lay, without adding Sin to Sin, and therein they report their Cure to be compleated; and this brings on them a white Leprosy, not incommoding the Body with Illness, but disgracing it with Spots in the Face, Arms, Thighs, Breast, and other parts about them. Children have frequently Scald Heads, which makes them keep close shav'd.

The Plague has not been known among them this Eighty Years and upwards, but the Spotted Fever kills them presently, yet is not contagious: the Bezoar-stone in this Case is highly approved.

The Gout afflicts few here, the Pox commonly securing them from it; however as painful as that proves to their Bones, or rather Membranes surrounding them, they applaud all provocatives in Physick, and will purchase them at any Rates; which are sometimes so strong, that they create a continued Priapism to these Goats and Satyrs, and by the Bows being always bent, are brought to an Inability of reducing them.

To divert their Care and Labours, they are great Devourers of Opium, and Koquenar (which is Poppy-heads boil'd), which they quaff when they have a mind to be merry; for which reason Hemp is sown among our Fens and Fields, so they sow Poppies, and when ripe, make incision for the Juice, which gathering, they inspissate, and eat; to do which, those unaccustomed adventuring unadvisedly upon too large a Dose, instead of the expected effect of cheering the Spirits, chain up the Vitals so that they are never loosed more, for they never awake from the Lethargy it intrances them in: so that they begin gradually, and then arrive to great Quantities; as from a Grain to half an Ounce, without any Harm, besides a frolicksome sort of Drunkenness; by means whereof, without any other Sustenance, they are qualified to undergo great Travels and Hardships: But having once begun, they must continue it, or else they dye; whereby it becomes so necessary, that if they mis-time themselves, as in their Ramzan, or on a Journey, they often expire for want of it: Yet those that live at this rate are always as lean as Skeletons, and seldom themselves; but such is their love towards it, that they give themselves up to the study of infatuating themselves by all the ways they can, never smoaking a Pipe without the Leafs of the intoxicating Bang, and flowers of the same, mixed with their Tobacco; besides which, they contrive many more Medicines to put a Cheat upon the Pungency of their Cares, and drive Sorrow from their Hearts; which indeed diverts them for some few hours, till they return with a more fixed Melancholy, burthensome to themselves and others: While the Operation of their forced Mirth lasts, they are incapable at that time of any Business; Whence they proverbially say, Belque Teriac ne resid, to any Trifler, or Fiery Spirit; that the Force of your Treacle you have eaten, still remains.

Moreover, they have other Treacles, such as are taken notice to be sold in the Markets, by Apulcies, and the Circe of Homer, prepared as Counter-Poysons, which are compounded of Garlick, Mother of Thyme, and other Herbs beaten together: that Rich one made use of only by Nobles, is adventitious, and is brought by their Merchants from Venice, the Poor not being able to go to the Price of such Medicines or Physicians as exceed the common Rates; and therefore it is that their great Towns and Buzzars are full of Mountebanks, Charmers, and Quacksalvers, to gull them of their Cash.

It is interesting to compare this very satirical account with another estimate, also written by an Englishman, but not a doctor, just 50 years before.[1]

Their physicians are great admirers of Nature [he wrote], doting so much thereon as they make that oft-times the first causer which indeed is but instrumental or secondary. Moral men they be, humane in language and garb, both which beget esteem from all that converse with

1 Herbert, *A Relation of some Yeares Travaile* 1638 (republished in Broadway Traveller series), pp. 244–5.

them; and did not avarice (a vice predominating there, and by occasion of sickness in me full dearly experimented) and magic studies too far sway them, I could value them above the rest. They have degrees transcending one another in title as their skill and seniority merits. So well as I could apprehend, these are learned in the sciences, and few but are philosophers; nevertheless, their libraries are small; their books usually Arabic, but choice and useful, commonly such as advance their practice and profession; and in their proper art I perceived that they prefer plants and other vegetables before minerals. Some schools I visited and observed (as I formerly mentioned, near Lar) that, according to the old adage necessarium est silentium ad studia, they affect silence, and sitting cross-legged wag their bodies, imagining that such motion advantages study and serves for exercise. The doctors are named hackeems, mulaii in Arabic. But a mountebank or impostor is nicknamed Shitan-tabib i.e. the Devil's Chirurgeon. They are masters of much knowledge, and not a little delighted with judicial astrology. Many Arabic writers, learned both in natural philosophy and the mathematics, have flourished in those parts, most of whose books they read, namely Hippocrates, Galen, Averroes, Alfarabius (al-Farábí), Avicenna, Ben Isaac (? Ḥunayn ibn Isḥáq), Abbu Ally, Mahummed Abdillah, Ben-Eladib, Abu-Becr (I cannot identify these four), Rhazis, Alghazzallys (al-Ghazálí), and Albu-mazar (Abú Ma'shar al-Balkhí).

With the departure of Fryer for India there is again a gap in the medical records of the Agency. The factory Diary contains frequent entries of illnesses, deaths, and petitions for sick leave, but no doctor is mentioned by name. But from other authorities it is known that a doctor named Engelbert Kaempfer was in practice for a short time in Gombroon. This man, born in 1651 at Lemgo in the county of Lippe, had reached Persia in 1684 in the capacity of secretary and physician to the Swedish ambassador to the court of Sháh Sulaymán. On the return of the ambassador to Europe Kaempfer went south and became physician to the Dutch fleet in the Persian Gulf. He made Gombroon his head-quarters and here he stayed until driven out by fever.

On his return to Europe he published his impressions of Persia in a work which he called *Amoenitatum exoticarum politico-physico-medicarum fasciculi V quibus continentur variae relationes, observationes et descriptiones rerum persicarum et ulterioris Asiae multa attentione in peregrinationibus per universum Orientem collectae.* An interesting sidelight is thrown upon the origin of this work by a manuscript now kept in the British Museum.[1] It is entitled *Descriptio Persiae communicata Dno. Engelberto Kaempfero, Ispanae* 1684, *cum grammatica linguae turcicae.* At the beginning of the description of Persia is found a dedication which runs: 'In obsequium clarissimi viri et Domini Engelberti Kempfer, medici peritissimi necnon ejusdem fidelissimi amici D.D. pristaue. In Hispan., Persidis regia, 22 Sept. 1684. Humillimus servulus Raphael du Mans residentiae nostrae 38 anno.' Fr. Raphael was the superior of the Capuchin Mission in Ispahan whose work *Estat de la Perse en* 1660 I have had to quote more than once.

The next mention of any Englishman practising in Persia, that I have been able to discover, occurs in the Gombroon Diary for 1727. A certain doctor, Anthony Forbes, was now in charge of the health of the factory. By this time a small hospital had been built upon which there was a monthly expenditure of 160 shahis. As the expenses of the house amounted to 5487 shahis a month the treatment provided for the sick can scarcely have been lavish. The scandal of the high cost of living was apparently realized by the authorities in India, for a few months later a command to reduce it was received. The doctor was one of the few who thereby suffered.

It being now near the end of the month and the chief for sundry good reasons inclinable to brake off the continuance of the Publick Table the principall motive inducing him to it being a letter he had the honour to receive from the Honourable the Resident of Bengall Palley wherein he is pleased to recommend the same to him and having observed that the monthly expce. thereof to allways exceed the stated allowance wh. he and Councill thought fit in their commands to Fort St George Palley to reduce it to and most of the Gentlemen (except Mr May, the Doctor, and Mr Pack) frequently absenting themselves from it He directed the Steward to signifie to those Gentlemen that it would not be continued longer than the last day of the month when they were to provide for themselves on the allowance of thirty rupees per month Diet money.

1 British Museum, Sloane Collection, no. 2908.

The spirit of economy which the directors, both in India and in London, were continually urging upon the factors in the Persian Gulf, appeared at its worst in the treatment of their sick, and in the meanness of the hospital allowance. A letter from Dr Forbes to the supervisor runs:

Pursuant to your order I have examined ye chests of Physic that came by ye Fort St George Galley and was much surprised to find most of it useless all ye Elect. Pills, Vol. Sp. & Salts being quite dry'd up and perfectly mouldy. The Volats. without any manner of smell the corks being entirely rotted all ye roots herbs & seeds being in ye same condition, only some few emollient oils and other chemicall preparations yt. are any ways serviceable, sevl. other medicines being only such as are the reall produce of this country, as senna, roses, bole, Dragons Blood likewise several seeds as anise cummin &c: all ye medicines in genl. being very old, so that we are now under the greatest straits imaginable, as there is many of the Garrison very ill.

Again two years later occurs the entry:

Gombroon Friday December 13th. 1728

The Doctor representing to us that he wanted spirits for sundry uses in the Hospital ordered the Linguist to deliver him a chest of Persian Brandy for that purpose.

Apparently the doctor was sometimes compelled to purchase the necessary drugs out of his own pocket, for the following entry occurs, dated Gombroon, July 1730:

Mr Tomlin our Surgeon gives in a petition to us complaining that Mr Clift has not paid him for sundry Medicines used in the Hospitall & charged in his stewards accots. to the amount of 1617 in March and April and Mr Clift being now become bankrupt & not in a condition to pay him, humbly prays his case may be taken into consideration, & he reimbursed said sum as he objected against Mr Clift for a Paymaster before he delivered in the Vouchers of his accounts, & as the surgeon did actually apply to the Chief before either of those months accounts were made up & desired they might be pass'd singly & the amt. paid to him declarg. he would not accept Mr Clift as a Paymaster, & the Medicines etc. having been used for the Company's servants & soldiery it appears to us reasonable that the surgeon should be reimbursed what he has expended on that account, agreed therefore that the Broker discharge the same and that the Accompt. debt Mr Clift for it.

By 1734 the meanness of the Company had reached such a pitch that all the officers were compelled to protest. The minutes of December of that year contain the detailed protest of the chief of each department. The general price of living in Persia had apparently risen, for the prices of wheat, butter and oil show large increases. Under the heading of Hospital and Medicines, the doctor wrote:

This depends on ye supplies from B.bay wch. has lately been so neglected that wee have not had any good or proper medicines in the Factory for the whole season particularly Bark and every man in the Factory sick of Feavers but have been obliged to purchase them from the Dutch and Eur. ships at Extravagant rates not withstanding wch. these Articles have not exceeded above per mensem 100.

Life was very thrilling and very vivid in those parts and in those days. Apart from the purely technical details of the price of various bales of merchandise and the methods of disposing of the stock, the greater part of the minutes of the monthly transactions of the Agency at Gombroon is taken up with detailed accounts of fighting against marauding Arabs and hostile Persians, intrigues against the Dutch, and diplomatic missions to the Persian court to secure some trade advantage.

Occasionally the fighting came very near their headquarters. For instance, in October 1733 the 'Ballooches' attacked the town of Gombroon in such overwhelming force that the English and Dutch joined up in order to hold the town for their companies. In the fighting the British doctor was killed.

Monday October 8th. About four this afternoon Doctor Tomlin dyed and was buryd in the Armenian Church Yard—it not being safe to venture to carry him without the Town wall.

That month the hospital expenses rose to the unprecedented figure of 977 shahis.

Dr Tomlin was succeeded by a Dr Patrick Oliphant, who on the pay list ranked second to the agent. The European staff at that time quartered in Gombroon consisted of an agent who, although a young man between 30 and 40 years of age, was in control of all the trading stations of Persia, the Gulf and Mesopotamia. He received a salary of £150 per annum. Second to him came the doctor with a salary of £60 per annum. Then came the senior and junior merchants who received respectively £40 and £30. The two junior civilians, called factor and writer, received respectively £15 and £5 a year. To protect the Gombroon factory against robbers, the Afghans and Arab pirates, the Company kept in barracks within the factory an ensign, two sergeants, one corporal, one drummer, twenty-nine British private soldiers and twenty sepoys. This was the total of the Company's servants, exclusive of the Persian staff for whom the surgeon was responsible. In his spare time he was allowed to treat those outside the factory. His collection of his fees from these outside persons was difficult and again and again the Company, realizing the value of such work, made good to him his bad debts.

Our Doctor having several times mentioned the trouble he has been at in attending the People in Government especially in the time of Tockey Caun and having allways Expended his own Medicines humbly requests we will take the same under our Consideration, and as we are sensible what bad Pay Masters the Gentlemen in Government are upon all Occasions Agreed that we allow him the sum of four thousand shahis which he seems satisfied with out of the Cash and entered accordingly.

Although all the records seem to show that only one surgeon was supplied for the whole of Persia, yet it is clear that other physicians were sometimes available who must have been either surgeons to ships or adventurers. For when the agent went on tour he took his medical adviser with him and a locum tenens attended to the needs of the factory.

April 13th 1734. The Agent having been dangerously ill for some months past and the Heats coming on apace, He finds himself to grow worse & is so faint and weak, the Doctor declares he should despair of his life, if he continued here. The Agent therefore set out this day, to retire into a cool climate....Doctor Oliphant, Mr Smith & Mr Savage attended the Agent.

In the winter of the next year the agent made another tour, this time to Baghdad, in order to stimulate trade and correct abuses. On his return he wrote to Bombay to complain that he was out of pocket on the trip and to ask for a special 'allowance for a Doctor' because Dr Oliphant had accompanied him again. The following entry occurs in the balance sheet for that year:

Doctor Russell as a Gratuity for staying at Gombroon till the return of Doctor Oliphant from up-country with the Agent 3,000 shahis.

In the year 1738 occurs a very interesting entry in the Diary, for it may be the earliest reference to the crippling effect of plague in the Gulf which was henceforth to play such an important part in the relations of Persia with India and Europe.

February 1738. Monsieur Vigoreux Commander of this Ship gives a miserable account of Bussorah, half of the inhabitants being carried off by the late sickness and no manner of trade stirring.

In the spring of this year Dr Oliphant, complaining of 'having served the Hon. Company five years in Persia & being reduced by many sicknesses to a very bad state of health, desires that We will give him leave to go up to Bussorah on the Expedition... with his request to be relieved'. He obtained leave to accompany the expedition, but apparently was not allowed to return from there to England, because four years later he was being employed on a mission to Mosul.

His resignation of his post at Gombroon was, however, accepted and a Mr John Rose was appointed in his place. He did not serve the Company long in this capacity for on the morning of 28 October 1740 he died of a 'Putrid continual Fever'.

In the following year Robert Herriot was appointed surgeon to Gombroon and again a severe epidemic, almost certainly either plague or cholera, broke out.

June 7th 1741. News is come from Cong of a pestilential sickness having raged there to such a degree that there were hardly found people in Health sufficient to bury those that died, amounting as some say to forty & fifty a day.

The Diary relates that so fever-stricken was Gombroon in the year 1743 that after the death of Mr Hugh Bidwell 'of a Bilious Fever after an illness of Five Days' there was no European civilian left alive in Gombroon excepting the agent himself. In the autumn the ensign died 'after a fever of three days'. In the winter the sergeant went off his head and shot himself. The surgeon performed the necropsy.

I was yesterday between three and four of the clock in the morning called up to see our Sergeant George Batterson who I was told had shot himself. I found him upon his cot, lying upon his back speechless and deprived of all sense and motion only breathing short and seemingly with difficulty, his Pulse hardly perceiveable. I found a large space upon the right side about the cartilages and anterior ends of the short ribs next to his stomack and also a little below the Cartilages upon his Belly very black and scorched with Gun powder, and a round wound in the middle of the black space like unto a gunshot wound entering his body, grasing upon the Inferior Edges of the Cartilages and about the region of the Liver. I also found near the Spine of the Back another wound answering to the former almost in a Direct line thro' the Cavity of the Bellye. My information from the Corporal and Sentinel that immediately before I was called they heard the Report of a Pistol and found his shirt burning upon his body and likewise the condition of both wounds makes me of opinion that they were at that time received from a bullet and the Cause of his Death and by all Circumstances it appeared he must have fired the Pistol himself. All which I certify to be true. In testimony whereof I have signed the present Report.

Robert Herriot

During the past 20 years Persia had been through the throes of the Afghan invasion, as I have related elsewhere, and was now groaning under the tyrannical rule of Nádir Qulí Sháh. Naturally the Diary of the Gombroon factory could not keep silent about the rumours which reached the town. Within a few years of his ascending the throne people began to talk of his cruelties and his desire to obliterate all reminders of the past greatness of Persia. He was said to have given orders that all the remains of the works of S͟háh 'Abbás the Great should be destroyed. On his return from India in 1739 stories of wholesale murders and impossible demands began to become current talk. The rewards of the Indian campaign were squandered upon dancing girls and, when his treasury was exhausted, he called upon his Persian subjects to supply him with funds. His conduct, of course, gave rise to a general discontent throughout the land. At first, however, his power was so absolute and the fear of his name so great that he could crush all opposition.

October 8th 1742. Was brought into Town upon a Camel a person who from a Travelling Dervize took upon himself the title of Shaw Ihmael pretending he was of the late Royal Family & got a few people to join him at Coghilloe a place near this Government, but was quickly overtaken in his Grandeur & been made to pay for his Presumption with the Loss of his Eyes as well as his Followers with their Lives. He is brought hither 'tis said to be kept a Prisoner in Ormuze Castle. This is the only instance of a Competitor Shaw Nadir has met with since his Usurpation.

An attempt upon his life caused the shah to suspect that his son Riẓá Qulí Mírzá aimed at assuming the crown in his place. Whether his suspicions were justified or not is unknown. Both Br. Bazin, the Jesuit, and Dr Lerch, a German physician attached to a Russian diplomatic mission, believed in the prince's innocence. Certain it is that he had put to death Ṭahmásp the ex-shah (although according to some authorities even in this he did not act upon his own initiative but under orders from his father), and had afterwards set himself up in Meshed in regal state.

January 4th 1743. The Agent had a letter from the Linguist at Spahaun, who gives a very Extraordinary piece of News of the King having punished his eldest son (the same who governed as Vice Roy while he was in India) with the loss of his Eyes and cutting off his Feet for that he had killed Shaw Thomas who he said was their King & Master and the Occasion of their Grandeur & furthermore had lately attempted his (the King's) Life.

It has been remarked that Nádir's outbursts of sadism corresponded very closely with his physical state of health and it is suggested that had his regular medical attendant been available, his mental health would never have been such as to allow him to commit this crowning act of cruelty. During his youth and middle age Nádir had enjoyed good health. But in later life having lost all his double teeth he seldom ate food that required mastication and was in the habit of swallowing without chewing. This set up a gastritis. The symptoms which contemporary writers describe, suggest that a gastric ulcer, or even a cancer, supervened.[1] During his attack on Delhi his feet began to swell. Nádir was so alarmed at this that he summoned to his presence Mírzá Muḥammad Háshim 'Alaví Khán, the physician-in-chief to Muḥammad Sháh, the emperor of Delhi.

It is impossible to pass over 'Alaví Khán without a little more notice, for he is one of the great physicians of this decadent period. His personality and his attainments recall most forcibly the famous physicians of the Golden Age of Baghdad. His grandfather had been a physician and practised in Shiraz. Here he gained considerable fame in more than one line. He was a teacher of renown and reckoned among his pupils Shaykh Muḥammad Ḥusayn Ḥakím-ul-Mumálik (who was even better known as a poet under the pen-name of Shuharat), Muḥammad Isma'íl (who settled near Agra and hence became known as Akbarabádí), and many others whose names it would be tedious to mention. He was also famous as a surgeon, as a penman and as a poet. When declaiming his poems in the coffee-house he would assume the dress of a *qalandar* or ascetic and hence he is sometimes styled Mírzá Hádí Qalandarí.

Mírzá Hádí died in 1695 and was buried at Shiraz. He left behind him two sons. Both became doctors. The younger apparently remained in Persia and wrote a commentary on the

1 Bazin, *Lettres Édifiantes et Curieuses* (Paris, 1780). Dr Cook states definitely that Fr. Damian cured Nádir of an ulcer. *Voyages and Travels* (Edinburgh, 1770), vol. II, p. 421.

Qánúnchi and another work called *Majma'-ul-Jawámi'* or 'Collectio Collectorum'.[1] The elder having made his studies under his father left for India in 1699, being then 34 years of age. He clearly had influence, for he was at once presented to Aurungzeeb, the emperor of Delhi, and was given a post on the staff of his son. Here he married the daughter of another Persian doctor who had settled in India. In the following reign he was given the title of 'Alaví Khán, and when Muḥammad Sháh came to the throne he was given the further title of Mu'tamid-ul-Malúk or 'The Trusted Servant of Kings' and a salary of Rs. 3000 a month.

Such was the man to whom Nádir turned. His choice was justified, for in a short time he found his symptoms relieved. Having got thus far 'Alaví Khán attempted to go further and administered to the shah good advice as well as good medicine. This recalls the days of Sinán and Bachkam. So successful was he that 'by a proper medical treatment the shah's disposition was so much improved that for a fortnight together he would not order the discipline of the stick, much less command any one to be deprived of his eyes or life'.

'Alaví Khán had only accepted office under Nádir Sháh on condition that he should ultimately be allowed to leave his service in order to make the pilgrimage to Mecca. He accompanied him on the return journey from India to Persia and when he reached Qazvin two years later, he claimed the fulfilment of the promise. Nádir allowed him to go and from that moment his health began to deteriorate once again. Distrusting even more than before his Persian medical advisers he persuaded Fr. Damian of Lyons, the Capuchin, to replace 'Alaví Khán.

Fr. Damian did his best for five years. But his real interest was not in medicine and he was in no sense a fitting successor to 'Alaví Khán. He was eager to return to the evangelizing of Persia, the work for which he had left France. So the shah was

1 Fonahn in *Quellenkunde d. Per. Med.* (Copenhagen, 1910) summarizes this work. But he is wrong in saying that it is founded on the author's great-uncle. Surely his famous elder brother is his chief authority.

forced again to look for another doctor to whom he could entrust himself. There can have been no European doctor resident in the capital. For had there been, Nádir would certainly have selected him. The Russian minister was the only diplomat in permanent residence there and as Nádir apparently made no request to the Legation, there cannot even have been a qualified Russian doctor there. However, the mission which arrived under Prince Golitzin in 1734 had two medical men on its cadre. These were Dr Schnese and Dr Lerch. Prince Golitzin stayed in Persia only one year and returned to Russia with his entire suite. Dr Lerch returned with the second mission of Prince Golitzin, accompanied by the English doctor John Cook. They reached Resht in April 1747. They were still on the road when news of the murder of Nádir was announced to the ambassador, who promptly returned to Russia.

In despair of securing the services of a doctor already in his capital Nádir turned to the English factor at Ispahan, who reported to his superiors that he had done his best to fill the gap.

June 26th 1746. The King having sent to this place for two Doctors, one European and the other Armenian, and the Linguist's Father having been a doctor and a European, the People in Government imagined him sufficiently quallifyed for the design, and tho' their endeavours had not in the least been wanting to prevent his going, yet a Denial might have been of ill Consequence & he was accordingly to set out in a few days and that his stay might be as short as possible in the Camp, the Resident had wrote letters to the Head People about his Majesty, whose indisposition was so much, that he was obliged to be carried in a Pallanqueen.

On 28 October 1746 the authorities at Gombroon received another letter from Ispahan, written a month before, in which it was stated that

they advise the return of their Linguist from the Camp where he had met with a favourable reception the King ordering him a Tent near his own & Servants to attend him, and all the Enquiry he made was to know the quantity and the quality of spiritous Liquors proper for him to drink and in what manner we used them which the Linguist to the best of his judgement informed and he seemed satisfied.

His Majesty had been pleased to receive a Petition from us and returning favourable answer with a Rogon exempting the Ho. Company from the Duty Goods pay on going into any Town Road Custom and Havage throughout the whole Kingdom, tho' the Customs Master endeavours had not been wanting to prevent our success having offered one hundred tumans to obstruct its passing through the several offices, and for this purpose the Linguist had been obliged to disburse two thousand nine hundred sixty shahees which was impossible to be avoided where no business was carried on without expectations of Gain tho' this they hoped would be made up by the Benefit & Credit it would be to the Honourable Company and his Majesty being timorous of his own Doctors had sent a Rogon for a European to go to the Camp which could it be done he would be well rewarded and in great favour with his Majesty.

The linguist thus sent to serve the shah must have been, I think, Joseph Hermet. He was the elder of two sons of a French doctor, who had married and died in Persia.[1] With his efforts in a medical role the Honourable Company were well satisfied and they voted him a robe of honour as an outward token of their appreciation of what he had done for them. And yet, even though the king himself asked for a physician to be attached to his person, they still failed to realize how greatly it would be to their interests to comply.

His Majesty having wrote to us to Provide and send a Doctor to the Camp, which at present is out of our power though were it otherwise it might be of infinite service to us in getting renewall of our former Grants, Mr Savage proposes writing a petition acquainting his Majesty our Endeavour shall not be wanting to comply with his Orders and at the same time entreat his Majestys countenance in carrying on our Ho. Masters affairs in his kingdom and it is Agreed that we likewise mention this in our advises to Messrs Peirson and Blandy and in case a person can be got at Spahaun to undertake such an Expedition that we permitt of their sending him to the Camp as we judge privileges might be got by this means without putting the Ho. Company to any great Expence.

1 Bazin, *Lettres Édifiantes*, vol. IV, p. 377.

In spite of the linguist's efforts the king's illness continued. His native physicians advised him to stay in Ispahan and to take a course of infusion of China Root. But this did not help very much. Next Nádir turned to the Dutch factory, but they were equally unable to provide him with the European physician whom he demanded. By chance there arrived at this moment a Jesuit lay-brother, named Bazin. Him the English Company persuaded to transfer his services to the court of Nádir Sháh instead of looking after the missionaries.

The spelling of the name of this Jesuit physician varies with different authors. The standard work on the Jesuit Order (*Catalogue de la Compagnie de Jésus*, by Frs. Augustin and Aloys de Backer, vol. I, p. 1069, Paris, 1890) spells it as I do. I consider this the best authority. A recently published work on the Carmelites in Persia (*A Chronicle of the Carmelites in Persia*, pp. 651 et seq., London, 1939), a work based entirely on contemporary sources, invariably inserts an *r* and calls him Brazin. In the *Lettres Édifiantes*, vol. IV, pp. 277–353, Paris, 1780, there are two letters from the brother himself. Here too the name is without the *r*. Dr Lockhart in his *Nádir Shah* (London, 1938) also spells the name without any *r*, but he is probably following the *Catalogue*. He is wrong in styling him Père, for he was never anything more than a lay-brother.

The *Catalogue* gives the following details of his life. He was born 24 May 1712; left France for Persia 1735; went to China 1767; and died in Pekin 15 March 1774.

In a letter to his superiors Bazin described his first physical examination of the shah. He announced to his royal patient that his case was not hopeless, but that he required two months in which to prepare the necessary remedies. Nádir gave him 30 days. In spite of the jealousy of the Persian physicians and the accusations that they made against him, Bazin was as successful as 'Alaví Khán. In consequence the shah was able to throw off his illness and carry out during the winter the tour that he had planned for the autumn. But his recovery left him more cruel and more rapacious than ever.

March 22 1747. A Chappar arrived this day from Carmenia who says his Majesty has left that place seven days and is to go by way of the Desert to Mushat. He has killed and blinded a great number of people whose only fault was not having money to pay the Exorbitant sums put upon them; they sold their Wives and Children to the Tartar soldiers for five and six rupees each which somebody acquainted the King of, but his answer was he was surprised they bore so great a price.

At Meshed his cruelties seem almost incredible.

The most unheard of and extraordinary cruelties that the King has been guilty of them, has put an entire stop to all Trade and nothing is done but collection of money for him which the Callentars are very severe in burning women on their breasts to make them confess their husbands' Wealth and at last selling them and their children to the Tartars who now make a trade of it; the City is much worse now than when it was besieged by the Afghoons nine months.

Most fortunately the Company had an English representative at Kerman during the time of the shah's visit, a Mr Danvers Graves. He has left a vivid record of the shah's activities there, of his meeting with the new French doctor, and of an audience with the shah himself. It was on 27 February 1747 that Nádir reached Kerman. Two days later Br. Bazin called on Mr Graves.

March 2nd 1747. Last night had a visit from Fryar Bazin, who attends the King as Physician, he has given his Majesty Physick ten or twelve days and says he is much better, but the poor man is in a precarious station, as the Persians who attended before are jealous and endeavouring to play tricks, he says his only inducement to enter into this mans service was in hopes he should be able to forward the European affairs, but on the contrary as soon as he offers to speak a word to the King he immediately orders him away and at last told him never to meddle with any business but what related to Physick. The Doctor is very facetious, Discreet, good sort of a Man.

March 4th. Fryer Bazein came again to the Comp. House and was asked to present a petition to the King but he said it would not be worth his life to do so, but in the evening of the 6th came again and said he would do his best.

March 8th. Before sunrise sent my Petition to European Doctor who with Mirza Abdul Baukee, the Kings old Physitian agreed to deliver it which is the only hopes I have left of getting over these affairs with Creditt; for the Mullah Bashee is only putting off from Day to Day notwithstanding I have offered 130 tumans for himself.

And a little later he continues:

The King being in an ill humour the Doctor has not as yet delivered my Pettition. This morning the King strangled six people, beat two Indians to Death and has ordered two hundred of the Carmenia people to be cut off, and a Pillar to be erected of their heads. What mercy can be expected from a mad Tyrant?

At noon the King ordered all the Camp People out of the Town and Gates to be shut, by which we judge he designs a general Massacre tonight, in which case God defend us, for the wild Aphgoon know no Distinction of Person.

In the Evening received another letter from the Doctor Bazein who says, the King is in such an ill humour that he durst not deliver my Petition; but has promised to do it tomorrow morning when he feels his Pulse.

March 9th. At Eight o'clock this morning Fryer Bassein sent for me, told me that after he had felt his Majesty's pulse he acquainted him that the Europeans here had met with great impositions from the people and that I had endeavoured several times to get a Petition delivered, that no one would do us that service. The King answered that we were his Guests, and would not allow of our being affronted and immediately sent for Mirza Abdul Baukee Hakeem Bashee and ordered him to enquire into our Complaints and he would do us justice.

I stayed at Fryer Basseins tent upward of an hour. When the King passed from his Public Tent to that of his Women which was about two hundred yards distance I had a full view of his Person crossing within Musquet shot of the place where I satt. He seems to be about five foot ten inches, and very well sett and notwithstanding his Age or fatigue of life he has gone through, walks very upright, and to appearance if no accident happens to him may live this twenty years.

March 11th. While at dinner received a letter from Fryer Bazein to advise me the King had again made a promise of what Rogons I wanted, immediately sent Joseph with a list of what the Right Worshipfull the Agent and Council had given me orders to obtain, but judged it not proper to mention anything about our being Customs free, as at this time it might put his Majesty upon making enquiries to the Honble. Companys Disadvantage.

This evening Joseph returned from the Camp, not having been able to do anything relating to the Rogons by reason the King was in a very ill humour and its said has fined his own servants 500,000 tumans. However Mirza Abdull Baukee Hakeem Bashee has promised to get our affairs finished tomorrow morning.

March 12th. Early this morning received a latter from Fryer Bassein to advise that everything was ready for writing the Rogon, and desired the Linguist might come directly to finish that affair. He says that a Choppar is arrived from the Dutch Chief at Gombroon, who is likewise sending a European Physitian to attend upon the King which has greatly pleased the Fryer being in hopes of obtaining his Majestys permission to return to Europe, tho' as he received so much advantage from his Medicines I rather believe he will carry him to Callaut and there detain him.

March 13th. In the Evening the Linguist who I sent to the Camp in the morning, returned but not yet finished our Rogon, the King being so excessively enraged that there is no such thing as speaking to him.

At night received a visit from Fryer Bassein, who tells me his Majesty begins to be mightily pleased with his Physick and promised to follow any directions he may think proper to give regarding his diet etc.

March 14th. In the morning sent Joseph again to the Camp to endeavour at finishing the Honourable Companys Rogons which they have promised me this Day.

In the evening Linguist Jos. Hermet returned from the Camp with one of the best Rogons the Honourable Company ever obtained in Persia, properly sealed and attested to. Answers the end: it is to protect our Banyan Brokers & other servants all over Persia; to exempt us from Mustarade and all other impositions in selling of Goods; and to prevent the People in Government from obliging us or our servants to sell them Goods against our own Free Will etc.

I hear the King has changed his melancholy humour into raging and killed twenty-four of his own people this afternoon.

March 21st. In the evening arrived one Mirza Tar (Kings Physician) in his way to Spahaun, his desire was to have stayed here till a Caphila offered, but seeing the miserable condition the place was in, especially our House from where he Expected assistance, he went back again to the Camp.

In June of this year having reduced both Ispahan and Kerman to utter ruin by his extortions and massacres, Nádir drew upon himself the destruction which he so richly deserved. Believing that he owed his position to the Afghans and having no faith in the Persians, he invariably oppressed the latter and favoured the former.

He had in his camp [wrote Bazin] a corps of 4,000 Afghans; these troops were entirely devoted to him and hostile to the Persians. On the night of the 19th/20th June he summoned all their chiefs. 'I am not satisfied with my guards', he said to them. 'Your courage and loyalty are known to me. I order you to arrest all their officers tomorrow morning and to place them in irons. Do not spare any of them if they dare to resist you.' No doubt he meant to put them all to death.

This time the net was spread too wide, even for a nation cowed into submission. The conversation was overheard and reported to the Persians. Seventy of their leaders determined to murder the shah that very night. The fatal blow was struck by Muḥammad K̲h̲án Qájár. 'The cause of his end', wrote a Carmelite friar who was in Julfa at the time, 'was nothing else than his tyrannical fits of madness, which in the last year of his life it was his whim to exploit to the utmost.'

After the death of Nádir S̲h̲áh until Ágh̲á Muḥammad established himself as *S̲h̲áhins̲h̲áh* in 1796, the internal history of Persia is one of robbery, risings and uncertainty. The Company's agent wrote month after month complaining that the roads were impassable owing to brigands and that the towns were dead owing to the exactions of petty princelings. Among the European doctors who arrived in Persia during these years were two Germans, one a physician and one a surgeon. On their way to Ispahan they were stopped on the road and stripped naked by robbers although travelling in a caravan of 3000 persons. Whether they were mere adventurers or whether they were engaged to work in the royal service is unknown, for neither their names nor their later history are recorded in the Diary.

In the meantime Dr Herriot had been succeeded at Gombroon by a Dr John Hardcastle. An interesting note on an obscure and fatal case, characterized by bleeding from the nose and the urethra, mentions that he called in his Dutch colleague for a second opinion. But the Dutchman could make no more of the case than could Dr Hardcastle.

It seems clear, too, that the surgeon at Gombroon was still the only doctor whom the Company employed in the whole of Persia. A certain Mr Dalrymple was ordered to proceed to Ispahan to join Mr Graves, who had been transferred there from Kerman. On the road he fell ill and Graves recommended that he should return to Gombroon for treatment as he could get none at Yezd or Ispahan. But the agent at Gombroon hardened his heart and would not hear of any return:

In regard to Mr Dalrymple being obliged to stay in the road we are much concerned at it, but as he may by this time be fitt for travelling we cannot permitt of his returning here as Mr Graves will be in want of his assistance and we think his proceeding is absolutely necessary, and more so, as being ordered by the Honourable President & Councill.

The years 1751 and 1752 were particularly terrible for the health of the Europeans. Dr Hardcastle had been replaced by a Dr Isaac Fullerton who died in September of 1751. Next there broke out some severe sickness on board one of the Company's ships.

October 28th 1751. The Detachment of Soldiers on board the Mamoody daily falling down with fevers, which the Officers represent is owing to their Way of living being only allowed Rice, Doll and Ghee which is very improper Food for this Season of the Year, ordered them a small Quantity of Pepper, and other Spices to mix with their Food.

In December of that year orders came from Bombay that the place of Dr Fullerton should be taken by Dr George Forbes, who was then physician to the Mamoody. He was not now the only British physician in the Persian Gulf, for at some time previous to this appointment (the Diary gives no hint as to when the Company had been guilty of this extravagance) a certain Dr

Hanmer had been sent to Bandar-i-Rig, a port near Basra, for the Diary records that the secretary to the factory there fell ill.

Mr Robert Went, who has been ill of a Nervous Fever for this long time past, having at length lost his Understanding, the Doctor is of opinion that he ought to be put under close confinement, but as we are yet in Hopes he is not really mad, an European Seaman is only order'd to give him constant Attendance.

April 12th 1752. Mr Went now seems to be somewhat worsed than before, having considerably recovered his strength of Body, but not his Understanding in the least, so that he is likely to prove troublesome to us, unless we confine him to some Part of the Factory, where he cannot have anybody to talk with him so conveniently as in his own Apartments.

April 30th. Mr Robert Went whom we have suspected of Madness all this month, has now become more outrageous than ever, and refuses to wear any Thing to cover his Nakedness, singing aloud and talking to himself all Day long, so that we have at last been obliged to bind him down upon his Bed, to prevent any Mischief happening either to himself or those that look after him.

Further down the Gulf at Gombroon the hot weather was playing havoc with the British residents. At the end of April the writer of the Diary says that 'The Air is very thick and unwholesome, every European in the Factory, excepting the Agent, being taken ill of Fevers'.

On the first day of May one of the staff managed to escape on sick leave.

May 1st. Mr Francis Wood being extremely ill of a Nervous Fever, which at Times deprives him of his Senses, was removed this day to Naban in a Palanquin for change of Air, as he finds no Benefit from either Bleeding or Blistering both which he has allready undergone.

Twelve days later the agent fell sick and the work of the factory ceased.

The Agent is this day taken ill with a heaviness at his Breast, attended by a slight Fever. Mr Wood also remains very ill at Naban, and Captain Kerr, Mr Wilson and Doctor Forbes continue very bad so that they are obliged to keep their Rooms.

On the night of 16 May the agent died at Gombroon and Mr Went at Bandar-i-Rig. On the next day died a 'Mr William Perceval who has been ill of a Fever for some Time past, being taken speechless about 3 this afternoon and dying before sunset'. Unfortunately at this point the Diary is wanting for two years. It is entirely fitting that the next page, dated September 1754, should contain a complaint from the doctor of a shortage of drugs.

In the following year Dr George Forbes died and was succeeded by Dr John Parker.

Again news from the interior showed that a physician was doing more for the protection of European lives and interests than any of the merchants could do. Yet still the Company did not realize that their interests would be far better served by the employment of a tactful and intelligent doctor than by a dozen linguists and secretaries. It had by then become almost a tradition that a physician should be at the right hand of the shah. But it was neither a Dutchman nor an Englishman who held this very useful post.

December 21st 1755. Letters from Spahaun of the 22 november mention that Azad Caun left that City the 13th and that he had carried with him all the omrah and leading men that he gave out that he was going to the assistance of his general Fattally Caun who had been twice defeated at Casshoun by Mahomet Caun Zand and Shaikh Ally Caun, that some of his troops who were between Cum and Casbin fled from Hossain Caun Cadjar, the same advices mention that before he left Spahaun he took from the Armenians of Julpha between six and seven hundred tomaunds, yet the Missionarys and Europeans paid nothing entirely owing to a French Man who is a physician having about a month before Obtained a Rogum from Azad Caun that all Europeans who put themselves under the French protection be exempt from all Taxes and Impositions whatever.

The French man above mentioned was threatened to be put to death by the Turks at Mossoul and that in order to save his Life he turned Mahometan, that his Christian Name was Simon de Vercheville but now Mirza Mahomet Reza.

22nd. Receiv'd a letter from the above Mirza Mahomet Reza

advising that he had wrote Consul Drummond at Aleppo that he had sometime ago been in favour with Azad Caun he could have saved the lives of many Christians, that he now verified his letter was not altogether compliment, as the priviledges he had obtain'd for all Europeans dwelling or travelling in Persia will be sufficiently low; that he does not transmit a Copy of the said priviledges being well assured I shall receive them from other hands, that the chief design of writing at present is to show his zeal and esteem for the English with some of whom he had been honoured with Respect, and he concludes his letter with saying that he hopes I will put a favourable Construction on his late Change, and in a postscript thereof mentions to enclose a Copy of the Rogum, the purport of which is that he (Azad Caun) had given to Mirza Mahomet Reza thirteen houses for the Conveniency of all European merchants who put themselves under his protection, that the said houses which used hitherto to pay Taxes be exempt in future.

Like so many of his predecessors Doctor John Parker went down before the prevailing fever and applied for sick leave. Before he left, he made some attempt to investigate the cause of the high death rate and sickness incidence at Gombroon among the Company's European staff. Dr Boerhaave of the Dutch East India Company held that it was due to the intense heat of the sun being reflected by the salt encrusted in the soil. Local unscientific opinion attributed it to the stink of decaying blubberfish which were cast up on the shore in great quantities in the hot weather. Ives, a surgeon in the Royal Navy, who visited the Persian Gulf about this time, claimed that it was malaria. In this he was probably right.

In 1773 Ives published the diary of his travels in these parts under the title of *A Voyage from England to India.* The third appendix to this book is an account of the diseases incident to Gombroon 'contained in a letter from an ingenious physician who resided several years in that settlement'.[1] This letter, although unsigned, is, I am sure, from the hand of Dr Parker. For in it the writer states that he was 'a living witness of an Autumnal Fever which

1 Ives, *Journey from Persia to England by an unusual route* (being Book II of *A Voyage from England to India in the Year* 1754), p. 498. London, 1773.

began and continued almost perfectly regular for thirteen months in my own person'. This agrees with another letter dated 19 May 1758, written and signed by Dr Parker at Gombroon, in which he applies for leave on the grounds that he has been 'attacked about ten months ago with a violent Bilious Inflammatory Fever which continued for fifteen days & then terminated into a Quotidian Ague, which remained with me several months...and scarce had I recovered from that but was siezed with a slow Continent fever which now hangs on me'.

It is quite clear that Ives drew his views about malaria from Parker, for the latter writes that he was compelled to use large quantities of 'the Bark', that is quinine, which he speaks of as 'this noble medicine'. This brought about, as usual, a shortage of drugs and almost in the words of his predecessors he wrote and complained to the directors of their parsimony which was starving his hospital. The better health of the Dutch factory he ascribed to other reasons.

May 1756. A Hundred Europeans is the established number of soldiers allow'd from Batavia for the defence of Carack fort: what I have seen, I take to be about sixty including 7 or 8 petty officers & they are all neat handsome fellows kept under strictest discipline. Besides these Mynheer has above one hundred Coffree slaves well arm'd according to the Country manner with Swords and Targets, who (from his manner of treating them) are likely to remain faithful & contented under the bondage: he takes care to supply them with plenty of dates, fish & bread, gives them decent Cloathing, cools the natural ferver of their Constitutions by allowing a considerable number of coffree women to live among them in common & never Controuls or even advises them in regard to Religion: but when they commit a fault he punishes them very severely and whenever he has Occasion to drub any of the Arabs or Country people he orders two or three of the slaves to take him in hand which service seems to be peculiarly adapted to the capacity and in my Life I never saw people acquit themselves in a duty of this kind with greater dexterity and judgement.

On his departure in May 1758 Parker was presented with Rs. 200 as a present for his attendance upon the Persian nobility of the town of Gombroon. He was succeeded by a ship surgeon, Mr Richard Mainwaring (or Mainwarring, for the name occurs in both spellings), whose duties he undertook on the return journey to Bombay.

Mainwaring was the last surgeon at Gombroon. The place was unhealthy, the station was unpopular, and the capture and sack by the French troops in 1759 forced the agent to recommend its abandonment. The excessive demands of the Persian governor of Lar two years later made the court of directors come to an immediate decision to close the factory. In 1763 it was moved to Bushire.

There were three available sites for a new factory, Bahrein, Bushire and Basra. The second of these three towns was selected. The hospital of Gombroon also was moved to Bushire and Mr Mainwaring became the first residency surgeon. But this factory, although encouraged by privileges granted by Karím Khán-i-Zand, failed to flourish. It was abandoned in 1770 and the whole staff was again moved, this time to Basra. Bushire was reoccupied, though, three years later, the Company's agent being a Persian. The hospital of the new factory at Basra was formed by appropriating part of an old warehouse. This was so inconvenient and ill-situated that the agent in a letter home described the building as being 'of no other use than as a hospital and a warehouse, not having proper accommodations in such a sultry climate as this is for your servants'.

In 1772 the resources of this very inadequate hospital were strained to the uttermost and, incidentally, the courage of the Europeans was tried as by fire, for during the winter one of the severest outbreaks of plague on record broke out in Baghdad. In April of the following year it spread to Basra. The agent and the senior servants of the Company retired to a house some four miles outside the city; the remainder shut themselves up in the factory, hoping that the approaching hot weather would put a natural end to the epidemic. Two frigates were kept at anchor over the bar and all communication between the factory staff and the native population was forbidden. But the heat, instead of checking the disease, rather encouraged it. The deaths were said to number more than a thousand a day. The nerves of the agent became more and more frayed. His food supplies were running short and he could see no means of replenishing them. When the Arab servants fled, he could resist no longer and boarding a man-of-war set sail with all speed for Bombay.

His juniors were forced to stay in Basra and with them stayed Surgeon Michael Reilly, who in the absence of his superiors acted as Company's agent together with an Armenian merchant named Petrus Mellick.

The epidemic continued to spread. It travelled down the coast and soon Bushire was infected and all the Persian littoral. The Persian authorities in Shiraz acted as though the town was besieged and allowed no one from the south to enter. By these means all the interior of Persia escaped. Along the Arab side of the Gulf the coast became infected as far as Bahrein. The casualties in the epidemic were enormous. Basra is said to have lost nearly a quarter of a million inhabitants. The French resident died; so did all the Catholic missionaries, all of whom stayed at their posts. Of the Company's servants who remained in Basra, three Europeans died and several sepoys. The agent on his return from Bombay in January of 1774 estimated that the total fatalities approximated to two million. The doctor and the Armenian merchant both escaped and the agent was good enough to point out to the directors in England that it was largely owing to the skill and the courage of Mr Reilly that the European casualties were so few. Each was presented with Rs. 1000 to express the gratitude of the court of directors.

With the cessation of the epidemic and the return of the full staff to Basra there were hopes of a revival of trade. But all such hopes were frustrated by a war which broke out between the Turks and the Persians. Karím Khán, then Shah of Persia, jealous of the importance of Basra, which was diverting the trade of India away from the Persian ports, made the capture of that city the principal object of his campaign. A state of war was only one degree less harmful to trade than a state of virulent epidemic. Again the greater part of the factory servants evacuated Basra and this time the hospital staff moved with them. They settled in Bushire and the sum of two thousand rupees was expended in installing the hospital in suitable accommodation.

Basra fell after a blockade of 13 months and the agent returned to the factory. The hospital, however, did not move back, but stayed at Bushire. Mr Reilly apparently did not return to Basra, as it is recorded that he died in Bushire in 1778 and was succeeded by a Mr Durham. Basra was not left without a doctor, for the Diary states that a surgeon named Mr Robson was sent by the agent into the desert to meet a Mr Bonnevaux, who had been attacked by a band of marauding Arabs on his way from Aleppo. But the old hospital remained closed and the premises reverted to their original use as a warehouse.

No attempt was made by the Turks to recover Basra, but on the death of Karím Khán Sháh the Persian governor voluntarily abandoned the town in order to look after his own domestic affairs in Persia. Perhaps his decision was influenced by the outbreak of some unknown epidemic, which the Diary calls epidemical fever. Possibly this was influenza.

Since June 1st 1780 an Epidemical fever has raged in Bussora, but though scarcely one of the inhabitants have escaped the infection, it has hitherto proved fatal only to the Mussaleem, and a very few more.

Among the Europeans also, scarcely one has escaped severe attacks & we have had the misfortune to lose Mr James Robson, Surgeon of this Factory, with Mr Francis Palmer from Bengal and two of the seamen belonging to the *Eagle*; and to heighten the melancholy scene Mr William Browne, owner of the *Yarmouth* from Bengal, whether through disorder of body or mind, Shot himself the 12th and expired immediately.

The fever spread down the coast, for the death of another Englishman was reported from Bushire at the end of the month, the diagnosis again being epidemical fever. The place of the late surgeon at Basra was taken by a Mr Ross, who was probably a ship surgeon, for his appointment was only temporary, and in July 1781 a Mr Williams came out to occupy the post.

Constant epidemics which their science knew no method of checking, constant wars which no diplomacy could prevent, made the trade of Basra grow less and less, until finally in the spring of 1793 the greater part of the staff was translated to Grain, an island on the Arab side of the Persian Gulf, now known as Koweit. A Dr James Small was nominated factory surgeon at Grain. In 1795 he moved back to Basra both to attend to the skeleton staff which was left there and to prepare the way for the return of the agent. For in spite of sickness and war Basra was the key of the Persian Gulf. Repeated attempts by the English, French, Dutch and Portuguese failed to divert its trade to any other port.

On Dr Small's departure to Basra his place at Grain was taken by a Mr William Cleland, who arrived in May 1795. Four months after his arrival the whole factory moved back to Basra again. Dr Small accompanied Mr Harford Jones to the recently established Residency at Baghdad in 1798 and Mr Cleland assumed charge of the health of the factory at Basra.

In this year there was again a widespread flooding of the Euphrates, followed by the usual outbreak of plague. Mr Cleland had been superseded by a Mr David Carnegie, who in the winter of this year had returned to Bombay and was succeeded by a Mr John Milne. The dreaded disease did not show any great virulence this year nor did it the following year. But in 1800 it again appeared with almost as great a violence as in the great plague of 1772. Mosul was the first city to be attacked. From there it spread south and soon the villages which lay along the road between Baghdad and Constantinople were infected. The Turkish Pasha of Baghdad took no steps whatever to protect his city. Yet, although Mr Harford Jones from Baghdad and Mr Manesty, the agent, from Basra wrote expressing the utmost fear that their cities would soon become infected, the epidemic reached neither.

In the autumn of 1799 there had been a change of doctors at the Residency at Baghdad, Dr Small returned to Bombay and a Dr James Short was appointed in his stead. Unfortunately during the interval between the departure of the one and the arrival of the other Mr Harford Jones contracted gonorrhoea. There was then no European doctor in Baghdad, with the exception of a French physician, named Outrey, who was attached to the staff of the Pasha, and whose services on behalf of an Englishman international politics rendered out of the question. Turkish or Arab doctors did not appeal to Mr Harford Jones. As soon as his infection began to give rise to unpleasant symptoms, he put himself under the treatment of a German Carmelite, who knowing more theology than medicine, treated the case with quinine. When his symptoms abated not one whit by this treatment Mr Harford Jones wrote down to Basra for the loan of the services of the Company's doctor. Mr Milne refused to leave his work and come up to Baghdad, a course of action which led to some very bitter letters between Mr Harford Jones, London and Basra. In his defence Mr Milne gives an interesting exposure of the duties which the surgeon at Basra in those days was supposed to carry out.

The establishment of the factory at this time consisted of the Resident, the Assistant Resident, one Indian native officer and thirty sepoys. Mr Milne, the surgeon, was the sole medical officer and was responsible not only for the upkeep of the hospital and the health of the establishment, but also for the treatment of any seamen, lascars and sepoys who might be landed sick from the monthly mail vessels which came up from Bombay.

As soon as Mr Milne received the application for his services in Baghdad, he replied that he had five seriously sick men in his hospital and that he would go as soon as his patients in Basra were sufficiently well to be left without a medical officer. Unfortunately, five days later four seamen were landed sick and a week later three more. It must be remembered that at this time the journey from Basra to Baghdad and back took about three weeks

With the very limited medical service which the Company provided, it was therefore highly desirable for Mr Milne to stay in Basra. He accordingly sent to Mr Harford Jones an elixir of vitriol, some camomile flowers, and a letter explaining that he probably had a stricture and that this would require the passage of a bougie and the application of a caustic to effect a radical cure and that he would do all these things at a more suitable moment.

The unfortunate Mr Harford Jones had to be content with this. Until he had a clean bill of health or until a ship surgeon came to relieve him, Mr Milne would not quit Basra. During November and December the *Antelope*, the *Viper*, the *Comet* and the *Alert* all arrived at Basra; but none of these ships carried a doctor. It was not until 11 January of the following year that the *Panther* arrived with a surgeon on board. But she had only stayed in port six days, when the captain, finding the wind suitable, returned to Bombay.

Mr Harford Jones lost both hope and patience and now reported Mr Milne to London for a refusal to attend a servant of the Company in need. Long before the answer could come from England the symptoms began to abate, and in March Mr Harford Jones himself came down to Basra. Mr Milne attended him, treated him, received 'a very elegant diamond ring' as a fee, and accompanied him back to within two days' journey of Baghdad.

On 12 July, weeks after Mr Harford Jones had recovered and when he had probably quite forgotten that he had lodged the complaint, came a letter of severe censure from London upon the inhuman conduct of Mr Milne in refusing to attend a sick officer. Mr Milne promptly returned the ring. Mr Manesty, the Resident at Basra, was no less astonished and disgusted. He at once wrote to the court at London, expressing in unequivocable terms his high esteem of the factory surgeon. The unpleasant situation was, however, brought to an end by a fresh outbreak of plague in Mosul and Baghdad, and Mr Harford Jones was in far greater danger than he had been during the past winter. The plague raged in Baghdad.

> The greatest part of the Persian merchants [he wrote] have already returned (i.e. to Persia). Most people are thinking of moving.... I cannot give your Honourable Board a better idea of the success, which is likely to attend the Precautions taken by the Government for the prevention of Infection entering the Town than by mentioning that the Persons appointed to fumigate the Letters which arrive from the pestiferous places, performed for some time untill I heard of it this operation by holding the letters in their hands.

The frequency of these epidemics, the interruptions to trade caused thereby, the cutting of the road between Constantinople and Baghdad and the consequent delay in the arrival of diplomatic dispatches between London and Fort William, and the danger of the spread of infection to India, at last caused the Gulf authorities to take some action beyond flight. Mr Manesty's standing orders of 1802 represent the first quarantine measures to be taken in the Gulf and can be looked upon as the seed from which sprang the quarantine services of the Gulf. In the first place he moved the whole of the factory staff to Maghil, a village about four miles outside Basra. All communication between the staff and the native population was cut down to the minimum. In the second place a sanitary cordon was drawn around the factory house at Maghil and extended to include all shipping within the Shatt-ul-Arab, which flew the Union Jack. Crews were to be confined to their ships: all intercourse between ships and the shore was to be reduced to a minimum. Finally, a cruiser was to lie at anchor off Maghil House to enforce these orders and to stand by to evacuate the staff in case of 'personal or political necessity'. The medical services were further reinforced by the government of India sending to Basra a Hungarian physician named Eross, whose duties were primarily the prevention of any non-British subject passing from the infected areas to India via the Gulf.

In Baghdad itself Mr Harford Jones adopted the best course that he could. All British subjects, together with their personal effects and any dispatches which they might be carrying, were made to undergo fumigation by Dr James Short, now surgeon to the Residency. Nor were they allowed to proceed on their journey until they had received a certificate of immunity signed by Dr Short and countersigned by Mr Harford Jones. Not content with this Mr Harford Jones succeeded in persuading the Pasha to recommend to the Pasha of Mosul, where the plague was also rife, to carry out a general purification of the houses and furniture by fumigation and aspersion of anti-pestiferants. Knowing that the Turks would put very little heart into their work, he asked the Catholic missionaries in the city to superintend the carrying out of these measures.

Inadequate though these regulations undoubtedly were compared with modern prophylactic measures, they were nevertheless effective. For now for the first time in any epidemic of plague reported in the Diary no loss of life occurred among the European staff.

CHAPTER XV

THE EARLY QÁJÁRS

WITH the death of Luṭf 'Alí Sh̲áh modern Persian history may be said to begin. For his successor, Ágh̲á Muḥammad, was the first of the Qájár dynasty, a line which ruled over Persia until 1925 and which saw the transition from the medicine of Galen and Avicenna to the medicine of Harvey and Pasteur.

The Qájár claim to supreme power was disputed for many years. Muḥammad Ḥasan Kh̲án, one of the Qájár chiefs, had fallen under the displeasure of Nádir Sh̲áh, the conqueror of India. On the death of that tyrant he attempted unsuccessfully and with Turcoman aid to secure the throne for himself. Although he captured Gilan and Mazanderan he ultimately suffered defeat at the hands of 'Adíl Sh̲áh; and his eldest son, Ágh̲á Muḥammad, then aged five, was captured and castrated. Ágh̲á Muḥammad survived the operation and a little later escaped from his prison. He rejoined his father, but was recaptured. Karím Kh̲án had by then become the ruler of Persia. With a mercy rare in those days he treated the young eunuch with kindness, married his sister, and even condescended to consult him upon many matters of State.

At the time of the death of Karím Kh̲án, Ágh̲á Muḥammad was away in the country hunting. As he approached the gates of Shiraz, his sister warned him of the change in the kingdom. He straightway loosed a hawk and on pretence of going in search of it rode north with all possible speed. He was soon at the head of an armed force. A little later he captured Mazanderan. He then laid claim to all Persia as his own kingdom.

In 1783 he captured Teheran. But he held the city only for a single night and was driven back to Astrabad with great loss. Soon he returned, captured once again all Mazanderan, and again advanced upon Teheran. The city fell and Ágh̲á Muḥammad established it as the capital of the Qájár rule. From then until to-day it has remained the capital of Persia. In 1787 he extended his kingdom southwards by capturing Ispahan, which fell to his forces without the firing of a shot. Two years later he attacked Luṭf 'Alí in Shiraz, but without success. In the following year Luṭf 'Alí rashly attempted to regain Ispahan and in his absence with the army Ḥájjí Ibráhím, his *wazír*, betrayed him and his city to Ágh́á Muḥammad.

Ágh́á Muḥammad now adopted the usual methods of making his position secure. He put out the eyes of his brother Muṣṭafá Qulí, slaughtered another brother who was attempting to escape, and attacked and captured Sh́áh Rukh, the grandson of Nádir Sh́áh, who was living quietly at Meshed. To make him reveal where the remainder of Nádir's loot from India was lying hid, he caused a ring of paste to be set around his head and on this he poured boiling oil. All the male members of the family of Sh́áh Rukh were castrated; the females were divided among the mule drivers of the army. So great was his ferocity and so cruel had he now become that it is said that he seldom said his prayers without giving a signal during the performance of his devotions for the striking off of someone's head.

His cruelties grew more and more abhorrent to all around him so that at last his own ministers doubted his sanity. He was afflicted by strange fits which seem scarcely to have been epileptic for they rendered him unconscious for as much as two hours at a stretch. During these attacks his face, which in normal times was beardless, would shrivel and become horrible and distorted like that of an old hag. One of his guard, who happened to find him in a fit, was so fatally fascinated by his countenance that he could not refrain from gazing upon him at all times when on duty. Ágh́á Muḥammad was so enraged at this that he ordered the man's eyes to be put out.

His end came when he was at the height of his glory. He foolishly allowed two of his personal servants whom he had condemned to death for quarrelling within his hearing, to remain on duty until the following morning. Despair gave them courage and they murdered him in his sleep. So died one of the cruellest, but most able, of all the monarchs that had ever sat upon the throne of Persia. He was buried by some Armenians in the common sewer of the town.

In spite of the hatred which the very name of Qájár aroused, he was succeeded almost without dispute by the young Fatḥ 'Alí Khán, whom he had nominated as his successor many years before. With Fatḥ 'Alí Sháh upon the throne a completely new era opened in Persia. He was no tyrant like his uncle. He retained in power all the ministers of the former regime; and of his enemies many he pardoned. In his reign intercourse with Europe became diplomatic rather than mercantile. In consequence he was the first sovereign to endure the bullying and coaxing of the European powers, a state of affairs which Persian nationalism has tried in vain to check. The first to interfere in internal affairs were the English and the French. British power in India was by this time firmly established. Bonaparte's dream of an Eastern Empire demanded the conquest of India for the French. For that the passage of his troops through Persia was essential. To gain permission for this a French mission was dispatched to the Court of Fatḥ 'Alí. To frustrate it the British Government and East India Company sent a rival mission. With them came European doctors attached to the ambassadors. Thus was Western medicine insinuated into the strongholds of Galenic practice.

The French were the first in the field. In March of 1799 a French mission was reported to have reached Yezd on the way to Teheran. The Honourable East India Company replied by dispatching in the following year Captain Malcolm at the head of a small band of followers. He travelled via Muscat, where he dropped one of his suite, Assistant-Surgeon Bogle, who being promoted to the rank of full surgeon, was made Company's Agent in those parts. This was at the request of the Pasha of Baghdad, who found that the Imam of Muscat was defrauding him of his legitimate dues on vessels plying between Muscat and Basra. The Turkish Government took the matter up and invited the British

Government to aid them to regulate the matter. Mr Harford Jones, writing from Baghdad, suggested that Surgeon Bogle should be given ambassadorial powers to conclude 'under the guarantee of Bombay a specific adjustment of the Imam's intentions'.

Malcolm then passed on to Persia, accompanied by a staff, which included Assistant-Surgeon Briggs. On reaching Teheran a satisfactory political and commercial treaty was speedily negotiated, and in the following year the Mission returned to India, passing back through Baghdad and Basra. All French diplomatic efforts to undermine this treaty were unsuccessful. The Franco-Russian alliance in 1804 threw the shah yet more decidedly into the arms of England.

Upon the departure of Lord Wellesley from the post of Governor-General in Calcutta, the Persian policy of the Company changed. The defeat of Napoleon in Syria and Egypt reduced the fear which his name had formerly inspired in Indian official circles. So it was that when Fatḥ 'Alí Sháh approached them for aid against Russian encroachments, he appealed in vain.

The French Government, seeing the turn in affairs, sent out in 1805 an envoy named Romieu with 'three other Frenchmen in long Cloaths'. These were joined by George Outrey, a son of the French doctor to the Pasha of Baghdad, who acted as interpreter. The premature death of Romieu (said to have been brought about by poison administered by agents of Harford Jones) brought the mission to an abrupt end. Another quickly followed under a M. Jaubert, which in 1807 was replaced by a more definitely military mission under General Gardanne, who arrived in Teheran, accompanied by twenty-five officers, two priests, a physician, and a staff of soldiers and servants.

To the success and far-reaching influence of these three missions is to be attributed the ascendancy which French science obtained in Persia and which has never been replaced by any other non-Persian system. The records of the East India Company do not even mention the name of the physician who came out in the suite of General Gardanne and whose work is still bearing fruit to-day.[1] It is only in the novel, *Hajji Baba*, that any account of him, at least in the English language, exists.[2]

With the physician came the clergy. The doctor opened a dispensary, the priests a school. With the first the English authorities attempted to compete: to the latter they left the field open. The two sowed the seeds of French friendship among the educated classes which has coloured their outlook until to-day. In the court it was not difficult for the French diplomats to belittle the English. The Russians, the chief enemy and terror of the Persians, were also the enemy of the French. Bonaparte showed a superiority over the English which no argument could gainsay, when he beat the Russians so decisively that even Moscow was left in flames. The English, so the French diplomats could argue, were weak and without allies. It was idle for the shah to call upon them, whereas manifestly the power of France was on the rise. Only England remained to be conquered and then all Europe would own the sway of the French emperor.

Persian politicians became openly francophile. The politicians were followed by the scientists, who, as far as their conservatism allowed them, simulated French methods of medicine. So it followed that, as Colonel Garrison remarks, Persian medicine for the last hundred years has been Arab viewed through French spectacles.

All this seriously alarmed the procrastinating governments in Calcutta and London, and a second mission under Malcolm, now promoted to general's rank, was fitted out and sent from India in 1808. This second mission accomplished far less than the first had done. Malcolm, on reaching Bushire, demanded that the French mission should be dismissed before he presented his letters of credence in Teheran. The answer was that he should negotiate with the Prince-Governor of Shiraz and that his presence

1 But see also Keppel's *Personal Narrative*, vol. 1, p. 201. The general's name is spelt with only one *n*.

2 Morier, *Adventures of Hajji Baba of Ispahan* (London 1824), pp. 97 et passim.

was not welcome at the central court. Malcolm, holding that this was an insult to the Company and the country he represented, refused to negotiate on these terms and returned to India, where he urged immediate war upon Persia. He left behind him Captain Pasley as chargé d'affaires, who established himself at Mohammerah with Briggs again as surgeon to the mission.

In the meantime a very awkward situation had arisen. Mr Harford Jones, leaving Surgeon Hine to deputize for him as Resident in Baghdad, had gone to England on leave and while there was selected by the Home Government, ignorant that the Company had already sent a mission to Persia, to head another mission to the Court of Fatḥ 'Alí Sháh. Harford Jones, now a baronet, reached Bombay very soon after Malcolm had sailed on his second mission. Though he delayed some days to learn the will of the Governor-General, he finally sailed without any orders from Calcutta. A few weeks later the Persian court received the astonishing news that a second English mission had reached their country. With Sir Harford Jones was a suite of about one hundred persons. His private secretary was James Morier, author of that great satire upon Persian life, which he called *Hajji Baba*. His medical officer was Assistant-Surgeon Campbell, who was at that time on duty at Bushire.

Luckily for England, General Gardanne had promised the shah rather more than he was capable of performing. The Russians continued to encroach upon Persian territory: the French did nothing to check them. The battle of Trafalgar had been fought; the future of the French did not appear so rosy as it had appeared a few years before. Even the Persian ambassador in Paris sent back unfavourable reports. 'These people', he wrote, 'are deceitful and liars and do not speak the truth to anyone; so that all the foreign ministers here are at a loss what to do. The true disposition of the French emperor is to conquer the world and he is constantly saying that in the same manner as Alexander and Amir Timur conquered the world, I will follow in their steps and even exceed them.'

Sir Harford Jones was therefore invited to go up to Teheran.

On 18 December 1808 he left Bushire, taking with him in his suite Dr Andrew Jukes. Jukes was originally a surgeon on the Bombay Establishment. His first appointment in Persia was as permanent assistant to General Malcolm on his second mission. On the return of Malcolm to India, Jukes remained behind in the Residency at Bushire; his duties being mainly political. At this post his official title was Surgeon to the Residency, Acting Assistant and Translator. For these additional services he received an extra allowance of Rs. 400 a month. The precedent thus set has survived until to-day. For the surgeon to the Residency, usually an officer of field rank in the Indian Medical Service, has also the pay, status and privileges of a vice-consul.

The mission reached Teheran on 14 February 1809; the French mission had left on the 13th. A treaty was now speedily negotiated, and Morier, accompanied by Mírzá Abú ul-Ḥasan Khán as first Persian chargé d'affaires at the Court of St James, set out for London with the freshly negotiated instrument. Dr Jukes then returned to Bushire. In April Surgeon Briggs at Mohammerah fell ill and had to return temporarily to India. Jukes was bidden to take his place. His final departure from Bushire was made the occasion of a spontaneous display of affection on the part of all classes of Persians towards him. Even the Prince-Governor of Shiraz wrote to him a highly complimentary letter.

During the negotiations the friction between Sir Harford Jones and Lord Minto, now Governor-General in Calcutta, became insufferable. Jones had succeeded where Malcolm had failed. The Company therefore decided to annul the diplomatic authority of Sir Harford Jones and to send another mission of their own. General Malcolm therefore got ready to sail to Persia for the third time. The nucleus of the mission was already in Persia, encamped at Mohammera. In order to avoid the risk of a rebuff, such as Malcolm had received on his last visit, it was decided to send up a small party in advance to report on the reception which Malcolm might expect to receive. Captain Pasley was therefore bidden to go to Teheran and discover the feelings of the shah.

Captain Pasley before going expressed a wish that he might take Jukes with him as his chief assistant.

This arrangement [he wrote] will secure me the benefit of his advice, local knowledge, and experience in the performance of my duties and combines the advantages of providing effectively for their due execution in the event of any indisposition or temporary disqualification on my part, which circumstances with reference to the late precarious state of my health, be deemed not improbable. His Lordship in Council will, I hope, therefore be pleased to assign him the allowance of Rs. 500 per mensem with his expenses as has been previously fixed in the event of his having proceeded alone and I beg you will bring to the notice of His Lordship in Council in forming his decision on this subject the circumstances that Mr Jukes will have to perform a double duty in taking charge of the Medical duties which obviates the expense attendant upon the appointment of a Surgeon without whom the Mission could not under other circumstances have proceeded.

This letter was answered by the chief secretary to the government in Bombay, replying that not only was his request granted but that if Captain Pasley thought it unnecessary for him to go to Teheran in person, the duty might devolve upon Jukes. Pasley, however, preferred to go himself, and his report being favourable, instructions were ultimately sent to General Malcolm to set out on his third mission.

On this occasion, perhaps taking a leaf out of the French book, the Company recognized the immense political value of medical propaganda. A policy of British self-satisfied superiority, backed by presents which a parsimonious trading company cut down to the lowest possible value, had caused their prestige to fall low and had already given both to the Russians and to the French an opportunity to score diplomatic triumphs. The third mission was to suffer from none of these things. Malcolm's suite was larger than any that had yet appeared in Persia. The presents he carried were more valuable than any yet offered to the shah. And to extend the respect which all Persians, both high class and low class, ought to feel towards England and the Honourable Company and at the same time to safeguard the health of such a large retinue, a second surgeon was attached to the suite, Mr Surgeon Cormick. At the same time the services of Mr Surgeon Campbell were lent to the army at Tabriz under the heir apparent, while Andrew Jukes awaited the arrival of his chief at Teheran.

It must be remembered that Sir Harford Jones was still in Teheran, claiming to be the official ambassador of the King of England. For a short time the government in India attempted to discredit him and even withdrew from him his diplomatic status and refused to meet his bills. His confirmation in office by London caused the Governor-General to modify his opposition and during the third mission of General Malcolm, Sir Harford Jones was accorded the primacy in Persia as the representative of King George III, although Malcolm also enjoyed diplomatic status as representative of the Governor-General. With the exception of a short period when Mr Campbell, medical officer to Sir Harford Jones, was lent to the army at Tabriz under the heir apparent, there were therefore three British doctors in Teheran in the year 1810.

In the following year Sir Harford Jones was recalled and replaced by Sir Gore Ouseley, who was the first to introduce European female society into Persia. For he arrived with his wife and children. Campbell was, at the time of his arrival, at Tabriz, serving with the army of 'Abbás Mírzá, the heir apparent. On his return to Teheran he resumed his post as surgeon to the mission. His death in 1818, while still on duty in Teheran, must have been a grievous loss to the British community. He was a man highly esteemed by those who knew him. Sir Harford Jones on leaving Persia had written that 'Campbell conducted himself highly to my satisfaction; and the medical duties both of the Mission and the more troublesome and fatiguing one of attending Persian patients have been zealously performed by him'.

Mr Willock, the British chargé d'affaires, after the departure of Sir Gore Ouseley, in December 1817 wrote recommending him to the notice of Lord Castlereagh, because 'his long residence in Persia and his accurate knowledge of the language, combined with the confidence and regard extended towards him by the

Prince Royal and all the Persian Ministers, enable him at all times to afford valuable aid to the public service at this court'. In March of the following year Campbell died and again Mr Willock wrote: 'The distinguished qualities of this gentleman throw a lustre on his native land in a country where the general character of a nation is estimated by the conduct of individuals.'

He was succeeded by a young graduate of Edinburgh named McNeill. John McNeill, destined to be the greatest of all the East India Company's doctors who served in Persia, was born in 1795. He graduated in 1814 and two years later was appointed Assistant-Surgeon to the factory in Bombay. The untimely death of Campbell left a vacancy in Persia and to it McNeill, although still very junior, was appointed. He found two British colleagues already there. First there was Surgeon Cormick who after the withdrawal of General Malcolm's mission took Campbell's place with the army of 'Abbás Mírzá. The second was Jukes who remained in the British political service. The latter on the return of the mission to India went back to his old task of translator in Bushire.

The expedition to exterminate piracy in the Persian Gulf gave Dr Jukes a fresh opportunity to win diplomatic triumphs. The annoyance, even if no stronger word is used, of the constant attacks by Arab marauders, whose base lay on the southern shore of the Gulf, determined the Company to protect the smaller craft, who were engaged in legitimate trade. Appeals to the Persian Government were useless. The Persians were incapable of policing the Gulf and of protecting even their own shipping. The duty therefore fell upon the paramount power. The annihilation of the pirates was accomplished in two expeditions. The problem then arose of how to prevent a recrudescence of the evil. The most popular suggestion was that the Company should occupy an island at the eastern end of the Gulf which should act as a sentinel and base for punitive expeditions. Kisham was suggested as the most suitable. The idea was even mooted of transferring the factory from Bushire to Kisham.

When the shah learnt of the proposal, he protested most indignantly at the suggestion of transferring any portion of the Persian Empire to foreign rule. In the British design he saw the thin end of the wedge. He suspected that it was but the first nibble which would finish by the swallowing of his whole empire. In the meantime the Company went forward with their scheme, deaf to his protest. Their action was not in truth quite so high-handed as, put this way, it sounds. For the sovereignty of the island of Kisham was claimed both by the Sultan of Muscat and by the Shah of Persia. The former had given permission for the establishment of a settlement there; the latter had presented it as a gift to General Malcolm when he first came to Persia.

A report that the Governor of Shiraz was collecting troops to expel the British by force from the island caused the Company to take steps to settle by conciliation a matter which it appeared might endanger their main policy in Persia. In May 1821 Dr Andrew Jukes was appointed Political Agent at Kisham and bidden to go there with all speed to see the real state of affairs and then to proceed to Shiraz and Teheran to conciliate the Persian authorities. He was to explain that the holding of the island was in no sense a prelude to the occupation of any part of the mainland and that the troops stationed there were purely a police guard, designed as much for the good of Persia as for the good of British traders. The unlikelihood of his success seems to have been in the mind of the Governor-General, for at the same time secret instructions were issued to him, authorizing him to give orders for the withdrawal of the troops in the last extreme, if all efforts at conciliation failed.

To his great credit and contrary to expectation Jukes was successful. After visiting Kisham he returned to Shiraz in the autumn. The festival of Muharram and an epidemic of cholera delayed his seeing the Governor for many days. When at last he was given an audience, he succeeded in talking him over to the British point of view. The Governor wrote to the shah, urging that the settlement should be permitted. But the shah was still unmoved and continued to demand the withdrawal of the British troops. Jukes therefore determined to go on to Teheran to complete his work. Most unfortunately, before he reached the capital, he fell sick and died. Thus died at his post the most popular doctor and one of the most successful diplomats whom the East India Company ever sent out to Persia. To this day his tombstone can be seen in the Armenian Monastery of Sourp Amenaprgich, New Julfa. It is now used as a paving to the churchyard, but the inscription is still legible: 'Sacred to the Memory of Andrew Jukes, Esq., Political Agent in the Persian Gulf, who departed this life at Ispahan on the 10th November 1821, Aged 43 and lies interred here.'

The rest of the story is briefly told. At first the Governor-General tried force. The garrison at Kisham was augmented and in the autumn of 1822 the Governor of Shiraz signed an agreement with the British Resident at Bushire that troops should be allowed to occupy Kisham for five years. A severe epidemic of cholera again swept through the Gulf in the autumn of that year. The shah denounced the act of his Governor and in January 1823 the Governor-General gladly capitulated, withdrew the troops and announced that they would be replaced by a 'naval equipment'. The storm over Kisham died down until the question of a sentinel post was raised once more, 50 years later, when the enemy was plague, not piracy.

The death of Andrew Jukes coincided with a change in British policy towards Persian affairs. The French attempt to hurt England by the threat to India raised Persian prestige to an undeservedly high level. The Persians with their typical egoism and pride of those days accepted all European advances as a tribute to their might, about which they had never had any doubts themselves. The shah, looking upon himself as the Umbilicus of the Universe, was glad to find that at last the infidel nations recognized his claim. To his disgust the interest which Great Britain had so suddenly shown in Persian internal affairs, equally suddenly died down when it became clear that Napoleon was no longer a menace to British trading adventures. The shah was therefore considerably piqued when it was announced to him that the British representative at his court in Teheran would no longer hold his commission from the British sovereign or speak in his name, but would in future be appointed by the Governor-General in India and be the representative of the East India Company.

At first he categorically refused to accept such an envoy. Persian ministers in London had made him well aware that the East India Company was a trading company. As a sovereign he claimed, and with some justice, to treat only with a sovereign. The Prince Royal, 'Abbás Mírzá, who was in receipt of a large annual allowance from British coffers, professed the deepest friendship for the English and urged his father to accept the new status of the envoy. Much was to be gained, he pointed out, by dealing with an English power that was close at hand rather than with a bureau of officials many days' journey away. But the shah was adamant; he would not hear of the proposal.

The Company took no notice of this objection and in March 1824 proceeded to appoint Colonel Macdonald as their envoy with Assistant-Surgeon Magrath as his personal physician, and bade them both proceed with an escort to Teheran as soon as possible. A report of the unfavourable reception which they might expect to receive caused the mission to halt at Bombay. For six months all parties tried to persuade the shah to change his attitude. In November he so far modified it as to agree to allow the Indian mission to land, but stipulated that the envoy should reside at Shiraz, not at Teheran.

This did not satisfy the British authorities. The Company was unwilling to be represented only at Shiraz and the Foreign Office was unwilling to continue their representation at all. Another year passed in arguing and persuading and it was not until July 1825 that the shah yielded and sent a messenger to Lord Amherst, then Governor-General, to solicit him to send an envoy to his court.

In the meantime Surgeon Magrath had found other employment, and the mission at last left without a medical attendant. Macdonald reached Bushire on 11 March 1826 and with all dispatch set out for Teheran. He took with him Surgeon Riach, who was then acting Resident at Bushire, to attend to the needs of the party on their journey into the interior. Dr McNeill, who had been acting as physician to the mission since 1818, was confirmed in his post when they reached Teheran. Willock was reduced to the rank of first assistant. Thus continuity between the Foreign Office and the Company was guaranteed.

The journey was not uneventful, for at Shiraz a 'malignant fever' broke out in the caravan and many of the Europeans were attacked. The envoy decided to push on, thinking perhaps that the fresh air of the country would do more to restore health to his suite than rest in the town. But affairs grew so serious that at Yezd-i-Khwast he was compelled to halt. The doctor was so ill that he could scarcely attend his patients. Two of the suite, a nephew of General Malcolm who was secretary to the envoy and the English head clerk, fell sick and died. Their bodies, together with those of two other Englishmen who had died here previously, been buried and their tombs neglected, were transported by the sad and sick party on to Ispahan. Here they were reverently interred in the Armenian cathedral at Julfa, and the whole party sat down to await the arrival of fresh medical aid from Teheran.

With Dr McNeill's help full health was soon regained. At the end of August, 5½ months after reaching Bushire, Colonel Macdonald assumed charge of the British mission to the court of Fatḥ 'Alí S͟háh.

The leading question of the day he found to be the Russian war. For many years the exact frontier between the empires of Persia and Russia had been in dispute. Raids upon Russian villages were frequent; semi-official reprisals upon Persian territory were the answer. The shah, confident in the strength of his arms, which the flattery of his courtiers increased, and misinterpreting the import of the French and English diplomatic advances, was all for war and for driving the Russians behind the Caucasus. 'Abbás Mírzá, as Governor of Tabriz, was the commander most interested in the question. Speaking to Dr McNeill he professed himself in favour of peace; in the presence of his father he displayed a warlike attitude. But his army was no longer a match for the Russians. When in 1815 the British Minister was recalled, with him had returned all the British military officers with very few exceptions. Their replacement by French officers had not proved a success, and 10 years later the regiments under the command of the Prince Royal found themselves ill fed, ill armed and without enthusiasm.

A series of incidents provoked the inevitable struggle. A Russian veterinary officer, who went to Teheran to buy horses, was ill-treated by the Persian officials. A Russian colonel in Tabriz was robbed and his house looted and could get no satisfaction from the Persian authorities. The Russian offer to provide an armed escort for the Prince Royal was refused. Finally, a boundary commission under Prince Menichikoff reached Teheran and was dismissed without accomplishing anything. In the very month in which Colonel Macdonald reached Teheran, hostilities opened. War was preached from every mosque throughout the land. To fight the Russians was now taught to be a holy war. Deputations of the clergy visited the shah to urge upon him a resolute and bellicose policy. One such detachment of holy men under a certain *sayyid* of Meragha reached the court dressed in winding sheets. The shah was so much impressed with their fervour that twice he came in person to visit the *sayyid*. On the second occasion he remarked that he was anxious to shed in the holy cause the spoonful of blood which his weak body contained and begged the *sayyid* to write down this statement and vouch for it with his signature. This precious document he ordered to be enclosed in his coffin when he died in order that the Angels of Judgement might recognize at once his zeal in religion, forgive his sins and admit him into Heaven without further delay.

For the British the situation thus created was difficult. Individually the relations with the Russians were excellent. Dr McNeill was sent by the chargé d'affaires to offer an official welcome to Prince Menichikoff. Doctor Cormick in Tabriz was appointed the medical attendant to his suite and on their return to Russia received a valuable ring as an expression of the thanks of the Russian Government. But it was impossible to deny that secretly British officials wished success to the Persian arms. The bogey of the Russian threat to India had now taken the place of the French bogey. It was therefore with considerable pleasure, and certainly with surprise, that they saw the army of the Prince Royal carrying all before it.

The Russian steam-roller works slowly. It took several months before the Russian forces realized that this was more than a border foray. It was not until July of the following year that the first big Russian successes occurred when Nakhchivan and then Abbasabad, the key town to Tabriz, fell into Russian hands. To prolong the struggle was useless. The very approach of the Russian troops to Tabriz caused the Persian soldiery to desert. In the defence of the city only three guns were fired, two of them being loaded with blank and the third while the approaching cavalry were still out of range. The Russians thus captured Tabriz without loss of blood on either side. 'Abbás Mírzá retreated in haste along the road to Teheran, accompanied by Dr Cormick, who was especially instructed to do his utmost to prevent him from taking any rash step in his despair at his complete defeat.

Negotiations for a permanent peace then commenced. These proved exceedingly tedious, for the Russians in return for the evacuation of the captured Persian territory demanded an indemnity of 15 crores of tumans, that is, about £30,000,000. To meet this demand the shah had to dive very deep into his treasury, and this was precisely what he was unwilling to do. The long protracted negotiations were carried on through the medium of the British mission. In Teheran Dr McNeill had almost daily interviews with the shah, to whom he pointed out that if he wished to save his country from complete dismemberment, the Russians must be bought off at any cost. In Tabriz Colonel Macdonald hovered between the camp of 'Abbás Mírzá and that of the Russian commander-in-chief. To the former he begged for haste; to the latter for patience.

When the Russian time limit expired, this sum was still unpaid. A further Russian advance proved to the shah that the threat to his throne was no idle one, and again he called for a parley. Very unwillingly and as though it were the blood of his heart, the shah now disgorged five crores of tumans, which he handed over to Dr McNeill and which were stored in the house of the British mission. On the receipt of this information the Russian commander-in-chief called a halt, and in December 1827 the first instalment of the indemnity left Teheran for Russia under the protection of a British escort. To the last the Russians feared treachery. Stories were rife that the bags said to contain gold, in reality held only lead and stones. The Russian general's faith in the British word was not misplaced, however, and the treasure was satisfactorily handed over to the victors in February 1828 and peace with Russia was signed.

At the end of the year normal relations with the Russian court were again opened. A Russian mission, which consisted of Prince Grebaiodoff as Minister Plenipotentiary, two secretaries, two attachés, a surgeon, a chaplain, and a large number of clerks and cossacks was welcomed in Teheran. Scarcely had the minister presented his letter of credence when the diplomatic world was shocked to hear of the murder of the whole of the staff of the mission. In the general massacre perished the doctor. It appears that the envoy received into his house a certain Mírzá Ya'qúb, an Armenian eunuch and a steward of the shah's harem, who claimed to be a Russian subject. With him he took some jewellery and a good deal of cash which belonged to the palace. In consideration of the status of the ambassador the shah relinquished all claim to the man, but demanded the return of the property. The ambassador was unwilling to make any return until a legal tribunal had settled the rights and wrongs of the case. In the meantime the eunuch, finding himself secure, abused the Law and the Prophet, vilified the clergy, ridiculed the government and cursed the Persian people. This infuriated the populace of Teheran, who could scarce restrain themselves from attacking the Russians when they passed them in the streets.

During this time of ferment it came to the ears of the ambassador that in the house of a certain Persian grandee there were held prisoner two Russian-Armenian women. The ambassador demanded their immediate release. In vain the owner answered that they were Turkish-Armenians and had no connection at all with Russia. The ambassador refused to believe it and repeated his demands with urgency.

To settle the question the shah ordered the women to be sent to the house of the ambassador so that he might examine them himself and thus find out the truth. To him they were therefore sent and he, ignorant of Persian customs, detained the women for the night in his house. For no woman in Persia can remain in the house of a stranger and keep her reputation intact. Having already a eunuch in the house, well used to the care of women, he entrusted the care of these to him.

Unfortunately, on that night Mírzá Ya'qúb thought fit to have a drinking party in the room in the ambassador's house set apart for him and furthermore thought good to introduce a prostitute into the company. The two women, who were forced to spend the night there, seeing what was going on, raised a cry. The people of the town, already sufficiently inflamed against the Russians, now had a double reason to demand satisfaction. A mob began to collect outside; the Russian guards began to use violence. A pistol shot brought down one of the townsmen and the riot began. The door of the house was soon broken in and before the extra troops, hurriedly sent from the royal barracks, could arrive, all the members of the mission from the highest to the lowest, with the exception of three, were murdered.

The shah, fearful that the mob would next turn against him, shut himself up in the 'Arq, the central citadel of Teheran, and took no further steps until the fury of the populace abated and fresh troops arrived to keep order. He then took such measures as he could to mollify the Russian wrath. The chief *mullá*, whom he accused of fanning the hatred of the mob against the infidels, he banished from the kingdom. A great host of others, less dignified in rank and more or less guilty, he punished by cutting out their tongues, slitting their noses and tearing off their ears. Russian honour thus appeased, a Persian mission of apology was sent to St Petersburgh and a new Russian mission was received in Teheran.[1]

To a very considerable degree the blame for the failure of 'Abbás Mírzá in the late Russian war must be ascribed to the shah himself. His avarice prevented him from using any of his treasure to equip the Persian forces; his senility caused him to vacillate and misunderstand. Fatḥ 'Alí was now 60 years of age. He had lost his physical strength as well as the vigour of his mind. He allowed himself to be swayed by his hopes and by his fears. His temper, never of the best, had now become liable to vary without warning. Even the members of his own family, who once had had most influence with him, now only desired to avoid all communication with him. The confidential servants about his person even entertained apprehensions of his sanity. One of them remarked that if his mind continued to decline as rapidly during the coming month as it had during the past, it would be impossible for him to transact business any longer.

In the midst of his troubles he turned to Dr McNeill and for the first time consulted him about his health. Up to this moment the shah seems to have shown no confidence in the European practice of medicine. McNeill's success with his favourite wife Táj-ul-Doula convinced him that the system was not so fallacious as his *ḥakím-básh͟hí* claimed. From that moment McNeill became the regular physician to the harem and to other members of the royal family.

1 The shah's letter of apology is quoted in full by Browne as an example of good Persian prose in his *Literary History of Persia*, vol IV, p. 312.

'Abbás Mírzá, on the contrary, had long believed in the superiority of Western medicine. Dr Cormick had for many years been stationed in Tabriz. There he attended the Prince Royal whenever he required him. Once, when taken ill upon the road between Tabriz and Teheran, he refused all native medical aid and insisted on McNeill riding out to visit him, and then and there he swore that he would never again travel unless attended by an English physician.

He must have been a difficult patient, for in the following year he was again taken ill. In one of Willock's dispatches occurs the following paragraph:

> The Prince Royal, having long indulged in the immoderate use of spiritous liquors, has at length been attacked by a violent inflammation of the liver, which endangers his life. He has improved on a course of Mercury, but Dr Cormick has so little confidence in the promises of His Royal Highness to relinquish his pernicious habits and has so little hope of His Royal Highness's progress in amendment and recovery under these circumstances that he has resigned the medical charge of His Royal Highness to a physician lately sent by the Shah from the capital.

In 1829 the shah for the first time felt too weak to leave his palace and go to the camp either for hunting or for military exercises. A dread of approaching death was uppermost in his mind. He ordered a tomb to be prepared for him in Qum and he sent to Meragha for a very large slab of marble which was, he instructed, to be laid upon his burial place to prevent his ashes from being disturbed after his death. In August of that year he had a severe heart attack and his life was despaired of. The conference of doctors around his bed was rudely disturbed by the inrush of Táj-ul-Doula and another favourite wife, who assured the dying monarch that the illness was a punishment from God for sending the chief *mullá* into exile and begged him to recall him. But even in his weakened state Fatḥ 'Alí retained enough sense to remain unpersuaded by this appeal.

The Persian doctors in charge were convinced that nothing except madeira and champagne were suitable for the royal stomach in this low condition. Having neither of these available, they applied to the British and Russian envoys. These were willingly supplied. The physicians' treatment was justified, for the shah rallied.

Unfortunately, the situation was further complicated by the illness of 'Abbás Mírzá, the heir apparent. In addition to the cirrhosis from which apparently he was suffering, he also complained of a fistula and more than once Dr McNeill was called to Tabriz to operate upon him for this condition. The senility of the shah and the uncertainty that the heir apparent would outlive him made this question of the successor to the throne a subject for speculation. Although the male offspring of Fatḥ 'Alí ran into dozens, no one showed any marked superiority of character or intellect over the rest. Ágh́á Muḥammad, the late shah, when informed that ten or twelve children had been born to his nephew in the course of 24 hours, remarked: 'Fain would I change them all for one Luṭf 'Alí.'

Of the many claimants to the throne the most deserving was his eldest son Muḥammad 'Alí Mírzá, a young man whose figure and features were coarse and vulgar, but who encouraged men of learning, was himself something of a poet, and who delighted in the society and conversation of men versed in history and literature. Unfortunately he died of dysentery in 1821.

After his death the next most suitable was 'Abbás Mírzá, who, backed by the British, had been nominated heir apparent after the demise of his elder brother. Though weak and a man who preferred the society of the low-born and illiterate, yet he was far more tolerant and up-to-date in his views than were his brother princes. He endeavoured to introduce the arts, the sciences and the manufactures of the West into Persia. These merits were recognized in England and to the great disgust of the shah, who thought that any form of distinction should be reserved to the reigning monarch, he was presented with a diploma by the Royal Asiatic Society of Great Britain. To him, even more than to Náṣir-ul-Dín Sháh, should be ascribed the introduction of Western medicine into Persian circles.

Among the many other claimants, near or distantly related to the reigning monarch, it is only necessary to mention two. Of these two the most vigorous was Ḥusayn 'Alí Mírzá, who in 1825 held the governorship of Shiraz and who three years later became the leader of the patriotic party which urged the shah to withhold the Russian indemnity. Although it was clear that the chief object of his government was to fill his own treasury, yet he was a man of action and resolute character. In the disturbed days which followed the signing of the Treaty of Turcomanshahi with the Russians, the southern provinces rebelled against the central government and to Ḥusayn 'Alí Mírzá was given the task of reducing them to obedience again. For this purpose he was created Governor of Kerman. In his suppression of the revolt he slaughtered some hundreds of men, levied some bushels of eyes from among the disaffected, and caused the bellies of the ring-leaders to be ripped open after they had been hung up like sheep in the market-place.

Two years later the Prince-Governor of Fars, the Farmán Farmá, his brother by the same mother, rebelled and this time Ḥusayn 'Alí Mírzá sided against his father and himself laid siege to Yezd. Yezd fell and Ispahan was threatened. To meet the emergency 'Abbás Mírzá was given command of the royal forces and an opportunity to regain the reputation which he had lost in the Russian campaign. In this capacity he was completely successful. Yezd was relieved and Kerman was reduced without a battle. Through the complete success of the heir apparent the shah could afford to be generous and Ḥusayn 'Alí Mírzá and the Farmán Farmá were allowed to retain their governorships with their reduced prestige.

Another claimant to the throne was never taken very seriously. This was a certain Muḥammad Taqí Mírzá, a minor prince and governor of Burujird. Hearing a report of the shah's death in 1821, he hastily collected all the armed men he could find and marched upon Teheran. On his arrival at the gates of the city he was mortified to hear that the shah was enjoying his usual health. Together with his army he slunk back to his remote governorship. When his very premature move came to the ears of the shah, he observed that as Muḥammad Taqí had shown such grief at his demise, he must take upon himself the expenses of his burial and mulcted him of 20,000 tomans.

In the midst of this confused and uncertain state the British envoy, Colonel, now Sir John, Macdonald, died at Tabriz after an illness of a few months. This was in June 1830. The charge of the mission then devolved upon Captain Campbell, who at once asked for the services of Dr McNeill to be given to him both as his physician and as his chief assistant. McNeill was by now far the most knowledgeable European in Persia. His long residence had made him a perfect master of the Persian language and had given him a knowledge of the customs and manners of the court, which no other European possessed, not even excepting Dr Cormick, who was his senior by two years.

For a while the Government of India hesitated in their choice of a successor to Sir John Macdonald. Captain Campbell continued to act as chargé d'affaires and Dr McNeill to act as his chief assistant. During this interregnum another office fell vacant, that of Political Resident in the Persian Gulf. For this post McNeill became a candidate and was duly appointed. As he had also been appointed assistant to the chargé d'affaires, he was officially informed that he was not expected to proceed to Bushire until some definite arrangement should be made to fill the vacancy caused by the death of Sir John Macdonald.

In August 1831 letters from India announced to Captain Campbell the intention of the Governor-General to nominate a Major Stewart as envoy, adding that he would be sailing from Bombay in November or December. Captain Campbell thought it essential that the new envoy should receive accurate information about the political situation in the courts of Tabriz and Teheran and therefore ordered McNeill to proceed to his new post without delay and to try and reach Bushire before Major Stewart's arrival.

McNeill therefore, a few days later, left Tabriz, moving his family with him. It being now the depths of winter, he chose to travel via Baghdad and Basra. His difficulties on the road were enormous. The passes were filled with snow; plague had reappeared in Baghdad and broke out among the crew of the boat which was conveying him down the river; the state of the country was everywhere unsettled and he was attacked by marauding Arabs. To crown his misfortunes he was informed, when he was within one day's sail of Basra, that his appointment as Political Resident was cancelled on the grounds that he was not a civil servant.

After years of toil, having travelled on government service at his own estimation 22,000 miles, all on horseback and often at the rate of 80 to 100 miles a day, he found himself not merely deprived of a high post to which his merits entitled him, but reduced to an office which gave him, he thought, no prospects of further advancement. On his return journey he wrote a letter of bitter complaint, somewhat mollified it is true, when on reaching Hamadan he found that Major Stewart's appointment was cancelled, that Captain Campbell was nominated envoy, and that he himself had been appointed permanent chief assistant to the mission. But his pay as assistant was less than the pay of the political resident; for the command of an Iberian Residency he was to play second fiddle in a Roman court; for a fixed and luxurious home he was to continue his life of travel and forced marches. A parsimonious and ungenerous government gave him no medical assistant, and after 16 years of hard labour the most experienced and most popular diplomat in Persia was only a chief assistant and medical officer combined on a consolidated allowance of Rs. 1250 a month.

Nevertheless he accepted the office with a good grace, for it was a post not without honour. His first task was to arrange the reception of the new envoy by the shah. A servant sent by Campbell to the court of the shah with a letter intimating his promotion was kept a prisoner and the letter was unanswered. McNeill was therefore sent from Tabriz to Teheran to make a satisfactory arrangement. He found, as he expected, that the real trouble was that the shah was doubtful whether the envoy would offer him as large a present as the last envoys had brought with them on their first arrival in the court. His doubts were justified. Malcolm and the envoys of those days were authorized to spend enormous sums as bribes to confirm the shah in his anti-French policy. Even Macdonald was allowed to announce his arrival with a very handsome present which might help to soothe the shah's conscience in accepting an envoy accredited by the Governor-General in India instead of by the King of England. In Campbell's case there was no reason why his favour should be bought.

The ministers of court, be it said to their credit, were extremely displeased at the part they had to play in this haggling over gifts. At last McNeill requested an interview with the shah himself. As long as he could, the shah kept the conversation away from the subject which was uppermost in the minds of both, and before McNeill could come to the point, gave the signal for the conclusion of the audience. McNeill, with a complete breach of court etiquette, ignored the order to withdraw and boldly informed the shah that should he be unwilling to receive Captain Campbell without any stipulation as to the value of the present, he would recommend the withdrawal of the whole British mission from Persia.

McNeill then withdrew to his own quarters to see what effect his words would have upon the shah. Very soon he was approached by the Minister of Foreign Affairs, who offered to compromise and accept only Ts. 5000. But McNeill would have none of this. That evening the shah capitulated; the envoy's reception was to be unconditional. Low though his motives undoubtedly were, yet the action of the shah is not altogether to be condemned. He felt the failure of the Russian campaign very acutely and looked for a snub in every diplomatic move. 'They do what they like now', he said, with bitterness. 'They think that the waters have passed over me.'

CHAPTER XVI

THE MISSION OF SIR JOHN McNEILL

DURING all these years of political disturbance, plague and pestilence, which had been the curse of the early traders, continued to take their toll of lives and merchandise. To recount year by year the various outbreaks would be unprofitable and monotonous. Persia herself, with her chief towns at an altitude of 2000 ft. or more, was rarely the primary focus. But on every side of her epidemic disease raged and usually was carried into one or more of the great towns of the plateau or to the ports along the Gulf. In 1829 cholera appeared in Teheran, having spread from Herat, where two of the royal Afghan princes had caught the disease and died. The following year it appeared in Tabriz, having spread across the Russian frontier. In the same year cholera again appeared in Teheran and spread from there to Qazvin, Kashan and Ispahan. In the autumn plague broke out in Tabriz with a mortality estimated at 30,000. 'Abbás Mírzá was obliged to move his court to Ardebil for the winter months through fear of infection; and the lower classes, flying in terror into the country, spread the disease to the villages around. By the following year the whole of Gilan was infected.

On the western frontier Kermanshah reported a severe outbreak of plague imported from Baghdad. In the latter city and in Basra the plague was raging with a virulence which suggested the great plague of 1772. The pasha shut himself up in his palace and would see no one. Even so he caught the disease, and, though he himself recovered, two out of his seven wives died. The Catholic Bishop of Babylon, who was also in charge of French affairs, died at his post. The number of deaths in Baghdad city were said to number 30,000.

In Basra the virulence of the disease was even greater. Dr Baigrie, who was then Residency Civil Surgeon in Baghdad, was sent down to see what he could do to relieve the distress. Smearing his fingers with camphorated oil and sprinkling concentrated vinegar on his clothes to protect himself against infection, he moved among the victims. He reported that about 100 a day were dying of the disease. The Turkish Government took not the slightest precaution against its spread. Like the Pasha of Baghdad, the Governor shut himself up in his house and would see no one. When the infection got in and began to take its toll of the inmates, he callously threw the dead bodies over the garden wall into the public street there to rot and threaten the health of passers-by. So great was the number of deaths that merchants were compelled to supply their cloth gratis for use as winding sheets. The higher and middle classes shut their eyes to this state of affairs and disliked to hear the subject discussed before them. They folded their hands and awaited death. The lower classes, who had the means of moving, moved; before long all the Persian Gulf was infected.

Two years later, when the British political agent visited Basra, he reported that the plague had left the city nearly without inhabitants, that the date-groves, their great source of wealth, were left unattended for want of hands to affect the normal impregnation of the female trees, and that consequently the supply of dates, the main food and chief material of commerce, was almost entirely wanting.

The series of epidemics was felt by the Government of India not only in the loss of trade, but also in the increased expense of their mission in Persia. The extravagance of the envoy was the subject of an annual letter. Macdonald was reprimanded for the value of the presents which he distributed on his first arrival. The only economy which he could suggest was to stop the vaccinating allowance of the two British doctors. For these services Dr Cormick drew Rs. 100 a month and Dr McNeill Rs. 160. Campbell, whose presents were kept within the allowed value, was blamed for the large retinue which he maintained and for the number of pack animals which he hired or kept in his stables.

Beyond suggesting that the post which Dr Cormick held should not be filled when he retired, he could make no proposals. He defended his establishment, saying that the combined prevalence of plague and cholera had compelled him for the preservation of the staff to maintain a large establishment of mules in order to remove them at short notice from the neighbourhood of infection, when it approached his encampment; that he had been under canvas for nearly thirteen months out of the eighteen that he had been envoy; and that his measures were amply justified by the fact that not a single menial had fallen a victim to the pestilences which had depopulated the rest of the Persian Empire.

The increasing amount of political work which fell to McNeill and which necessitated his prolonged absence from the Chancery, left Campbell, who in 1832 became Sir Robert Campbell, frequently without the services of a doctor. His eyes, about this time, were giving him considerable trouble. Over and over again he had to consult Dr Cormick owing to the absence of his own doctor. Cormick had announced his intention of retiring in the winter of 1830, but was still at work in Tabriz. Campbell therefore applied for the services of another doctor and put forward the name of Dr Reach (or Riach, both spellings occur), who had been surgeon to the Residency at Bushire for several years. His request, for the moment, remained unanswered by the Government of India, whose policy from the early days of the Company had been to stint their health services.

'Abbás Mírzá, his position as heir to the throne secure by the victories in the south, now moved eastwards to attack Afghanistan. He first reduced to order the unruly province of Khorasan and made Meshed his headquarters. McNeill, who was accompanying him, reported that his affairs were so prosperous that it looked as though Herat would soon be added to the Persian Empire. A threatened Turcoman revolt, however, kept him for a time in Meshed, where he spent his leisure negotiating with the *amír* of Bukhara for the suppression of the *amír*'s trade in Persian slaves.

At the same time the *amír* approached the British authorities for the supply of a British instructor for his troops and for some British physicians.

In the summer of 1833, in obedience to the shah's request, 'Abbás Mírzá returned to Teheran on a short visit. He left his son Muḥammad Mírzá in command of the troops with instructions to push on the campaign against the Afghans. The sickly appearance of the heir apparent caused a general consternation in the capital. Dr Cormick was hurriedly sent for from Tabriz; Dr McNeill returned from Meshed. The two English doctors held a consultation with Mírzá Bábá, the prince's personal Persian physician. They were unanimous in recommending as a preliminary to all other treatment, the retirement of the prince to some quiet spot and the complete abandonment of the campaign against Herat. 'Abbás Mírzá would not listen to them. Sir Robert Campbell was still suffering with his eyes and, 'his system being much affected with mercury', he was too ill to go and urge upon the prince the desirability of following the doctors' advice. In the end a compromise was reached whereby the Prince Royal would take up his residence at Nishapur, which was cooler and more secluded than Meshed, yet near enough to the Afghan frontier for him not to lose touch with his generals in the field.

Before he finally left the capital, he determined to send an envoy to England to settle certain outstanding questions between the two governments. Chief among these were the guarantee of his succession to the throne, the payment of the annual subsidy and the supply of arms for his army. After much deliberation he finally nominated his physician, Mírzá Bábá, for the post, and after some delay the Mírzá set off. It would have been extremely difficult at that time to find anyone else equally qualified for the post. Mírzá Bábá had spent twelve years in England already studying medicine and could therefore speak English. He was moreover without that mercenary spirit which characterized most of his contemporary countrymen. And finally he enjoyed to the full the confidence of 'Abbás Mírzá.

On 7 August 1833, Dr John Cormick issued an official bulletin on the state of the health of the Prince Royal.

> His Royal Highness labours under a serious dropsical affection of the lower extremities, extending as high up as the hip joints, which has caused a diseased and obstructed state of his liver. This is the fifth attack he has had of this disease.

Two days later, in spite of his manifest ill-health, 'Abbás Mírzá set out for Khorasan, unaccompanied by any European doctor. By the orders of the shah Dr Cormick remained in Teheran for a final interview; by the orders of Sir Robert Campbell Dr McNeill was engaged elsewhere.

During the summer a strange epidemic, possibly influenza, had broken out in Teheran. It even pierced the boasted immunity of the staff of the mission. So many fell sick that Sir Robert Campbell decided to move down from Shimran, the hills behind Teheran, into the city. Even the shah was attacked. His doctors reported that he was suffering from a severe fever and ague. The state of the city was even worse than the state of the villages of Shimran. The deaths ran into many dozens a day. The dead and the dying lay about the street corners and a wretchedness existed beyond even that of the times of plague and cholera. With all this, bread became scarce, the meat uneatable, and the risk of a widespread famine by no means negligible.

The wildest of reports began to spring up. The fever from which the shah had been suffering for several days was reported to have assumed a serious form owing to the unskilful treatment of his physicians. It was generally believed that his death was imminent. In the midst of this state of anarchy and confusion came two further alarming pieces of news. First the death of Dr Cormick on the road to Nishapur was reported and then the death of the Prince Royal himself.

Among the official files of that year there is preserved a private letter from Dr McNeill, in which he describes the former melancholy event.

Poor Cormick died about the beginning of last month at a caravanserai on the road to Khorasan. There was no European near him and not even a confidential servant. He was travelling in haste to join the Prince and had scarcely a bed with him. These are the chances of this country. He had wealth and honour and the favour of princes and such was his end. The loss of so benevolent and useful a person will be sensibly felt at Tabreez where he did much good with little ostentation.

I too feel his death more than I could have anticipated. He was the only link between the old times and the new, except myself. I am now the oldest in years as well as the oldest servant of the Government and the oldest resident in Persia who is left.

Teheran
11th November 1833

Three weeks later 'Abbás Mírzá, too, was lying dead in Meshed of a ruptured liver abscess and the question of the successor to Fatḥ 'Alí Sháh became the prominent question of the day. His death found the British Government without a definite policy. Russia had already announced her intention of supporting the claims of Muḥammad Mírzá, his eldest son, to succeed to the status of heir apparent. England feared to follow that lead, for the Foreign Office foresaw that the claim of Muḥammad Mírzá would not be allowed by his brothers without a struggle. To support him without loss of prestige meant almost certainly to support him by force of arms. To withhold recognition of his title on the other hand meant that Muḥammad Mírzá would look more and more to Russia as his ally and would turn to that country for help and advice when established on the throne. This at all costs the Foreign Office were determined to prevent. It was therefore with considerable doubt that they read the letters from their envoy, urging them to recognize the pretentions of Muḥammad Mírzá, even before his grandfather acclaimed him.

The situation was indeed difficult. Should Muḥammad Mírzá be defeated before Herat, his chances of succession would in any case be nil. The power of his uncles in the south was paramount. The shah, though fond of him, was unwilling to take any definite step. He was now in his 72nd year, much debilitated and subject to relapses of fever. In his physically weak and mentally unstable condition it was hopeless to expect him to make any definite decision without considerable external persuasion. Clearly, in the mind of the shah the choice lay between Muḥammad Mírzá and his own son the Ẓill-ul-Sulṭán. As a matter of practical politics the ultimate decision rested with the governments of Russia and England.

Between the two rivals there could be no question which was the fitter. The character of the Ẓill-ul-Sulṭán was in every respect so contemptible, so devoid of principle and so destitute of energy and his habits so dissolute that no European government, or even the Persians themselves, could wish to see him on the throne. On the other hand, Muḥammad Mírzá, being still a youth, was free from the vicious and corrupt habits which characterized the Persians of those days and more particularly the royal princes. With all classes he was popular.

These qualities were not lost upon the shah. Immediately, but without committing himself to the right of succession, he named Muḥammad Mírzá governor of those provinces and commander-in-chief of the armies, which had formerly been entrusted to ʻAbbás Mírzá. Six months later, mainly through the instigation of the Russian ambassador, saying that Ágh͟há Muḥammad had appeared to him in a dream and had bidden him do so, he declared Muḥammad Mírzá the heir apparent and had him publicly vested as *Valí ʻAhd* in Teheran at the end of June 1834. Muḥammad Mírzá then abandoned all thoughts of his Afghan campaign and left for Tabriz to hold his court in that city, as had been the custom of his father.

During all this time it was a question whether the shah would live long enough for Muḥammad Mírzá to consolidate his position. In January he was seized with some internal complaint, which for several hours threatened his life. Application was made by his physicians to Sir Robert Campbell for a supply of strong wine, and again he revived. At the end of the month he was still so feeble that he was confined to one room. The supply of wine having run out, application was made for beer instead. Again the Government of India came to the rescue and the ailing shah grew strong once more. In February he resumed his public audiences. But his interest in the welfare of his country had gone. His frame was enfeebled by age, sensual indulgence, and frequent relapses of fever. Hence by midsummer he was glad to listen to his foreign advisers and to hand over the government of the land to his ministers and the heir apparent.

The difficulties which surrounded Muḥammad Mírzá might well have depressed a more experienced man. His treasury was empty; the pay of his army was in arrears; famine, pestilence and war had reduced the revenues of his provinces to a mere pittance. There was still the balance of the war indemnity to be paid to Russia. His European advisers were all new. 'Abbás Mírzá had a Major Hart as commander of his army and Dr Cormick as his physician and friend. All three died within a few days of one another. Colonel Pasmore and Major Sir Henry Bethune were now with his army; Dr Griffith and an adventurer named Clarke were his European medical advisers. It was with considerable gloom therefore that the British envoy, who had accompanied Muḥammad Mírzá to Tabriz, heard the rumour that on 28 October 1834 the shah had suddenly died. It appeared that he had been in reasonably good health and had gone down to Ispahan to collect the arrears of taxes which were owing to him from the Ẓill-ul-Sulṭán. After a fiery interview with his son he lay down in a state of complete exhaustion, fell into a gentle slumber, from which he passed without any sign of distress into the sleep of death.

On his journey to Ispahan he was accompanied by about fifty members of the royal family. As soon as his death became known to them the utmost consternation prevailed. They were at a loss how to act, not knowing where best to spend the night, fearing that they might each and all be murdered before the morning. During the night the greater part of the court disappeared. Those that stayed behind found to their great relief that their lives were in no immediate danger, for the fury of the townspeople was being vented solely upon Sayf-ul-Doula, the Governor of Ispahan, in revenge for his many and various acts of tyranny and oppression. He, wise man, had already fled and had barricaded himself with a few followers in the palace of the Chár Maḥal. Ispahan then became a scene of great disorder and confusion. No opposition, however, was made to the transport of the body of the late shah to Qum, where he was buried with all the honour and ceremony that the men of the city could devise.

From Qum the Ẓill-ul-Sulṭán hurried on to Teheran and there proclaimed himself shah. Seated upon the marble throne in the Gulistán he assumed the outward status of the ruler of Persia and, seizing the royal treasury, he sent word to Muḥammad Mírzá that he should stay in Tabriz and still consider himself heir apparent.

Fortunately in this crisis the English and Russian envoys were prepared to act in unison. Winter was now drawing on. Tabriz is separated from Teheran by a series of not inconsiderable mountain passes, and the Ẓill-ul-Sulṭán, knowing the dilatory methods of his countrymen, naturally expected that the army of Azerbaijan would remain inactive until the passes were clear of snow. In this he failed to count upon the energy and activity of Muḥammad Mírzá's European advisers. In less than a month the army of Tabriz was on the march for Teheran. The English and Russian envoys, proclaiming Muḥammad Mírzá as Muḥammad Sháh, accompanied the forces on their long march. The petty chieftains along the road everywhere swore allegiance. Qazvin was entered by the advance guard under Sir Henry Bethune without firing a shot and Rukn-ul-Doula, the governor, who had actually placed the Ẓill-ul-Sulṭán upon the throne and had received the governorship of Qazvin and Gilan as his reward, rode out to welcome the new shah.

Qazvin is barely 100 miles from Teheran. The Ẓill-ul-Sulṭán, seeing that his cause was hopeless, determined to set fire to the city and escape to the south. A promise of free pardon for him saved the city. A few days later Muḥammad Sẖáh arrived and received his submission. Thus the succession to the throne, which had hitherto always been decided by the sword and which had in previous times led to murders, bloodshed and torture, was perhaps for the first time hereditary and peaceful.

At first Muḥammad Sẖáh took up his residence in the Nigaristán palace outside the city. There he publicly placed the royal tiara in his cap, the belt of pearls around his waist with the sword of State, and the royal bracelets upon his arms. Taking his seat in the gold-enamelled Peacock Throne he received the formal acknowledgements of the court as their sovereign. His reception of the Ẕill-ul-Sulṭán was more friendly than might have been expected; he might without injustice have deprived him of his eyes or even of his head. In his defence the Ẕill-ul-Sulṭán stated that it was never his wish or intention to touch the treasury or to assume the title of king, but that Rukn-ul-Douleh and others had compelled him by actual force to sit upon the throne and place the crown upon his head. So gracefully did he yield to their force that during the month of his occupation of the throne he spent just over a million tumans.

Muḥammad Sẖáh did not at once enter Teheran. He awaited a day which the astrologers should declare to be one of good omen for him. So long were they discovering an auspicious day that the two European envoys remonstrated with him for his failure to follow up his initial success. The shah excused himself on the grounds of expediency. 'My late father', he replied, 'had no faith in astrological predictions. Neither have I myself. But the prejudices of the people must be consulted. Every person is said to be born under some particular star or planet. Mine is said to be Mars, the most unfortunate of all, and anyone is said to be unlucky over whom it presides.'

At last the astrologers predicted that sunrise on 2 January 1835 would be a good-omened hour. January in Teheran is an extremely cold month. In the pale light of dawn the troops could scarcely hold their muskets: his retinue could scarcely sit their horses.

The weather froze the spirits of the townsmen. And thus, without a royal welcome and without any panoply of sovereignty, Muḥammad Sh̲áh, a young man of twenty-five, entered his capital to take up the office and duties of *Sh̲áhinsh̲áh* of Persia.

The new shah owed his position entirely to Russian and English help. It was mainly to the latter that he should have addressed his thanks. It had been the traditional policy of the Government of India for many years to give military aid to the heir apparent. A few months previous to the death of the shah a new relief, consisting of seven officers, a medical officer and several sergeants, reached Bushire. These made their way with considerable difficulty to Tabriz and took part in the march to Teheran. To the mission the services of Dr Griffith, the medical officer, were very welcome. Dr Cormick was dead; Dr McNeill was on leave; and the Government of India had not yet sanctioned the transference of the services of Dr Riach from Bushire. Sir Robert (who now called himself Sir John) Campbell was still in a not very good state of health. The short-sighted and miserly policy of the Company still prevailed. Sir John again and again wrote pointing out that 'the presence of a medical officer, whose duties were exclusively medical and whose time, unemployed in other duties, could be devoted to the influential personages in Persian society, would be productive of solid good to British interests and would be calculated to improve and maintain the existing friendly intercourse between the English on one side and the Court and Persian peoples on the other'. But no notice was taken of his letters.

So bad was his health in the summer of 1835 that he found it impossible to endure the heat and dust of the city. He therefore left his house in the town and pitched his tents at the village of Gulahek. This village had been granted to the British mission by the late Fatḥ 'Alí Sh̲áh as a summer residence.

It consists [wrote Sir John Campbell] of about twenty houses. The revenues are a mere bagatelle and, if given to the ryots, as I have notified my intention of doing, to enable them to bring more water from the hills and to improve the land, they will be comfortable. As master of the village I receive nothing but a small piece of ground to cultivate a few potatoes for home consumption and have informed the inhabitants that they are to be paid for everything which they furnish to my camp.

In this village the British Government built, and still maintain, a summer residence for the staff of the mission. It was a wise plan which other powers and the Persians themselves soon followed. Four miles from the city and 1000 ft. higher, Gulahek is fanned by a cool breeze while the city is sweltering. More than once it has served as a place of retreat when the city has been swept by cholera. Such an occasion occurred almost immediately after the gift was made.

Although Muḥammad Sháh succeeded in the north without bloodshed his authority was not unchallenged in other parts of Persia. The south, always notorious for its independent views, was in a state of rebellion under the two governors, Ḥasan 'Alí Mírzá and the Farmán Farmá. To reduce them to loyalty the shah despatched a force under Sir Henry Bethune, who took with him Assistant-Surgeon Griffith as his aide-de-camp and surgeon to the troops. Ispahan fell at once and within a few weeks Sir Henry captured Shiraz and with the city the two governors.

With the successful termination of this campaign the new shah's position was fully guaranteed and freely acknowledged throughout Persia. Sir Henry Bethune, whose health had been suffering from continuous campaigning, returned to England. The shah, finding his position within his own dominions thus secured, determined to recommence his war against the Afghans. This step met with by no means universal approval. His desire to suppress the slave trade in Persian subjects was wholly laudable. His wishes to add Herat and Candahar to his empire were in a different category. The Indian Government could not connive at this and therefore, though they did not categorically forbid, they did not issue orders permitting the British military advisers to accompany the army. Even in Persian court circles, with the exception of Ḥájjí Mírzá Áqásí, the Prime Minister, there was a silent opposition to the contemplated expedition. The Russian ambassador supported the shah and it was hinted that Russian aid would be supplied provided that the invasion was begun promptly and without further delay.

For some time the shah hesitated. He seems to have felt that his move against the Afghans would not be either successful or popular. At last, stimulated probably by Russian promises, he suddenly gave orders for the army to move. When his command became known in the camp outside Teheran, where the troops were lying, consternation and confusion prevailed. Provisions and transport were lacking. For these the bazaars of Teheran were ransacked. Fruit merchants were plundered of their supplies; muleteers were robbed of their beasts. Thus inadequately equipped, the troops moved off and reached the village of Dulab. Here the scenes of violence and robbery were repeated in order that they might have the means to make the second day's march. When these doings were reported to the shah, he was infuriated beyond measure. 'If the troops', he cried, 'plunder a village within half a mile of my palace, where a ball from my fowling-piece would reach them, what will they do in more distant parts?' And he gave orders for the bastinadoing of all the colonels and for a tighter discipline to be kept over the rank and file.

On the next day the shah himself left Teheran to assume supreme command over the troops. With him marched Mírzá Bábá, the doctor to the late 'Abbás Mírzá, who was now promoted to the rank of *ḥakím-bás̲h̲í*. There also accompanied him Dr Riach, who had now been appointed to the post of physician to the mission and was also acting as secretary in the temporary absence of Dr McNeill. He now marched to Meshed, not in his capacity as secretary to the mission, but as a personal physician to the shah. There also went with him Captain Stoddart, who held the post of instructor to the military cadets, and the British sergeants who were trying to introduce military discipline into the rabble which constituted the Persian regular army. Sir Henry Bethune,

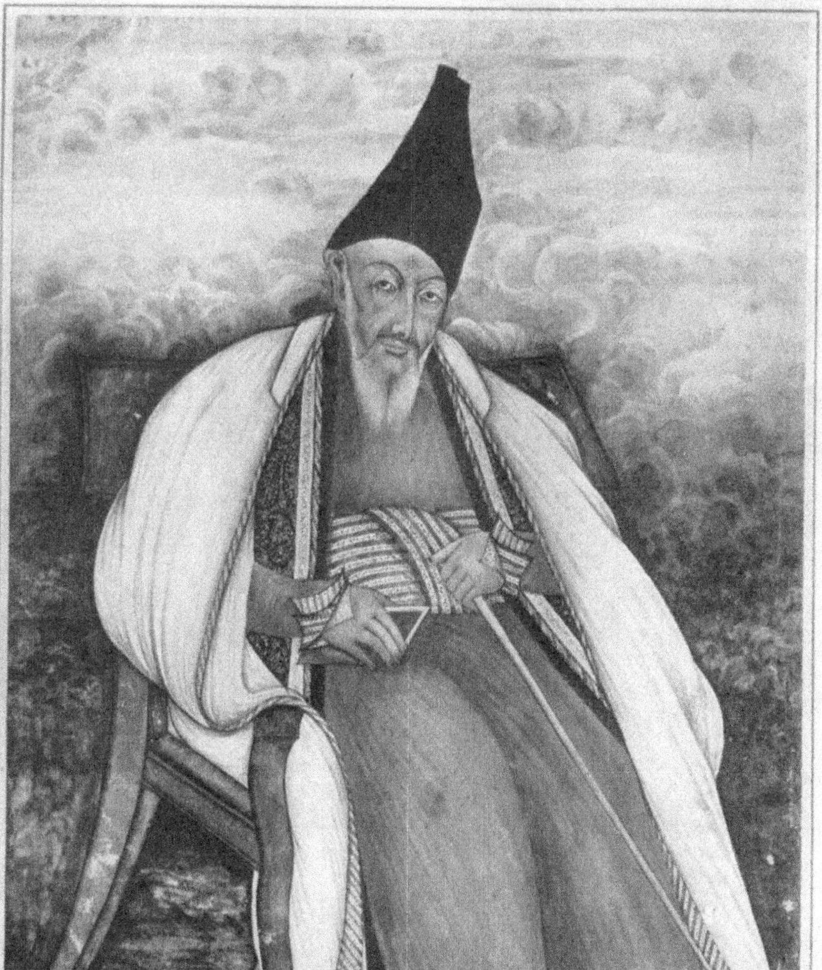

Plate V. Ḥájji Mírzá Áqásí

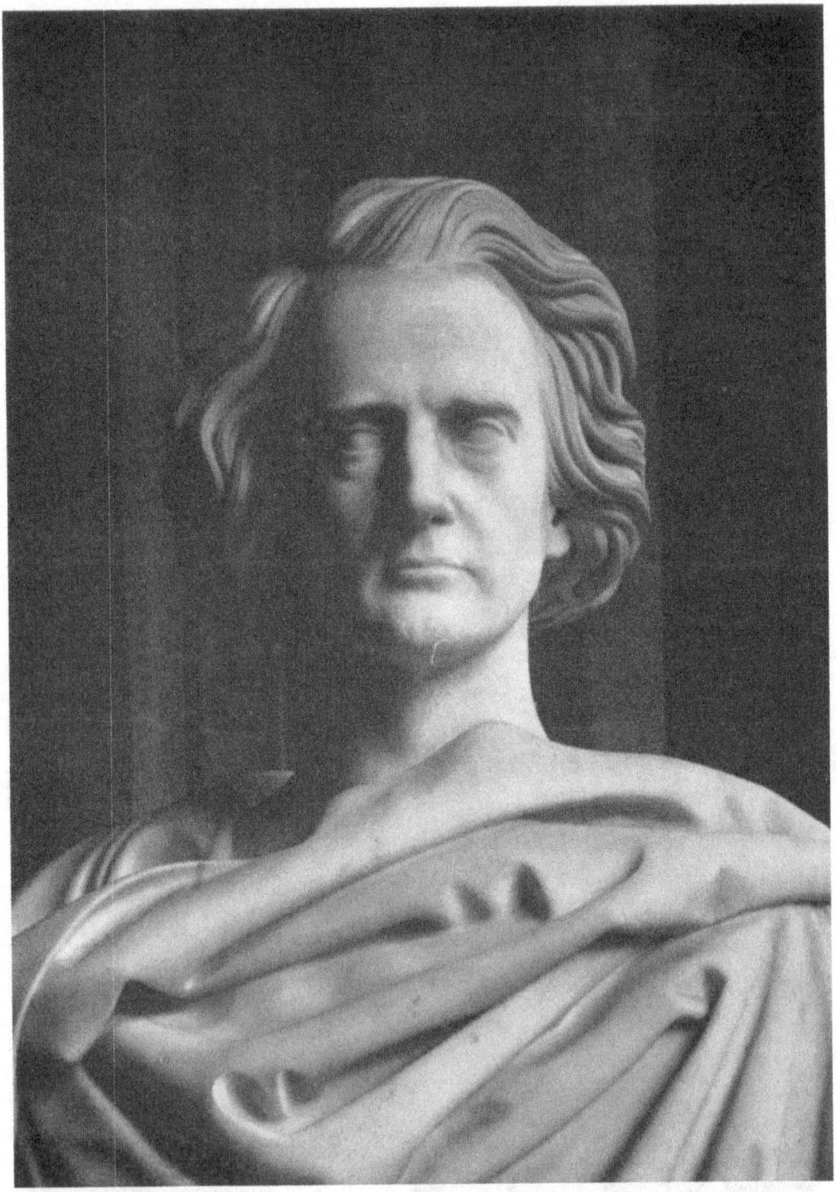

PLATE VI. Sir John McNeill

(*See p.* 492)

now promoted to the rank of Major-General, was on his way out from England and joined the column on his arrival.

The march towards Herat was beset with difficulties and dangers. The presence of cholera in the villages of Khorasan compelled the army to encamp in the desert rather than in the cultivated parts. Unfriendly Turcomans constituted a perpetual danger to the flanks and rear. The opposition of the Government of India to the expedition and the friction which broke out between the senior Persian officers and Sir Henry immediately on his arrival, made the position of the British officers in the camp wellnigh impossible. Time after time Sir Henry's orders were disregarded, until at last he was compelled to beg the shah to send him to another post on the grounds of ill-health. Not unwilling to be free from his criticism the shah transferred him at once to the Azerbaijan frontier, and making his plea of ill-health an excuse ordered Dr Riach to accompany him. Riach, holding that he had joined the expedition not as a British diplomatic representative but as a personal physician to the shah, obeyed the command. The two, together with all the British personnel excepting Captain Stoddart, returned to Teheran. Save an unemployed general, who wished to borrow money from Sir Henry, and Mírzá Bábá, no one came to bid them farewell before they left the camp.

Even with this source of trouble removed things did not go well. Firídún Mírzá, who had been dispatched to subdue the tiresome Turcomans, was defeated and returned in disgrace. The men of the army, ill-fed and ill-equipped, grumbled and deserted by the score. Riach, reporting on his return upon what he had noticed after several weeks of marching and encamping with the troops, said that he had not seen a single flint in a musket since he left Teheran, that with the exception of two battalions not a grain of powder had been served out to anyone, and that the knapsacks were empty and discarded.

There was widespread sickness, mostly bowel complaints and fever. True spasmodic Asiatic cholera appeared and a servant of

Dr Riach in the camp died of it. By a miracle it did not spread. The Russian ambassador, who accompanied the expedition with his wife and children, was loud in his complaints. His personal physician, Dr Yennish, was now the only European physician in the camp. The troops were in no mood to force their way across the frontier and attack the Afghans, who were prepared to defend their villages to the last ditch. The shah therefore *nolens volens* retired early into winter quarters and pitched his camp within a day's march of Astarabad.

To halt his army made the situation no better than to keep it on the march. Officers and men were compelled to undergo the greatest privations. The dearth of food was so great that the soldiers plundered even the provisions destined for the shah's own use. Barley sold in the camp for ten times the price at which it could be purchased in Teheran and wheat was not procurable at any price. A great number of the baggage animals were carried off by the Turcomans, whose light horsemen hovered around the encampment and kept up a continuous alarm from dusk till daylight. Among the animals carried away were 40 belonging to the shah and 180 which carried the baggage of the Russian ambassador. The troops at last became so dissatisfied that the shah was obliged to promise that he would abandon the campaign and return to Teheran without further delay. And so, early in December 1836, he returned to his capital, having accomplished nothing, having fallen considerably in popular estimation, and having rendered the treasury completely bankrupt.

In the meantime the British Government had taken a step which they hoped would be both satisfactory to themselves and pleasing to the Imperial Persian Government. They had promoted Dr McNeill, who was then in England, to the post of Ambassador and Minister Plenipotentiary to the Court of Teheran. To the shah personally the appointment was welcome. McNeill had been a good friend of his father, 'Abbás Mírzá, and had enjoyed the confidence of his grandfather, Fatḥ 'Alí Sháh. He could speak Persian well; he was fully conversant with the ceremonial of the court, with the extraordinary methods of provincial governors, and with the current politics of the Russian Government. These very virtues, which made him *persona grata* to the greater part of the court, also made him a person highly undesirable to the Prime Minister and to the Minister of Foreign Affairs. The former, Ḥájjí Mírzá Áqásí, was not unnaturally afraid that McNeill, as a friend and confidant of the shah, might feel it his duty to point out to him the seriousness of reigning with an empty treasury, with an undisciplined army, and with two discontented southern provinces. Mírzá Mas'úd, the Minister for Foreign Affairs, was equally upset, for he was aware that McNeill knew well his devotion to Russian interests and his utter indifference to any improvement in his own country. Though these sentiments on the part of the two principal ministers of the shah could not, of course, make for easy running of diplomatic affairs, yet they were not of such importance as to nullify the advantages of McNeill's appointment. Personality now counted for more than political insight. The times were gone when the shah would consult the British minister or any other European about the state of his court or his country; and even had McNeill offered advice, unless it was accompanied by a lavish present or by pecuniary backing, such advice would not have been well received and would certainly not have been acted upon.

Dr McNeill, accompanied by Dr Bell as his surgeon, met Mr Ellis, the outgoing chargé d'affaires, in Tabriz. Hearing that Dr Riach had returned from the Herat expedition and was now in Teheran again, he left Dr Bell in Tabriz to attend to the health of the English stationed there. He himself proceeded in a leisurely manner towards Teheran. The British diplomatic mission was therefore in this year, with the exception of the military members, composed entirely of medical men.

By the time McNeill reached the capital the shah had abandoned once again the campaign against Herat. McNeill decided not to go and meet him on his return journey, but to present his letters of credence upon his arrival in Teheran. Previous to this he managed to utilize his former position to strengthen his new. The wife of Mírzá Mas'úd, the Minister of Foreign Affairs, was seriously ill. McNeill, who had formerly been acquainted with her, sent many polite inquiries after her health and requested Dr Riach to attend her. Finally, exercising his prerogative as a physician, he begged leave to enter the women's apartments and to attend to her himself. Such permission was readily granted and Mírzá Mas'úd was profuse in his professions of gratitude. It thus became difficult for him, Anglophobe though he was, to avoid showing to the British mission those little courtesies which he would more readily have withheld.

On 9 December 1836 the shah reached Teheran and on the following day Dr McNeill presented his credentials. The court of Muḥammad Sháh he found very different from that of Fatḥ 'Alí Sháh. Westernizing influences, the legacy of 'Abbás Mírzá, were beginning to be felt. Criticism of royal despotism and a new spirit of patriotism was abroad. Ḥájjí Zayn-ul-'Ábidín, sitting in Riach's consulting room, declared that the late shah was the ruin of the country and that all those who were educated in his court were selfish sensualists, who cared nothing for their nation. He even persuaded the new shah to pay for the re-establishment of a lithographic press in Tabriz. The sum required, and promised, was only Ts. 3000. After much trouble the owner of the press got a bill on the government, signed by the shah, for the sum required. It was taken to the Prime Minister for his counter-signature. He immediately tore the note in pieces.

It was now over 200 years since Persia had first become acquainted with the art of printing. Bishop John Thaddeus, the Carmelite, had stimulated the interest of Sháh 'Abbás the Great by showing him a printed version of the Psalms in Persian and the Gospels in Arabic, so that 'Abbás at once demanded a set of type for himself. The press did not arrive, however, until the year of his death. Fr. Dominic, writing, as he puts it, from 'the Desert of Arabia', on 6 December 1628 says:

It is 47 days since we left the city of Aleppo....The printing type, which we are bringing, costs a good deal of money, as it is so very heavy, to such an extent that one camel can hardly bring it. In the middle of the desert, according to what some friendly persons told us, little was wanting for the printing-press not to go any further; because some of the officials of the 'king of the Arabs' came to levy the dues which the caravans pay him, and at the same time they are wont to have a look at all the loads and merchandise. So, in order that they should not open up our loads with the printing-type, it was necessary to give them 10 piastres; if they had opened it and found the lead, they would have detained it, and even adjudged that we were carrying war material to the king of Persia, their enemy. So, to escape that inconvenience, we thought it well to make them some present.[1]

Whether any books were ever produced by this press I do not know. Fr. Raphael du Mans says that in his time, that is 30 years later, there were no printed works available for students in the University of Ispahan.[2] It is highly improbable that it was ever regarded as anything except a toy or a curiosity. For only 10 years later the Visitor-General wrote from Rome to ask 'what has been done with the Arabic and Persian printing-type sent from Rome to Ispahan—what is to be hoped from it—is any use made of it?' Much later General Malcolm declared that when he left Persia printing was quite unknown.[3]

In 1816 a fresh attempt to introduce the art of printing was made by 'Abbás Mírzá who set up a press in Tabriz. Among the first works to be printed there was a treatise on smallpox. About the same time another printing press was established in Teheran under the supervision of Mírzá 'Abd-ul-Waḥḥáb Mu'tamad-ul-Doula. All books printed in this press were known as the 'Edition of Mu'tamad-ul-Doula'.

About 1824 'Abbás Mírzá sent one Mírzá Ja'far Tabrízí to Moscow to learn the art of lithography. On his return the first lithographic press was also established in Tabriz and began to work there. Five years later the whole press was transferred to Teheran. On the death of 'Abbás Mírzá the typographic press

1 *Chron. Carm. in Persia*, vol. I, p. 305.
2 Du Mans, *Estat de la Perse*, p. 256.
3 Malcolm, *History of Persia*, vol. II, p. 582.

went out of fashion and did not regain favour until the end of the century.

The lithographic press of Teheran continued to function. A weekly newspaper, of which Muḥammad Sháh expressed his favour, did not begin publication until after his death in 1848; but a series of translations, mainly military, mathematical and historical, were produced by this press. But the disorders in the country's finances limited the shah's efforts in this direction and the peculiarity of his religious opinions made all his reforms unacceptable to orthodox Mohammedans.

Turning now from the printing press back to politics, a new feature is to be noted. The two leading nations in Europe no longer hold the Persian stage alone. There is a tendency for one of the protagonists to introduce a lesser ally. Till now the fight for Persian favours had been a straight one, first between the English and the Dutch, then the English and the French, and lastly the English and the Russians. Now by a more subtle stroke the Russian ambassador introduced an uninterested power into the arena and began on a small scale what has been practised on a large scale in our own times. Dr Riach had been curtly dismissed from his post of physician to the shah and shared the unpopularity of the Government of India and Sir Henry Bethune. The Russian ambassador therefore thought it opportune to introduce into the royal presence a Piedmontese physician, named Martingo, who had formerly been a physician to the Ẓill-ul-Sulṭán and who was afterwards in Russian service. Clearly the aim of the ambassador was the permanent displacement of the British Embassy doctor from his confidential position in the shah's *ménage*. At this inopportune moment Dr Riach fell ill and was compelled to seek the treatment of the hot springs at Tiflis. McNeill therefore summoned Dr Bell from Tabriz and set him in Dr Riach's place. Their united efforts were successful and Dr Martingo failed to receive the support of the shah.

The calls upon the services of Dr Bell were many, aided though he was by Assistant Apothecary Abraham Carapit. He was frequently summoned to attend to the health of the many British residents in the towns of northern Persia. In June 1837 the shah was again taken seriously ill while Bell was away. McNeill immediately offered his services as a physician; his offer was thankfully received. The illness began as a simple recurrence of the gout. After the first few days of the attack the pains left the joints and settled in the abdomen. For a short time his life was despaired of. To McNeill's anxiety as a physician were now added his cares as a diplomat. If the shah were to die, who was to succeed him? The British Government had no settled policy. McNeill had no instructions for his procedure in such an unexpected event.

Several years before this Sir John Campbell had recommended the nomination of the infant Náṣr-ul-Dín Mírzá as heir apparent and the shah had followed his advice. The prince was still only a child of seven and it was obvious that the Ẓill-ul-Sulṭán and others, who were still alive, who had claimed the throne on the death of Fatḥ 'Alí Sháh, would be even less likely to allow an infant to succeed than they had been when Muḥammad Sháh put forward his claim. To support the young prince and nominate a regent in agreement with the Russian Government or to remain completely indifferent to the internal strife, provided the Russians also remained neutral, were two possible lines of action. To remain indifferent while Russia actively supported one of the candidates was an impossible policy. McNeill wrote urgent dispatches to England urging the Foreign Office to respect the hereditary right of Náṣr-ul-Dín while the matter still remained in the balance. To the general relief a final decision became for the moment unnecessary, for the shah recovered and the danger of civil war disappeared.

Unfortunately, the shah utilized his recovered health to renew his attempt to add Herat to his kingdom. In July of 1837 the third expedition against Afghanistan was launched. To this expedition the Government of India could take no more favourable a view than they had of the last. Dr Riach was still in Tiflis and was not summoned to return and accompany the shah.

McNeill remained, as did the Russian ambassador, in Teheran. All the British military mission, with the exception of Stoddart, now a colonel, remained at their posts in the provinces. The shah therefore marched from Teheran with no European military advisers except Colonel Stoddart and no Western trained physician except Mírzá Bábá.

The general opinion was that the expedition was doomed to an early and ignominious failure. Within a month Colonel Stoddart wrote that though provisions were still abundant in the camp, money was very scarce. When the shah wished to send Ts. 6000 to Meshed, he was unable to obtain that sum from the public funds of the government and only succeeded in raising it by borrowing small sums from such persons in the camp as could be induced to lend it. Baggage animals were levied from the principal persons in the camp to their great inconvenience and disgust. Several battalions which had been raised in the provinces had already dispersed. Others had deserted in mass after their arrival in Teheran. Three more battalions had taken sanctuary in the mosque of Sháh 'Abd-ul-'Azím and one battalion had marched off to its home with their complete equipment.

The total Persian forces after reckoning up these losses consisted of 8000 infantry and 1500 cavalry, all in bad order and badly armed, with an advance guard of four battalions and thirty guns. To meet them the Afghans could raise at least ten times that number of horsemen and nearly three times that number of foot soldiers. To all onlookers it seemed madness to venture with such an inferior force into the hostile and barren deserts which lay between Meshed and Herat.

Nevertheless, the shah pushed on. No discipline was maintained. The troops feared the enemy, yet no precautions were taken against surprise, and it was the opinion of Colonel Stoddart that the shah and the whole camp were at the mercy of fifty horsemen. Soon provisions began to run low. The price in camp of all articles of food rose to five or six times the price of the same things at Meshed or Nishapur, which were only a few stages in the rear. There was still a march of nine days for the army through a country which had not one day's supply, before it could reach Herat. The whole of the provisions expected from the rear and from the districts on the line of the march did not exceed four days' consumption. Every mile the troops advanced, carried them so much the further from their means of subsistence. The cold was already so great that the men had begun to suffer from it. A Persian gentleman, writing to his father, stated that at night the cold was so intense that in the morning people could neither use their hands nor speak distinctly. The horses were weak from exposure, fatigue and want of provisions. The shah continued to suffer from gout which incapacitated him from mounting his horse and at times even from walking from his tent to his carriage.

A spirit of pessimism seems to have filled all hearts except that of the shah himself. It was whispered in the bazaars that Russia was secretly planning a *coup d'état*. Political prophets hinted that the Ẓill-ul-Sulṭán was making ready to reascend the throne. The more scientifically minded pointed with gloom to the eclipse of the moon which was due to occur in the autumn, which involved the constellation which ruled the shah's destiny. The singular accuracy with which the predictions of the astrologers were fulfilled in the deaths of 'Abbás Mírzá and Fatḥ 'Alí Shá͟h had confirmed every Persian's confidence in this science. It was firmly believed that some signal misfortune would befall the shah, possibly even his death. Actually, at the time of the eclipse the only misfortune from which he suffered, was to be confined to his tent for a few days with an acute attack of gout.

In the more responsible political circles the spirit of discontent found vent in a series of complaints against the British attitude towards the campaign. Even the prime minister was so indiscreet as to remark in public that McNeill had already once prevented the Persians from capturing Herat, when 'Abbás Mírzá was in the field, and that if again Persian arms suffered a reverse, he would raise all Teheran to murder the British mission, as they had murdered the Russian a few years before. When these words reached McNeill's ears, he could scarcely believe that they had been spoken. He at once sent to the camp for a denial and for safety withdrew his staff and all the British residents of Teheran to a villa at Sulimaniyeh, a few miles outside the city.

The city of Teheran, with the court absent and the British mission withdrawn, became the seat of the wildest rumours and the wildest behaviour. To exercise a steadying influence and at the same time to test the feelings of the populace McNeill determined to take the bold course of riding alone and without escort through the city. On 20 November, accompanied only by the military attaché, he rode in through the Shimran Gate, down through the bazaars, and on to the British Embassy. His return was welcomed with joy by all the upper classes; from the lower not a sign of hatred was shown or a discordant note struck. Finding that the voice of the prime minister was far from being the voice of the mob, much to the relief of the civil governor the mission returned to the city.

In the first week of December the Persian arms met with their first great success, when they captured the fortress of Goorian. Not only did the road to Herat now lie open to them, but also the provisions and ammunition, captured within the fortress, made a very welcome addition to their own scanty supply. The siege of Herat now began in earnest. The Government of India, who up till this time had in the light of McNeill's reports refused to believe in the possibility of the loss of Afghan independence, were compelled to take serious note of the threat to their north-western frontier. It was highly undesirable that any nation, so indebted to Russia and so swayed by the court of St Petersburgh, as was the Persian, should hold Afghanistan as a vassal state. They therefore instructed McNeill to leave Teheran with all speed for the shah's camp and to compel him by every means of diplomatic persuasion to come to terms with the Afghan monarch. Accordingly in March 1838 McNeill set out.

He found on his arrival in the camp that the state of the Persian army was just as bad as he had expected it to be. The country was nearly exhausted of its supplies; the troops were suffering great privations, many of them subsisting upon the herbs which at that season of the year spring up on the fertile soil around Herat. Yet they were continuing to do their duty in the trenches and evinced a devotion and a power of endurance which must be rare in the military history of Asia. Without pay, without sufficient clothing, without any rations whatsoever, the same troops remained day and night in the trenches, which were on several occasions knee-deep in mud and water and in which they were wont to lose a score of men daily from chance bullets and Afghan sorties.

The presence of McNeill in the camp was highly displeasing to the shah and he lost no opportunity of insulting him. Embassy servants were arrested and imprisoned on trifling excuses. Letters addressed to the English were opened and read. No redress was given. In the provinces governors were encouraged to belittle British officials and to hinder British trade. Matters came to a head when a drunken *sayyid* insulted Mr Gerald, the British apothecary to the Resident in Bushire. Gerald, having had his hat knocked off, thrashed the *sayyid*. At once the city was in an uproar at the attack of an infidel upon a descendant of the Prophet. The *sayyid* professed to be wounded and on the point of death. The governor demanded that Mr Gerald be given up to receive punishment from the Persian court; and he threatened in unmeasured terms to attack the Residency, if the demand was not satisfied.

The official answer to these moves came rapidly. McNeill himself not only withdrew from the royal camp, but on reaching Teheran also commanded the whole mission to withdraw to the frontier. At the same time the Government of India sent troops to Bushire, some of whom strengthened the garrison of the Residency. The remainder occupied the island of Karrack. The shah was then informed that the capture of Herat would be considered an act unfriendly to Great Britain and that diplomatic relations could not be resumed as long as any part of Afghan territory was held by Persian troops. The shah, very unwillingly, yielded to superior force, and having already accomplished what all observers, native and foreign, had considered the impossible, raised the siege of Herat and returned to Teheran.

Even then there could be no question of McNeill returning to the capital in person. Dr Riach and Colonel Shiel, who were sent up to represent the mission, reported that their reception was far from favourable. None of the British demands were satisfied. The Persian Government offered no apology for their treatment of the embassy couriers and for other diplomatic insults. The Persian troops continued to occupy Goorian and to hold a large slice of Afghan territory. In case it was now only prestige which prevented the shah from yielding, McNeill offered to resign his office in order to make the act more easy. His generosity produced no result. A further 'incident', when a Jewish banker, attached to the Residency in Bushire, was attacked and robbed, called forth another protest from McNeill, still at Tabriz, and the question of the Resident at Bushire also quitting Persian soil became acute. Diplomatic pressure availing nothing, in November Colonel Shiel and Dr Riach were recalled from Teheran and the whole mission left Persia. McNeill himself returned to England to give an account of his embassy. Colonel Shiel remained at Erzerum with Dr Riach to look after the affairs of the British Government and British subjects in Persia as best they could.

The Persian attitude towards the English now became violently antagonistic. Nor was it without some justification. The English had intervened and robbed the shah of his heart's ambition just when it seemed to be within his grasp; English troops had taken possession by force of arms of a part of the Persian Empire. The rioting which accompanied the visit of Admiral Sir Frederick Maitland to Bushire completed the case for the Persian Government. Denied permission by the governor of the town to use any except the public landing-stage for his re-embarkation, the admiral summoned three boatloads of armed sailors to enforce his demand to use a private landing-stage near the Residency, a privilege which he claimed his rank demanded. The result was an uproar, exchange of shots, and the pelting of the British sailors with stones and mud. The admiral embarked in safety and returned to his ship. The next day the Resident abandoned the Residency and the whole factory staff moved over to Karrack.

Wild accounts of this incident reached Teheran. It was said that an English admiral had arrived in a ship of 80 guns and that by a stratagem had obtained possession of Bushire, that the gallant Báqir Khán had defeated and driven out both the admiral and the Resident, and that the British flag and a large collection of heads had been sent to Shiraz to substantiate the story. The news of the victory caused great jubilation at the court. *Firmáns*, dresses of honour and decorations were dispatched to Báqir Khán the general and to other notables of Bushire. The garrison was ordered to be augmented and bastions and redoubts were to be constructed as rapidly as possible in preparation for the war against the English, which now seemed inevitable.

Opinions in England were very divided about what the next step should be. The old stagers, such as Sir Harford Jones and Sir Henry Bethune, considered that Persia had been ill-treated throughout. The Cabinet, however, sided with McNeill and marked their approval by conferring upon him a knighthood. This division of opinion was reported to the Persian court by their minister in London, who added as a postscript that he would 'speak in such terms to the English Government that McNeill should be for ever dismissed from the service'. Ḥájjí Áqásí could not conceal his delight. 'Do you see', he said to the shah one day, 'what my schemes have brought on the English? I have burned their fathers. They are quarrelling among themselves. Are the English fit to be counted as men? Not they: they are nothing more than knife-makers. They have subdued the wretched Hindees and they think that Iran is like India, without knowing that the Iranis have burnt the fathers of all mankind.'

Thus buoyed up, the shah gave orders for the reassembling of his army. Whether it was to lay siege to Herat again, as some avowed, whether it was to attack Baghdad in punishment for the Turkish seizure of Mohammerah, or whether it was to drive the English out of Karrack, can never be known, for repeated attacks of gout kept the shah confined to his room. It was not till nearly twelve months later, January 1840, to be exact, that he was well enough to put himself at the head of his troops and leave Teheran. An eyewitness wrote: 'The shah is off at last. He mounted his horse last Monday during a fall of snow. I was close to him. He looked ill and could not walk well, no doubt from his late attack of gout.'

He moved off in a southerly direction. He reached Ispahan and there executed some forty or fifty turbulent spirits, and then by slow stages came back to Teheran. He was not up to campaigning. The gout had travelled to the knees and the hip-joint and he could scarcely move.

The outlook for Anglo-Persian relations was still just about as bad as it could be when a most unexpected event completely changed the policy of the Imperial Government. Mírzá 'Alí, a son of Mírzá Mas'úd, Minister for Foreign Affairs, was found forging the shah's signature to State documents and granting posts, pensions and promotions in return for a corresponding present. Mírzá 'Alí was summoned to the palace and interrogated by the shah himself. After a brief examination the shah gave orders for him to be strangled there and then before his eyes. The intervention of the Russian ambassador saved his life. The death sentence was commuted to 500 strokes of the bastinado. This was at once carried out and both he and his father were degraded from their office. A few days later Mírzá Abú ul-Ḥasan K͟hán, formerly Persian ambassador in London in the days of Fatḥ 'Ali S͟háh, was appointed Minister for Foreign Affairs.

The new minister was frankly Anglophile. His policy of a rapprochement with England was supported by the Russian ambassador and by the new *ḥakím-bás͟hí* Mírzá Naẓar 'Alí. At the same time the British successes in other parts of the world were not unknown to the shah. In Afghanistan, Syria, Khiva, Naples and China, English policy and English arms had met with success. The internal state of Persia itself was more than enough to occupy the whole attention of the shah and his ministers. The public finances were in disorder: the privy purse was nearly empty. The province of Kerman was in rebellion: the Ẓill-ul-Sulṭán was hovering around Baghdad, waiting for an opportunity to strike for the throne again. The British Government, recognizing that the tide had turned, were not slow to grasp the opportunity. Dr Riach was sent back to Teheran to negotiate for the evacuation of Ghoorian and Afghan territory and for the subsequent return of a British mission. He reached Tabriz in the middle of January 1841. He found that public opinion had completely changed and the English were once more in favour. After a warm reception by the shah a few days later he set off for Meshed, carrying in his pocket an autographed letter from the shah himself, bidding the Persian general withdraw all his troops to within the Persian frontiers.

With astonishing promptness for that dilatory age and that procrastinating race, Ghoorian was restored to the Afghans on the last day of March, and Riach was enabled to return to Teheran in the spring with the first part of his mission successfully accomplished. On his return to the capital he found that once again the shah had changed his mind. An Afghan mission had arrived in Teheran, offering the whole of Afghanistan as a fief in return for protection against aggression on the part of the Government of India. It was added that should Persia refuse to take them under her wing, the mission was ordered to proceed to Russia and to make the same offer to the tsar. The shah was in a quandary. On the one hand only two months ago he had renewed his protestations of friendship with the English and had made a grand gesture in restoring a conquered fortress without any semblance of compulsion. In return he could well hope to receive financial and military aid and the restoration of Karrack.

On the other hand he was now presented with the accomplishment of his life's ambition. The revolt in Kerman, too, had been crushed and even the unruly Bakhtiaris had been temporarily subdued. The temptation was too great. The shah accepted the lordship of Afghanistan, reappointed the ex-king as his first viceroy, and broke with the English again.

Even so, Dr Riach held that the British were bound to restore Karrack. So thought also Sir John McNeill who, with the prospect of an immediate renewal of diplomatic relations, was waiting at Trebizond. This, however, was not the opinion of the Government of India. In the Persian suzerainty over Afghanistan their fears were reawakened. In addition, the health of the troops during their stay on Karrack having been none too good, the Government had gone to great expense to build permanent barracks. And Karrack had not only a military value; it had also very great commercial possibilities. The Government of India was still a trading company and had a duty towards its shareholders. Besides, it was very uncertain, they argued, that the Shah of Persia had any greater right to the possession of the island than they. The actual owner was a certain Shaykh Nafṣá, a Persian of Arab extraction, who was the hereditary chief and a semi-independent ruler. To compel him to sell the island and then to establish the factory there permanently instead of at Bushire would no doubt cause considerable annoyance to the shah and set back for a time all hope of re-establishing friendly relations. But the certainty of gain by such a step was better than the uncertain profit of the re-establishment of English popularity.

In spite of the obvious difficulties in the way the shah again and again invited Sir John McNeill to return to Persia. At last, even though the Karrack question was still unsettled, McNeill received permission to do so. He found the shah in the throes of another attack of gout. His reception in the capital was cordial; the Persian Government was out to take any steps to remove all traces of the hostility of the past two years. Within a few weeks a fresh commercial treaty was negotiated which gave Great

Britain the right to establish a permanent consulate-general in Tabriz and a consulate in Teheran. At the same time the shah guaranteed that if Karrack were restored, the islanders should suffer no disability for their friendliness towards the occupying troops. McNeill, having received orders from London to cause the island to be evacuated as soon as he had secured the royal signature to the treaty, sent down written instructions to the general officer commanding to return to India at once with all his force.

The protests and fears of the Government of India delayed the evacuation of the island for several months, and it was not until the middle of January 1842, that the first shipload of troops returned to India. By the end of April the island was free of sepoys, and Persian troops occupied the barracks, although the naval authorities continued to retain the agent and a coal depot there for several more months.

McNeill, having thus lived to see the restoration of friendly relations between Great Britain and Persia, decided that it was time to terminate his connection with the Middle East, and in May resigned his high office and returned to England after 25 years' loyal and successful service in Persia. Starting as a physician with no diplomatic status or qualifications he at once showed himself by his negotiation of the Russian Treaty on behalf of Fatḥ 'Ali Sháh to be a statesman endowed with a natural skill and tact. Honoured first by the confidence of the wife of the shah and then by that of the shah himself, aided by a facile tongue, a mastery of Persian etiquette and language and a power of drafting dispatches in clear and respectful English, he was promoted in turn Political Resident in the Gulf and Permanent Chief Assistant to the mission. His success in paving the way for the unconditional reception of Sir Robert Campbell, when on his own authority he took risks and broke the accepted rules of court etiquette, marked him out as the strongest man in Persia.

In spite of this, the appointment of a physician to the highest rank, that of Minister Plenipotentiary, was an experiment which met with only moderate success and which the Foreign Office has not, at least in the case of Persia, ever repeated. Ministers, other than members of the regular diplomatic corps, there have indeed been since the days of McNeill, but these have invariably been soldiers. The Persians are well accustomed to the elevation of physicians to the post of *wazīr*. Their past history gives no instance of a physician assuming the supreme power. It struck the Persians, even in those days, as slightly incongruous that one, who had once accepted fees for his services to them, should now walk among them as the representative of his king.

Besides his origin and his profession in McNeill's particular case there were other difficulties which militated against his achieving those victories which he had won as a first assistant. In the first place he found himself opposed during the greater part of his period as minister by two Persian ministers who not only distrusted England, but also feared, if they did not actually dislike, McNeill in person. And it is difficult for an envoy to carry out successful negotiations when both the Prime Minister and the Minister for Foreign Affairs are his personal enemies. The shah, too, was so under the influence of the former that whatever good relations might once have existed between himself and the British physician, they were completely annihilated when the physician became the British Minister.

In the second place McNeill had the misfortune to be minister at a time when the shah was determined upon a policy which was diametrically opposed to that of the Government of India and which was by no means approved of by the English Foreign Office. Over and over again he was forced to be the mouthpiece of sentiments which he knew would cause the utmost displeasure to the Court, to which he was accredited. He was further mortified by the quarrelling which went on behind his back between Whitehall and the Court of Directors. He could never be sure that the mild disapproval, which London bade him convey to the shah, would not be followed by the most dogmatic denouncement from Calcutta. He could not even be sure that he would not receive directly conflicting commands.

To have satisfied the Government of India by securing the independence of Afghanistan, to have pleased the Court of Directors by the negotiating of a commercial treaty, to have mollified Persian suspicions and wrath by the restoration of Karrack, and to have carried out his duties so satisfactorily that he was awarded by his sovereign a G.C.B., marks out Sir John McNeill as one of the most distinguished members of his profession and as one of the great diplomats of the Middle East.

He lived for another 40 years after his retirement from the East and during these 40 years received the honour of being created a Privy Councillor, a Doctor of Law of Oxford University and a Fellow of the Royal Society of Edinburgh.

CHAPTER XVII

THE INTRODUCTION OF WESTERN MEDICINE

ABOUT the same time that McNeill left Persia Dr Riach also resigned, having helped McNeill through his anxious years as envoy, just as McNeill had helped Sir John Macdonald and Sir Robert Campbell. On his departure the shah honoured him with the order of the Lion and the Sun of the First Class. This was the highest order that the shah could bestow. In the case of Dr Riach all men held it deserved. But when a little later it was bestowed upon a French doctor who had treated the shah for only a few months, Count Medem, the Russian minister, declared himself insulted and protested that unless some higher mark of favour were bestowed upon him, he would not wait upon the shah on public occasions. And in fact he absented himself from the next levee.

The repeated illnesses of the shah and the consequent question of his successor compelled the Foreign Office to decide upon a line of action, now that the mission was once again in Teheran. In the year that McNeill left Persia Náṣr-ul-Dín Mírzá, the recognized heir apparent, was thirteen. He was a slender youth and of a delicate constitution. There seemed every possibility that history would repeat itself and that he would die before coming to the throne. In that case the most suitable person to succeed was Bahman Mírzá, a full brother to the shah, a Qájár on both sides, and a man who had shown himself an experienced and capable governor. Supposing, too, that the shah were to die before Náṣr-ul-Dín Mírzá attained his majority, Bahman Mírzá was clearly fitted to act as regent. The real danger was that in either event Bahman Mírzá would usurp the throne for himself and kill or blind the three young sons of Muḥammad Sháh. Unfortunately, the young Náṣr-ul-Dín showed no signs yet of those qualities which were lying latent within him. He was exceedingly childish for his age. His education had been neglected. He had been brought up in seclusion and was entirely ignorant of public life. And he was completely under the sway of his mother.

At this moment the shah was not receiving the best possible medical attention. Ḥájjí Mírzá Áqásí, the Prime Minister, still retained that complete influence over him which he had now exercised for so many years. For a long time there had been a rivalry between the Prime Minister and the *ḥakím-báshí*, Mírzá Bábá. The Ḥájjí left no stone unturned to overthrow such influence as Mírzá Bábá possessed over the shah. At last he succeeded in securing his dismissal. The shah then confided the care of his person to a Jewish quack. The immediate result was a severe paroxysm of gout which so weakened him that reports of his death were prevalent throughout Teheran. He recovered, but found that he had lost the use of one leg. Through the influence of the Ḥájjí he still refused to see the English-trained Mírzá Bábá or any of the physicians attached to the foreign missions. He preferred to place himself under Persian practitioners and to receive treatment according to the native theories.

Persian remedies proved as useless as the Jew's, and Ḥájjí Mírzá Áqásí allowed him to place himself under a French doctor, named Labat, who happened to be in Teheran at that time. Under his care he recovered to a certain extent, although he remained so feeble that he was incapable of movement unless supported by two persons, and then only for a very short time. This infirm state of the shah was not without advantage to the country, for it completely checked his military ambitions and also prevented him from his frequent tours of inspection in the provinces. His presence on such occasions was a calamity owing to the damage to the country folk, caused by the troops and his followers, and to the gifts which custom compelled the more wealthy to present to him. A short time before, when he proposed to visit Qazvin, the inhabitants offered him a large contribution on condition of his not approaching the city.

Dr Labat, however, found it inexpedient to stay long in such circles and announced his intention of going before he fell from favour. Such was the fear or jealousy of Ḥájjí Mírzá Áqásí that he still refused to allow the shah to consult a Russian or British doctor, and asked the French minister to send to France for a suitable physician. While awaiting his arrival Count Medem, the Russian minister, and Colonel Shiel, the British chargé d'affaires, insisted that their own doctors should at least supervise the treatment which the shah was receiving. Dr Kale (or Cade) of the Russian mission and Dr Bell of the British, therefore, called daily at the Palace and had the consolation of seeing a great improvement in the shah's health.

This success had an astonishing result. The distrust of the English, which the shah and all the court had so often manifested, gave place to a display of marked confidence. Colonel Shiel was even asked to appoint a confidential person as interpreter to his majesty. He named to that office Mírzá Ibráhím, who had formerly been Professor of Persian at Haileybury College. Soon after his appointment Mírzá Ibráhím was asked also to superintend the food and medicine of the shah, and a year later, when the shah was very much better, his services were transferred as tutor to the heir apparent. The shah was delighted with the effect of the combined Russian and English treatment, and on the arrival of his permanent physician, Doctor Cloquet, he presented to each of them a sum of Ts. 1800.

The illness of the shah and the arrival of Dr Cloquet occurred in the spring of 1846. In the summer his tranquillity was again disturbed by an outbreak of cholera in Teheran. The first case occurred on 23 July. The appearance of the disease so much alarmed the shah, who was residing in his usual camping ground some miles from the city, that he departed with his court and his harem in the utmost confusion to a remote mountain village 20 miles distant. Though the mortality arising from the malady was still inconsiderable, not exceeding perhaps fifteen persons daily, his precipitate flight caused a panic in the city, which the inhabitants began to abandon in crowds.

The epidemic increased in severity and flight did not save the shah's camp. One of his sons, aged seven, died of cholera, as did also a daughter and two of his wives. The Minister for Foreign Affairs, Muḥammad 'Alí Khán, also fell a victim. It even spread into the camp of the British mission and claimed one victim. The European practitioners could make no headway against the disease and scarcely any one who caught it, survived. Had the shah himself become infected, escape would have been impossible for him in his exhausted condition. The estimated mortality in the city of Teheran was 12,000 persons and, as the city during the summer months is largely deserted by all who can escape to the hills and cannot have contained more than 30,000 souls in all, even after allowing for oriental exaggeration the epidemic must have carried off over a quarter of the whole population. The disease stopped as rapidly as it had begun and no town west of Qazvin became infected.

In the following year Dr Bell returned to England on leave, fell sick at Erzerum, and there died. But the shah lived on. He had already outlived all his foreign advisers, who had been so concerned about his successor. Colonel Farrant was now chargé d'affaires in the British Legation: Prince Dolgorouki had become Russian minister. Dr Dickson had succeeded to the post of physician to the British minister and Dr Cormick, a son of the medical attendant of 'Abbás Mírzá, was the second British physician.

The state of Persia was still unhappy and insecure. Bahman Mírzá, the brother of the shah, expecting his brother's death at any moment, had begun to collect troops at Tabriz, and then changing his mind resigned his governorship and came to Teheran and took refuge from the shah's displeasure in the Russian Legation. The young heir apparent had been married and appointed to the vacant governorship of Azerbaijan against the advice of the Russian and British envoys. Dr Cormick accompanied him to his province. The prince-governors of Shiraz and Ispahan were in Teheran, waiting to be confirmed in office by the shah-to-be, and in the meantime their provinces were in rebellion. The wandering tribes along the shores of the Persian Gulf had thrown off all pretence of allegiance to the Central Government.

Only Ḥájjí Mírzá Áqásí and his power remained unmoved. His influence with the shah was now greater than before, if possible. The shah had quite ceased to take an independent hand in the government of the country and even in the most trifling affairs took no action without first consulting his prime minister. Of late the Ḥájjí had become more avaricious and daily appeared less and less inclined to transact business. His mind during the greater part of the day was confused and excited by opium. He would take no advice, believing his own talents and knowledge to be superior to those of anyone else. He would brook no interference; he attempted to direct every department of State. Nothing warned him of his impending fall. The disturbed state of Khorasan, the shah's brother in sanctuary in the Russian Legation, the shah's mother his bitter enemy, an army unpaid, a ragged, undisciplined rabble without arms or clothing, an exhausted treasury, and every department in disorder; all these caused him no anxiety.

The shah through being a confirmed cripple and unable to undergo any exertion, was happy to find a person in whom he could place such implicit confidence and who he felt had no wish to usurp his power, yet who would relieve him of all the cares and troubles of governing. But the end of both was very near. The shah recovered from an acute attack of gout, brought on by eating excess of water-melons. A second attack of indigestion was followed by erysipelas of the left arm. Dr Cloquet hurriedly summoned Dr Dickson and the doctor to the Russian Embassy. But their efforts proved vain and at nine in the evening of 4 September 1848 Muḥammad Sháh breathed his last.

Dr Dickson hastened back to the Legation with the news. By midnight it was known throughout the bazaars. At dawn the Russian and British Legations were besieged by a rabble of townsfolk, demanding the dismissal and death of Ḥájjí Mírzá

Áqásí and swearing allegiance to any shah whom the British or Russians might name. The Ḥájjí had already left his house and shut himself up in the 'Arq, the central walled heart of Teheran, which contained the palace, the treasury, the late shah's harem, all the artillery and 1200 soldiers. Even here the Ḥájjí did not feel himself secure. At mid-day he left the city in disguise. He was recognized and pursued. His friends and servants deserted him to a man and with his foes literally at his horse's tail, he flung himself into the mosque at Sháh 'Abd-ul-'Azím, only five miles from Teheran, and there took sanctuary.

The lawful successor to the throne being now in Tabriz, many days' journey away, his mother and the chief priest of Teheran took charge of the government on his behalf. So ably did they conduct affairs that during the six weeks which it took for the news to reach Náṣr-ul-Dín, and for him to arrive in Teheran, only one rival claimant to the throne thought it worth while to assert his claim. This was Sayf-ul-Malúk Mírzá, a son of the Ẓill-ul-Sulṭán, who in similar circumstances had claimed the throne and had ruled for a month. Sayf-ul-Malúk Mírzá now addressed a circular to the different chiefs of the tribes in the vicinity of Qazvin, asking them to join his standard and to help him to upset the reigning dynasty. To provide for his immediate wants he robbed the courier of the Russian Legation of 3500 ducats, which he promised to repay on his arrival in Teheran. His small following was at once defeated and he himself was captured.

Náṣr-ul-Dín reached Teheran in the middle of October, but no auspicious hour presenting itself he did not enter the city until the 20th. At midnight, the astrologers having declared that hour to be the most propitious for the ceremony of the coronation, Prince Dolgorouki and Colonel Farrant together with the gentlemen of the two missions received special invitations to pay their respects to the new shah. The terrified Ḥájjí Mírzá Áqásí, still lying in sanctuary, received permission through the mediation of the Russian minister to proceed to Kerbela on a perpetual pilgrimage. But his numerous creditors would have none of that, even though the populace, whom he had maltreated and squeezed, had forgotten their desire for vengeance.

Náṣr-ul-Dín Sháh was just nineteen when he succeeded to the throne. Having attained his majority, there was no question of a regent. He at once decided that Bahman Mírzá should be allowed to live as an exile in Georgia. He then set about choosing his ministers. In this he did not consult the British or Russian envoys nor did they offer their advice. It was with some fear, though not with hostility, that they saw him elevate to his right hand Mírzá Taqí Khán, a man of courage perhaps and not wanting in ability, but slow, obstinate, and not well acquainted with the intrigue of the court. His promotion was rapid. He was at once given the title of Amír Niẓám and was soon married to the shah's sister. In his hands the shah became a mere cipher. Yet he was by no means a second Ḥájjí Mírzá Áqásí, for he was undoubtedly actuated by some desire for the good of his country. Neither the British nor the Russian missions gained from his appointment. He was adverse to Russia, yet he can scarcely be said to have been favourably disposed towards England. His great object was to diminish the influence of both missions. With that object he would take advice from neither. He is reported to have said that the slaughter of 20,000 of the inhabitants of Meshed (a city which was now in revolt against the new shah) was preferable to pacification affected through European intervention. Dr Cormick was therefore relieved of his post of medical attendant which he had held during the short time that the new shah was governor of Azerbaijan, and Dr Cloquet was confirmed in his office of senior physician to the court.

For good or ill therefore to the Amír Niẓám must be ascribed the reforms and advances which occurred in Persia during the first few years of the new shah's reign. Among these was the abolishing of the right of sanctuary which mosques and tombs had hitherto afforded to malefactors and those out of favour with the authorities. In the lawless state of the country which prevailed, it soon proved inexpedient to abolish completely these rights and ultimately these 'cities of refuge' were limited to the foreign missions, to the mosque at S͟háh 'Abd-ul-'Azím, and to the holy city of Qum. Through the Amír Niẓám's influence also a weekly paper was instituted, which chronicled the doings of the court and published all official news and regulations. This paper was placed under the management of an English merchant named Burgess and in spite of the opposition of the Russian minister, who claimed the right to have articles from his pen published at his pleasure, continued to appear regularly for many years.

Of far greater importance than these, from the point of view of medicine, was the foundation in 1850 of the Dár-ul-Fanún or École Polytechnique. The Amír Niẓám throughout his period of high office gave his first consideration to the army. For the first time officers and men were regularly paid, were properly clothed, and were contented and disciplined instead of being a menace to the civilians among whom they lived. To improve the higher ranks a college was now formed in which young Persians, destined for a military career, were to be educated. Instruction was to be given by military officers from Switzerland, Hungary and Italy; the teaching was to be broad and liberal; military science rather than military tactics was the objective. From being a purely military academy the college spread within a short time into an incipient university. Other faculties were formed to collaborate and aid the military college, the principal faculties being those of natural science, medicine and political economy. The interest of the shah was awakened. He paid such frequent visits and did so much to encourage the students that he is often said to have been the founder of the university.

All these specialized departments were placed under the charge of Europeans with Persian collaborators. The Faculty of Medicine was singularly fortunate in its European professors. A number of excellent teachers laid the foundations of what is still the only school of medicine and licensing body in all Persia. From Austria came Dr Polak who lectured on ophthalmology and did so much for the establishment of a Persian anatomical vocabulary. From Holland came Dr Schlimmer, who was to write his great *Terminologie Medico-Pharmaceutique*. This book, almost unobtainable to-day, was first published as a small dictionary of Persian equivalents for the commoner French medical terms. In 1874 it appeared considerably enlarged, in a lithographed edition, more terms being included and the more interesting of such terms forming the subject of lengthy notes. Its scope is sufficiently indicated on the title page: 'Indications des lieux de provenance des principaux produits animaux et végétaux, détails nouveaux sur le gisement de plusieurs minerais importants, sur les principales eaux minérales, sur la thérapeutique indigène et sur les maladies endémiques et particulières les plus intéressantes des habitants de la Perse.' It was indeed a gigantic attempt to make the transition from Avicenna to Harvey less abrupt, to fit the old nomenclature to the new ideas, and to standardize the technical terms of the new university.

The founding of the Dár-ul-Fanún provided an enormous stimulation for the printing press, and, though the lithographic press was still the method in favour, a large number of books appeared for the use of the students. The most important of these is the *Terminologie* of Dr Schlimmer, which I have just mentioned. Dr Polak wrote on surgery, Dr Albo, a German, who was attached somewhat later to the School of Medicine, wrote on physiology, Abú-ul-Ḥasan K͟hán on therapeutics and 'Alí Ra'ís-ul-Aṭibbá on anatomy. A scientific paper, called the *Rúznáma-i-'Ilmiyya-i-Dawlat-i-'Aliyya-i-Irán*, was founded in 1863 and appeared from time to time under the superintendence of 'Alí Qulí Mírzá I'tiẓád-ul-Salṭana.

Within a few years the first Persian students were ready to receive their diplomas. In 1858 forty-two left Persia for Paris. Of this number five were graduates in medicine. Of them the most distinguished was Mírzá Riẓáí, who having completed seven years of post-graduate study in Paris returned to Persia. At first he devoted his energies to work in the provinces, but he was very soon called to the capital and given a teaching post in the Dár-ul-Fanún. Here he worked until he died in 1877. He left behind him a translation into Persian of a work on pathology by his old French master Dr Grisolle. Another of this pioneer band was Mírzá Qásim, who became chief translator to the university, turning many of his French text-books into the common Persian tongue.

In the midst of these truly magnificent efforts the Amír Niẓám suddenly fell from favour. Unsuspected by himself and quite unforeseen by the court and by the public in the winter of 1851 a sudden command reached him to give up his seals of office. He was at once degraded from his rank and title and became again Taqí Khán, a private citizen. Not content with this utterly unmerited treatment of a servant who had conferred so many benefits upon him, the shah promptly threw him into prison at Kashan. There, at the instigation, it was said, of his mother and the new Prime Minister, the shah had him foully done to death. For several days previous to his murder the guards adopted the practice of summoning him out of his room under the pretence of ascertaining that he had not fled. On these occasions he was accompanied by the princess, his wife, the shah's sister, as a protection. After some days this ceremony appearing to be a mere form, she ceased to accompany him. This was the aim. The shah's *ferrásh-báshí* was then dispatched to superintend the execution. When he arrived, Taqí Khán was summoned, as usual, and appeared alone, as was anticipated. He was at once seized, gagged and dragged to an adjoining house, where he was thrown on to the floor, stripped and bound. The veins in both arms and legs were then opened. In this state he lingered for some three or four hours when he expired.

In his callous treatment of his right-hand man the young shah showed a side of his character of which his early behaviour had given no indication. He now began to display an arrogance and folly which rivalled that of the most dissipated of the monarchs who had preceded him. A member of his own household remarked that no faith could be placed in his word. His incalculable folly was shown in his attempt to persuade his new Prime Minister to appoint a lad of nineteen as his Minister for Foreign Affairs. His cruelties equalled those of the long-forgotten Nádir Sháh. His rapidly growing unpopularity among all classes provoked a desperate attempt on his life in the following year.

In August he was staying in his summer encampment a few miles outside Teheran. He had just mounted his horse to proceed on a hunting expedition, when three men went close up to him as if to present a petition. One of the party placed his hand on the shah's dress and on being repulsed drew a pistol from his girdle while one of his confederates at the same time seized the horse's reins. The animal, finding himself checked, reared, and the Minister of Finance, who chanced to be close at hand, pulled the shah from his horse. In falling the shot lodged in the loins of the shah; but the pistol being loaded only with partridge shot and a few slugs, the wound was merely skin deep.

So intent was the assassin on effecting his object that he immediately drew a formidable dagger and in spite of several desperate wounds persisted in attacking the shah. In his endeavour to get near him, he ripped up the entrails of one of the attendants, nor did he cease to struggle until he himself was slain. The other two assassins were captured alive and afterwards put to death by torture. In the fray both discharged their pistols at the shah, but both missed him.

The first intelligence of the assault was accompanied by the announcement that the shah had been killed. The panic was not stayed by the announcement of Dr Cloquet that he had extracted the shot without difficulty and that there was no cause for alarm. The royal camp began to break up and the crowd rushed towards Teheran. The shops were immediately shut. In a short time bread was not to be procured, everyone struggling to lay in a stock of food in preparation for coming events. But no pillage or violence took place. On the following day to reassure the minds of the people and satisfy them of the reality of the shah's safety, a salute of 110 guns was fired, the large body of troops encamped near Teheran were brought to the royal camp to view the shah, and a similar invitation was sent to the clergy and civic authorities. Order was given for the bazaars to be illuminated.

It is almost incredible that the assassins should have devoted themselves to almost certain death unless they were actuated by religious fanaticism. This was the view of the shah and his ministers. The two survivors did indeed declare themselves to be adherents of the new faith of Bahá'ism or Bábism, which had just been founded in Persia and which had already suffered ruthless persecution from the orthodox inhabitants. So convinced was the shah that the members of this obnoxious faith had plotted to destroy him and that they were determined to take his life that he did not venture outside his summer residence again and returned to the citadel within the city of Teheran a month earlier than usual. Nevertheless, he strongly suspected his mother, and his brother, now aged thirteen, who were living at Qum, of complicity in the plot and he determined to blind the former and murder the latter. The flight of these two to Baghdad under British protection saved them from his vengeance.

The attempted assassination afforded an excuse for a general round-up of all the known Bahá'ís and for the next few days the court presented the extraordinary and disgraceful spectacle of all the chief officers of State being converted into executioners. Each department of the government was found to be harbouring a supposed conspirator against the shah's life. The Minister for Foreign Affairs, the Minister of Finance, the son of the Prime Minister, the Adjutant-General of the Army, the Master of the Mint each was ordered to fire the first shot or make the first cut with a sabre at the culprits delivered over to them, who were then dispatched by the subordinates. The artillery, the infantry, the cavalry, and the camel artillery each had their allotment of victims. Even the priesthood were assigned a share of the butchery. The *ḥakím-bás͟hí*, Mullá Muḥammad Qiblí, when presented with his batch of prisoners, begged to be excused from acting as an executioner, because, as he said, it was the universal law for physicians to use their powers in saving life rather than in taking it away. Dr Cloquet, too, managed to avoid the horrible task by pointing out that in the course of his daily work he had already sent so many people into the next world that it was too much to expect him to add to that number.

Had this attempt been successful it is difficult to say into how great a state of confusion the country would have been thrown. Once again there was no recognized heir apparent. The shah had his full complement of wives allowed by the Prophet, but his children had a habit of dying in infancy. The birth of a male child in February 1852 therefore filled him with joy. The speedy recognition by the British Government of the infant Mu'ín-ul-Dín Mírzá as heir apparent completed his satisfaction. The astrologers were therefore ordered to consult the stars and to fix a fortunate hour for the public announcement of the infant as heir to the throne. A general illumination of the city for seven successive nights was ordered, the chief servants of the court as well as the troops, officers and men, were to be feasted, and invitations to attend the ceremony were issued to the foreign missions.

On this occasion the astrologers made a mistake, for the hour which they chose was anything but propitious. On the very day previous to the one appointed for the ceremony one of the chief officials at the court suddenly died of cholera. The infant prince, too, having fallen sick the fête was postponed indefinitely and the shah retired the same day to a palace some six miles outside Teheran to await events.

The departure of the shah was the signal for a general panic and for several successive days there was a continuous stream of persons flowing from the city to the villages and neighbouring mountain range. Nearly four-fifths of the inhabitants of Teheran fled from their homes. The cholera raged among those who remained. The official returns declared a mortality which exceeded a hundred a day. From Teheran the epidemic spread westwards as far as Zenjan, southwards as far as Shiraz and Hamadan, and eastwards to Shahrud and Mazanderan. The Prime Minister stated that the mortality was so great in many of his villages in Mazanderan that the peasantry, although the harvest had commenced, had left the crops standing and fled in a body, some of the villages remaining without a single inhabitant. It even appeared in the shah's camp, though his family all fortunately escaped.

The year 1853 was also an unfortunate year for Persia. Not only was the whole of the centre of the country ravaged with cholera, but the town of Shiraz was laid waste by one of the severest earthquakes on record. Ten thousand people are said to have perished, killed by the falling buildings. Nor was this all, for the country round was destroyed by a flight of locusts. In other provinces the crops were seriously damaged by a mildew caused by the unusual quantity of rain which fell that year. Great losses were also sustained in various districts by showers of hailstones of great weight. And the crop of opium, the staple product of Yezd, was destroyed by a violent wind off the desert.

During these years the autocratic spirit of the shah, which had shown itself in the summary dismissal and execution of the Amír Niẓám, grew yet more marked. He seems to have wished to free himself from control of any kind. The fall of the Ṣadr Á'ẓam, who had succeeded the Amír Niẓám, was due to the failure of his plots, which, as usual, were centred in the *andarún*. The shah very much preferred one of his temporary wives to any of his four permanent consorts. The new lady of his choice was ambitious and the form her ambition took was to see her son nominated heir apparent. The trouble was firstly that Mu'ín-ul-Dín, the *Valí 'Ahd*, was still alive. The second trouble was that the son of a *síga* or temporary wife could not legally succeed to his father's position. The first obstacle presented no difficulty, unless the Russian and British Governments were determined to compel the shah to keep his word. The second obstacle could only be overcome by the divorce of one of the legal wives and her replacement by the *síga*. For this the help of the Ṣadr Á'ẓam was required. Her plans fell not unagreeably upon this minister's ears and in return for her persuading the shah to disgrace his commander-in-chief, who was a political rival of the Ṣadr Á'ẓam, he in his turn promised to arrange the divorce and legalization of the union. It all fell out as arranged. The commander-in-chief was dismissed with ignominy, the divorce was carried through, and the son of the late *síga* became the heir apparent.

Most unfortunately in June of the following year the new heir apparent contracted meningitis from which he died. His death was certainly accelerated, if not actually caused, by the attendance and conflicting remedies of half-a-dozen Persian and two Jewish doctors. The shah was heart-broken. In August the Ṣadr Á'ẓam was dismissed from office.

The shah being now without a prime minister decided to rule without one and for seven years the government of the country was carried on by a council of ministers over whom the shah presided and who could take no decision in any matter in any branch of the State without his express permission. This state of things continued until the shah, tiring of politics and perhaps with an eye to the grand tour of Europe which he was soon to carry out, decided to delegate his authority to responsible ministers again. For the premiership there were two candidates. First came the Ṣadr Á'ẓam, who was quite willing to resume office. But so great was his unpopularity with his colleagues that the shah was forced to pass him over. The second was Farrukh Khán Amín-ul-Doula. So eager was he to assume the dangerous, though elevated, office that he even begged Dr Dickson to plead his cause on the next occasion that he was called in to feel the royal pulse. But the shah for some reason would not listen to the recital of his merits and when finally the ex-minister of war became the new prime minister, Amín-ul-Doula did not even have a seat in the cabinet.

For about a year after this the cabinet functioned. But in June of 1866 the shah wearied again of semi-constitutional government, reduced the prime minister to his former rank, and again ruled without a premier. The post of Minister of Public Works, a post which included the Presidency of the Royal Military College and Director of the Printing Press throughout Persia, was given to 'Alí Qulí Mírzá I'tiẓád-ul-Salṭana. To his duties a new directorship had been added, that of Director of the Telegraph Department. The introduction of the telegraph into Persia is a matter of some importance, both political and medical. The possibility of consulting Whitehall on any question and of receiving a decision within 24 hours clearly revolutionized diplomacy. It meant the end of the days when the most suitable person to be British minister was the man who knew most about Persian intrigues and Persian personalities. In other words the Legation doctor was no longer a candidate for the highest post in the mission. With rare exceptions the minister was for the future always chosen from the regular members of the *corps diplomatique*. For medicine, not only did it mean the immediate knowledge of the outbreak of any epidemic threatening Persia, but it also brought to Teheran a second British doctor. For the senior staff of the Telegraph Department being British demanded a British medical attendant. Thus the old traditions of the days of Fatḥ 'Alí Sháh and 'Abbás Mírzá were revived.

At first it was very doubtful which nation would have the honour of directing the Persian telegraphs. In 1860 a French company offered to build a telegraph line connecting Teheran to the Anglo-Indian line which was then being built via Constantinople and Basra. In return they asked for a monopoly of telegraphic communications for 60 years. Eager though the shah was to link up his country with the line to Europe he boggled at the high figure that was named for the concession. Accordingly he looked round for a better offer. In the summer of that year he definitely declined the French proposal and no other nation making him a suitable offer he succeeded in building his own line from Tabriz to Teheran. The opening of that line gave him immense satisfaction. He used to visit the office daily and converse with the authorities in Tabriz during the greater part of the morning on any and every subject to the great annoyance of the authorities of that city and to the stultification of the legitimate uses of the line.

In the meantime negotiations continued with the British Government for the linking up of Teheran with the telegraph line in the south. The discussions were carried on through Mushír-ul-Doula, a former Persian ambassador in London. In the case of the English it was not the length of the concession that caused the shah to hesitate, but their demand that the Persian Government should assume the duty of guarding the line against destruction by marauders and practical jokers. How could he spare the troops to guard 500 miles of wire, said the shah, when all his soldiers were occupied in fighting the Turcomans? At length, wearying of the protracted discussions Mushír-ul-Doula was dismissed from the post of negotiator and bidden to retire to Meshed to say his prayers at the shrine until further notice. The shah then took the matter in hand himself and a compromise was reached by which it was agreed that the British should superintend the line and that the Persians should build it. In 1865 Dr Dickson left for England with the initialled telegraph convention in his pocket.

In June 1867 Dr Dickson returned with the ratified convention and the Indo-European Telegraph Department in Persia began to function. Dr J. E. Baker was the first English doctor to arrive in Persia in the service of the new department; Dr A. C. Turner, still in Persia in the service of the Oil Company, was the last. For the department scarcely survived its jubilee. It committed suicide when Riẓá Sháh tore up capitulations and cancelled all foreign concessions.

The state of medicine in Teheran when Dr Dickson and Dr Baker began to work together was one of great activity. Westernization had been introduced into Teheran and had come to stay. Yet the Persians for the most part remained wholeheartedly conservative. The young graduates of the Dár-ul-Fanún had not yet produced any effect upon the medical practice of the country. The protagonist of the old school, Mírzá Bábá Shírází Malik-ul-Aṭibbá, in his *Risála-i-Jóhariyya* thundered against the use of European drugs and the Western methods which the foreign professors were inculcating in the young undergraduates of the capital. But the opposition against him was too strong. The shah was completely under the influence of his Western advisers. Of Dr Cloquet I have already spoken. His end was a sad one. One day he asked a servant to fetch him a glass of brandy. The servant by mistake filled the glass with tincture of cantharides. Dr Cloquet tossed off the contents. At once he realized what had happened and, despairing of his life, bade the servant give him a second glass of the poison so that he might die the quicker. Within a few hours he was dead.

Dr Cloquet was succeeded by Dr Barthelemey. He in turn gave place to Dr Tholozan, a surgeon of the French Army and subsequently a Professor at Val-de-Grâce. He reached Teheran in 1864 and became chief physician to the shah and the leader of the reforms in the public health services. With him was associated, as surgeon-in-chief to the army, a Maltese British subject named Stagno. In the Dár-ul-Fanún there was another British doctor in the employment of the Persian Government. This was Dr Dolmage, an adventurer who arrived in Persia in 1859 and having become proficient in the language applied for and obtained a post in the medical school. This post he did not hold for long. The Persian Government approved of him as little as did the English when he acted as Legation doctor in the temporary absence of Dr Dickson. He then made his way to Meshed where he got into financial difficulties through speculating in skins. But perhaps it is best to say no more about one who was a credit neither to his profession nor his nation.

In pursuance of his policy of Westernizing the medical services of the country a new hospital was founded in Teheran, which was opened in 1868. It is not quite correct to say that this is the first hospital in Persia in which modern medicine was practised. There had been a Portuguese hospital at Hormuz until the fort was captured by the combined forces of the Persians and English in 1622, though perhaps the medicine practised there was scarcely 'modern'. Fr. Eusebius in his *History of the Missions*, writes:[1]

In 1609 there was (in Hormuz) only one house of Augustinian Hermits, twelve in number, who were also in charge of the Royal Hospital: besides their own church, within the fortress there was the mother church with three chapelries on the royal foundation, and outside (the fortress) an Augustinian Hermit had to tend each of the other two little churches. Opposite the fortress there was the noted Hospital of the Misericordia, a place of pious devotion deserving remembrance and praise of the Portuguese nation....Under the management of some well qualified gentlemen by its insitutions it provided dowries for necessitous girls, in various hospitals it looked after the sick, foundling infants, weak minded adults, it ministered to the condemned, buried the dead and had masses said for their souls, and kept others on their feet by loans.

In more recent times, in 1848 to be exact, the Russians had established a hospital of fourteen beds on the island of Ashurada in the Caspian Sea and the shah had issued a *firmán* that year for the building of another hospital near Astarabad. His orders, however, were not carried out. The new hospital in Teheran was originally intended to serve the army. It was at first placed under the management of Dr Polak and Dr Schlimmer. On the return from Paris of the Persian graduates it was handed over to them. Twelve years later another hospital was founded for the use of the troops. The older hospital was then handed over to civilians and put under the charge of Dr Albo, a German who was lecturer in medicine in the Dár-ul-Fanún. It now became known as the Imperial Hospital or Maríẓkhána-i-Daulatí and led an uneventful but useful life until the time of the War of 1914–18 when it became the centre of a diplomatic 'incident' with which I shall deal later.

1 *Hist. Miss.* vol. II, ch. 3.2. See *Chron. Carm. in Persia* vol. I, p. 267 and vol. II, p. 1041.

Having accomplished thus much the shah decided to go to Europe to see for himself what the West was like. His first journey outside his own dominions was in 1870, when he left Teheran for three months on a pilgrimage to Kerbela. The journey was not without distress to his loyal subjects, anxiety to the Turkish authorities, and great discomfort to his retinue. He insisted upon being accompanied by a suite of 6000 persons, who together with the followers made a total caravan of nearly 20,000 people. There was cholera on the road and there was considerable difficulty in finding lodging and food for such a vast host. The Turkish health authorities begged the shah to reduce his following and to observe strictly the laws of quarantine which were then in force against pilgrims.

The shah returned to his capital in February of 1871. With his thoughts full of a grand tour of Europe, he made a tour through Mazanderan in the following year. He returned to Teheran infected with malaria and was treated by Dr Dickson. He was so grateful to him that he insisted that he should accompany him to Europe. In May 1873 the great day arrived and he set out, the first shah of Persia to do so since the days of Xerxes. Leaving Prince Mu'tamid-ul-Doula as regent he left Teheran in the beginning of that month. At Enzeli he divided his retinue between two ships. In the first boat sailed the shah himself with his principal ministers of State, his harem and Dr Tholozan. In the second boat sailed the rest of his suite and Dr Dickson. The story of his adventures in Europe is recorded in his own official diary. There are other stories of his doings and sayings on this and on his second journey to Europe that have never been and never will be published. The romance and mystery of his name and rank so caught the fancy of the British public that even to-day an imaginary portrait of him can be seen swinging in the wind outside an occasional public house. He was not long away from Persia. He returned in September of the same year and with him returned Doctor, now Sir Joseph, Dickson.

CHAPTER XVIII

THE SANITARY COUNCIL AND THE QUARANTINE SERVICE

THE danger of famine, which had never been far away, assumed alarming proportions in the second half of the nineteenth century. The year 1861 was the first of the great famine years which succeeded one another at irregular intervals until the advent of motor transport guaranteed that half Persia should not starve while food rotted through glut in the other half. In this first great famine there was wheat in abundance in Azerbaijan and Kermanshah; in Mazanderan there was no failure of the rice crop. But snow blocked the mountain passes which lead from these provinces to the towns of the central plateau and excessive rain destroyed the roads. Teheran thus found itself threatened with famine. In March of that year a clamorous mob of famished creatures beset the residence of the shah. He in terror summoned the Lord Mayor of Teheran to his presence and after a few words of royal censure committed him to the executioner. The chief magistrate of the city was thus put to death on the spot. His body was stripped and dragged through the streets amid the execrations of the populace and was hung up by the heels at one of the city gates. The shah then assumed a suit of red clothing, which implied that more blood was to be shed. But what was of greater importance, he also opened the royal granaries.

By May this supply was exhausted: the crop of that year was not yet ready: and the people were still hungry. The attitude of the mob again became threatening. The minister of war was hissed in the streets. A crowd of women forced their way into one of the mosques while the head *mullá* was at his prayers, and dragged him out, insisting upon his calling upon the shah to cause an immediate distribution of bread. On the same day another crowd of women attacked the British Legation and demanded that the minister should bring to the notice of the shah their distressing condition. One of the guards was wounded in trying to close the gate. In order to appease them the minister was obliged to write a note to one of the Persian ministers. When the women saw the note in Dr Dickson's hand and heard him order a servant to deliver it at once, they expressed their gratitude and peaceably withdrew.

With the summer came relief. The snow melted, bridges were reconstructed, and good harvests relieved the want. But the Government had learnt no wisdom. No provision was made against this calamity and five years later there was again a shortage of bread and again demonstrations against the shah and his ministers. The famine of this year was followed by a very severe outbreak of cholera in Teheran. In the next year cholera reappeared, starting this time in Meshed, where the deaths numbered between 100 and 120 a day. The death of Jalál-ul-Doula, a son of the shah and the Prince Governor of Khorasan, brought home to the Government the seriousness of the epidemic. The shah fled to the country, accompanied by his wives, eunuchs and court. The health authorities of Teheran did nothing to check the progress of the epidemic. A large caravan of pilgrims, numbering about 5000, arrived in Teheran from Meshed on 5 August. Although coming from a place where cholera was raging and actually carrying with them seeds of the disease, no precautionary measures of any sort were adopted before or after their arrival by the local authorities. Consequently cholera declared itself in Teheran on the 7th and spread through the poorer quarters of the city. The death-rate, however, was not high, although among the victims were I'tiẓád-ul-Doula, the general officer commanding the artillery, and several peasants in the British and Russian villages of Gulahek and Zargandeh.

In 1869 cholera appeared in Ispahan. From there it spread to Shiraz, where over 2000 persons are said to have died; and finally it reached the Persian Gulf. It now became a matter of importance to the Indian Government. The port of Bushire was about as insanitary a town as could be imagined. Intramural burial was practised. Sanitary arrangements were entirely lacking; quarantine regulations were non-existent. The town and sea-walls were in ruins through want of repair for many years. The space around the town walls was used as an open privy, which the flow of the tide, passing in through the cracks and gaps in the sea walls, converted into a pestilential swamp. The number of cases of cholera increased daily. Panic set in and the populace refused any longer to handle or bury their dead. The British ladies of the Residency and some of the establishment moved to the neighbouring island of Bassidow. The Resident himself and his doctor stayed in the city.

Pressure by the British minister in Teheran compelled the Central Government to take some action. The Governor of Bushire was then ordered to have all infected clothes burnt, to make burial outside the city compulsory, and finally to listen to the Residency and native doctors in planning the best means of stopping the epidemic.

From Bushire cholera spread along the coast, and Baghdad, threatened both by the pilgrim traffic from Teheran and by the coasting traffic along the Gulf, was soon infected. If quarantine was poor in Persia, it was worse in Baghdad. An attempt was indeed made. Accommodation outside the town was provided for about 1000 persons. As the number of pilgrims who arrived every month for Kerbela was in the region of 10,000, this accommodation was utterly inadequate. Those unfortunates who could not get a roof over their heads were exposed to the hot sun by day, to the bitter wind of the desert by night, and to the pilfering of lawless Arabs all the 24 hours. Fortunately, cholera is a self-limiting disease. Perhaps for that very reason the Persians were disinclined to take any serious steps to mitigate its severity or to protect themselves against recurrence. During the winter the disease died a natural death and when the shah proposed in the spring of 1870 to make a pilgrimage to Kerbela, it was not on the grounds of public health that his proposal was discouraged.

In spite of these repeated warnings the famine of 1871 caught the Government again unprepared. It was in the south that the worst conditions prevailed. During the hot summer months the streets of Bushire were filled with panic-stricken people, many in the last stages of starvation and not a few dead. Those that were still able to move about, busied themselves turning over the various collections of refuse to be found in every corner. Those who came across a fowl's entrails or a dry fish-bone considered themselves lucky. Those not so fortunate deadened the cravings of hunger by eating the droppings of the donkeys in the streets. Nor were conditions much better in Yezd. Here the Governor found it necessary to place a guard over the public burial ground to prevent the people from digging up the newly interred corpses. Between Bushire and Shiraz the villagers were living for the most part on grass. The ancient city of Kazerun was almost deserted. In Ispahan and Meshed the death roll to be attributed to starvation alone ran into hundreds a day. At Qum a man was executed for cannibalism.

To meet these appalling conditions a Famine Relief Fund was opened in London to which the shah and prominent Persians also contributed. Dr Dickson and Dr Baker were members of the Committee in Teheran. Reports by them of the state of the people, even of Teheran itself, make very sad reading. Dr Dickson states that he himself once picked up in the street a child whom he recognized as belonging to a once affluent family. The winter was particularly hard upon these poor undernourished people. Three hundred deaths a night are said to have occurred from cold and starvation. It was not long, of course, before typhoid fever broke out and those that hunger and cholera had spared, fell victims to the new epidemic.

The foreign medical advisers to the country did not fail to foresee that a nation, weakened by a series of famines, would fall an easy prey to the epidemic diseases which flourished in the neighbouring countries. Dr Tholozan, as Chief Physician to H.M. Shah, ranked as the doyen of the medical corps. By his influence and by his efforts a central sanitary bureau was at last founded, which was to be responsible for the internal health of the country. This body was at first known as the Board of Health and later took the title of Sanitary Council. It met in the Dár-ul-Fanún. The President was *ex officio* the Minister of Public Instruction, though the guiding hand for the first few years was that of Dr Tholozan. All the distinguished Persian doctors of the capital and all the physicians of the foreign legations formed the Council. Visiting physicians were occasionally allowed to attend. Professor E. G. Browne wrote: 'When I was at Ṭihrán in 1887 Dr Tholozan, physician to his late Majesty Náṣiru'd-Dín Sháh, kindly enabled me to attend the meetings of the Majlis-i-Ṣiḥḥat or Council of Public Health, in the Persian capital, and a majority of physicians present at that time knew no medicine but that of Avicenna.'[1]

Dr Tholozan was indefatigable. He established a Board of Health. He instituted a rudimentary quarantine system. He revived the public vaccination service which Dr Cloquet had initiated. He dispatched into the provinces physicians, trained under him in the Dár-ul-Fanún, armed with the necessary outfit to deal with epidemics in the villages. And he composed two books, one on cholera and plague, and one on auscultation, which he named *Badáyi'-ul-Ḥikmat-i-Náṣirí*, or the 'Wonders of Christian Science', and translated several French books into Persian.

One of the first duties of the new Board of Health was to undertake measures for the establishment of a frontier quarantine service. Negotiations were opened with Russia for the defence of the northern boundary of the Empire and with Turkey for the defence of the western frontier and the Persian Gulf. But the negotiations led nowhere and there being no funds available to render the Board of Health capable of producing any practical result the Board was allowed to die of inanition.

With an increase of knowledge in the method of prevention,

1 Browne, *Arabian Medicine*, p. 93. Cambridge, 1924.

it became more and more clear that neither the Avicennan system of Medicine as practised in Persia nor the defunct Board of Health were capable of dealing with the problem. Nor, indeed, was the International Sanitary Commission, which sat at Constantinople, more likely to guarantee the public health. Far-seeing medical officers viewed with apprehension the unsatisfactory measures taken by Mesopotamia and Persia to prevent or check an outbreak of any epidemic. Dr Colville, Surgeon-Major to the British Residency in Baghdad, was the first to raise the question of the desirability of a 'sentinel quarantine station' at the mouth of the Persian Gulf in order to protect India. In his official report to his Consul-General, dated 5 June 1875, he urged this need, adding: 'Should quarantine be determined upon, great care must be taken that the International Commission at Constantinople is not permitted to meddle in the matter, for I have had twice to submit to quarantine under its direction, and I do not desire to see the farce repeated when the health of India is at stake.'

In the following year an epidemic of diphtheria in Teheran, of cholera in Afghanistan and Seistan, and of plague in Mesopotamia called attention to the defenceless state of the interior of Persia. In order that adequate measures might be taken, the defunct Board of Health was replaced by a Sanitary Council, which met under the Presidency of Prince I'tiẓád-ul-Salṭana. Dr Castaldi was now Sanitary Officer in Teheran and Ottoman Sanitary Delegate in Persia and, taking the chief role in the discussion, urged the formation of a regular quarantine system and a permanent sanitary service. The state of affairs was serious. Already for three successive years plague had appeared within the frontiers of Persia, although so slight had the epidemic been, that many were inclined to deny that it was indeed the dreaded plague. Next year a fourth epidemic broke out with considerably greater virulence. In Shuster there were 8000 cases with more than 1800 deaths; in Mesopotamia the number of deaths was said to have exceeded 3000. So poor was the Intelligence Service that the Persian Sanitary Council was completely ignorant even of the outbreak of the epidemic until a report was forwarded to them from Dr Millingen. At the same time Dr Colville wrote to Dr Dickson, by then Sir Joseph, recommending in the strongest terms that joint action should be taken by the sanitary authorities of Turkey, Egypt and India to control the Gulf, as well as by those of Persia, if that should be possible.

The Persian health authorities rose to the occasion. A commission was at once appointed to deal with the subject, upon which sat Drs Tholozan, Castaldi, Dickson, Kuzmingi of the Russian Legation, Baker of the Indo-European Telegraph Department, and Hack, another English doctor practising in Teheran. They were assisted by Mírzá Sayyid Riẓá, Chief Medical Officer to the Army, Mírzá Riẓáí, lecturer in Western Medicine in the University, Mírzá Abú ul-Qásim, lecturer in Avicennan Medicine in the University, Mírzá Abú ul-Faẓl, Ja'far Qulí Khán, the Dean of the Medical School, Mírzá 'Alí Akbar, Head of the Imperial Hospital, and the shah's personal physician. Dr Tholozan was called upon to compose a pamphlet on the diagnosis and treatment of the disease for distribution among those in the infected area who could read. At the same time he was empowered to draw up fresh regulations for the establishment of a quarantine service and to set up a quarantine station at Khanikhin to prevent the passage of infected cases along the Baghdad-Teheran road.

The Government of India promptly sent an agent to investigate how best they too might participate in checking the spread of the disease. He reported by telegram to the Viceroy on the utter inadequacy of the Persian measures and pointed out that the task was beyond their powers.

With respect to quarantine in the Gulf it does not appear that any proper provision for performing quarantine exists on the Persian littoral and that such provision will have to be extemporised.... Moreover, before the proposed quarantine could be carried out, it is necessary to obtain the assistance of Great Britain, for Persia has no armed force by which obedience to her quarantine regulations could be enforced. The responsibility is in fact thrown upon England of enabling Persia to protect her littoral in the Gulf from plague.

In spite of this report the Government of India took no further action throughout the epidemic and professed themselves satisfied with the action of the Political Resident in Bushire who warned all Agencies, Persian authorities and merchants of the existence and dangers of plague and at the same time ordered the Residency Surgeon Dr R. M. Wall to make an inspection of all vessels passing from Basra to Bombay, to segregate all sick passengers, and to quarantine all boats and passengers calling at Bushire.

But the matter was not thus allowed to drop. The health of the Persian Gulf had become a matter of concern to the shipping of the world. The subject was next raised in London and this time by the Count Beust, the Ambassador of the Emperor of Austro-Hungary. In a letter dated from Belgrave Square on 27 June 1877 he thus wrote to Lord Derby:

> Le Gouvernement persan n'a rien fait jusqu'ici pour empêcher l'importation des épidémies. C'est un devoir impérieux, tant au point de vue humanitaire qu'à celui de la conservation personelle, que de faire cesser cette incurie en Perse; et comme il n'est point à espérer que le Gouvernement persan en prenne lui même l'initiative, c'est aux autres Puissances intéressées à apporter leurs soins à l'établissement des mesures nécessaires.
>
> Ce que le Gouvernement Impériale et Royal cherche à atteindre c'est le règlement du service sanitaire. Entre les mains du Gouvernement persan cette tâche ne sera jamais accompli. Une institution internationale devra aborder sérieusement cette tâche sous les auspices des Gouvernements étrangers.

His proposal was that the quarantine service of the Gulf should not be left in Persian hands, but should be directed by an international council sitting at Teheran, in the same way that the health of Egypt and the Suez Canal was directed by the International Board at Constantinople. This Council was intended to replace the newly formed Sanitary Council of Teheran and was to be armed with executive powers, have charge of all sanitary services, and be provided with a budget and power over its own essential expenditure. The President was to be a Persian. Representatives of their nations were to be furnished by the Legations of Austro-Hungary, England, France, Russia, Turkey and Holland; and there was to be a minority of Persian delegates.

The British Government accepted in principle Count Beust's proposals and the matter was referred to the Persian Government. On their part there was no objection. Persia of those days was always willing to accept any favour or advantage provided that it cost nothing. The proposals then went back to the British Government as the most interested party with a note that the Persian Government accepted all the proposals except the financial section. The British Government now looked into the question in greater detail and found that there were certain objections which had at first been overlooked. Egypt and Turkey, they claimed, were not good models and the proposed council must be free to adopt any sanitary measures they might hold desirable and should in no sense be tied by Turkish precedents. Finally, the British Government strongly objected to paying for any part of the proposal except the salary of their own delegate. The Persians sat back with hands folded and watched the wrangling of England, Turkey and Austro-Hungary. Nothing was agreed upon; nothing was settled. After a few months the whole proposal was dropped and the sanitary health of Persia continued to be administered by the Sanitary Council of Teheran which now admitted as members the delegates of the European legations and which had affiliated itself to the International Sanitary Council of Constantinople. In other words, the Persian Council became the protégé of the Turkish Council instead of its equal.

The next most pressing task before the Council was the setting up of quarantine posts along the northern boundary and in the Caspian Sea ports. And thirdly came the duty of forming an internal public health service and regulating the traffic in corpses and pilgrims. Pious Persians prefer burial in one of the holy cities of Mesopotamia to interment in their own land. A caravan of coffins winding down the passes towards Nejef and Kerbala is not a rare sight to-day. A tax on each corpse made the traffic profitable to the Turkish authorities. The risk of disease made it fearful to every village along the road. It was not until 1925 that the matter was finally and satisfactorily settled. In that year the Iraq Government agreed to accept only 'dried corpses', the criterion being a certificate of burial three years previous to arrival at the frontier.

For nearly 20 years the subject was allowed to lie dormant and there was no external interference in Persian health affairs. The year 1896 was a memorable one in Persian history both because Náṣr-ul-Dín Sháh was murdered in the mosque at Sháh 'Abd-ul-'Azím and because the outbreak of a severe epidemic of bubonic plague in India again turned the thoughts of the interested nations towards establishing an effective quarantine service in the Persian Gulf. The struggle between England and Russia for supremacy in Persia was now keen. The obvious interest of England in the Persian Gulf excited Russian apprehensions and two medical agents were sent down, ostensibly to study plague. Bushire, Bandar Abbas and Basra were in turn visited by these energetic physicians and reports duly sent back. Their real object was scarcely veiled and on their return the Viedomosti of St Petersburgh on 20 October 1899 (that is, 1 November, O.S.) wrote:

> Two months have not elapsed since the close of the Peace Conference when England violated the most sacred rights of the South African Republic and by her demands forced the Boers to declare war in order to defend her liberty, the most precious gift of man and State.... It is time for us also, taking advantage of the times which favour us, to realise our sacred dream and to pierce in the Near East also to the Ocean. We are speaking of the acquisition by us of the port of Bandar Abbas on the Persian Gulf.
>
> The English are spreading the rumour that the climate of Bandar Abbas is unbearable and that the Russians, if they took it, will be roasted. It is not hard to see with what object such stories are circulated. Many Russians (recently doctors sent to inquire into the plague and diplomatic agents) have been there and deny this.

In July 1899 one of the severest epidemics of plague on record broke out in the Gulf. Captain Rainier and two medical officers were sent to assist the British staff which was already established there. Neither the prime minister of the time nor the local authorities seemed to realize the supreme importance of prompt and effective measures. Sir Mortimer Durand, the British Minister at Teheran, informed the Persian Government that if they were unwilling or unable to take the measures recommended by the English doctors the British authorities had no further responsibility and that the Persian Government must justify themselves to other countries.

The hostility of the villagers and the *mullás* to any form of quarantine was unconcealed. Cholera was a disease which they knew and dreaded; plague was a form of death with which they were for the most part unfamiliar. All the odium for the discomfort caused by the sanitary regulations was thrown upon the English. The acting governor of Bushire informed the merchants at a prayer meeting that the Government was being forced to undertake measures by the foreign doctors and that they should appeal to the shah for redress. It was clear that without a considerable force it would be impossible to carry out sanitary measures. Above all money was necessary, as the acting governor refused to do anything unless supplied with funds.

So inflamed was local feeling that an attempt to take measures against the plague caused a riot, which broke out on 24 July. On 1 August the town of Bushire still seethed with excitement and Colonel Meade, the Political Resident, requested authority to land bluejackets, if necessary.

In spite of local opposition and central apathy the British quarantine officers continued to carry out their work. The only helpful feature of the Persian administration was the attitude of the Sanitary Council. Ḥakím-ul-Mulk, physician to the shah and leader of the Court Party, had resigned the office of President to Dr Schneider. Sir Joseph Dickson had given over his seat on the Council and his post in the Legation to Dr Oddling. On the recommendation of the Council a disinfector was ordered by the Bushire authorities. But as soon as it was produced it provoked the most intense apprehension among the natives. The people appeared to believe that it was an engine designed for the purpose of boiling children, who were required in that condition for certain occult purposes by the European doctors. After earnest warnings from the Governor and other authorities it was finally decided to place it on the Persian guardship for safe keeping.

More serious, had it been true, were the charges of unfair discrimination by the quarantine authorities between the different classes of passengers. Europeans, they claimed, were allowed to pass with no restrictions, Persians were kept back. Doctor Vaume, the Turkish delegate on the Sanitary Council, became the mouthpiece of these accusations. He complained about the precautions taken: he complained about the disinfection: and concluded by declaring: 'Une conclusion s'impose: l'insuffisance de l'organisation sanitaire actuelle sur le littoral persan du Golfe.'

The Government under the circumstances decided to send down to the Gulf an independent observer. Ḥájjí Zayn-ul-'Ábidín was chosen. In his report he asserted that the epidemic was grossly exaggerated.

I have seen [he wrote] no case of plague on the way down. Two persons are said to have died in quarantine in Bushire. One Ḥájjí Raḥím of Kazarun, a passenger from Jeddah, suffered from diarrhoea at that place and during the voyage. On disembarking a trunk fell upon him and broke his ribs. He died shortly afterwards.

Another person, a native of Shiraz, was suffering from diarrhoea in quarantine, when he was under the care of the English doctor. He died during the last night of quarantine and the travellers, fearing to be subjected to an additional ten days' quarantine, substituted another man for the deceased, who was buried secretly at night without the doctor discovering the trick which had been played. The passengers were admitted to pratique.

The Persian Government, backed by this report of their agent, showed a complete lack of interest not only in the work of the

British doctors, but also in the efforts which the Sanitary Council were making to suppress the epidemic. At the November meeting of the Council it was suggested that the members should themselves put an end to the farce by no further attendance. It was, however, finally decided to request Dr Adcock, Physician to the shah, to call on the Ṣadr Ā'ẓam and to represent to His Highness that unless the Persian Government showed some interest in the proceedings of the Council or paid some attention to their recommendations and requests, the Council would assume that their services were not required and would suspend their sittings. Suicide was not required, for the Persian Government informed the members that the sitting of the Council was adjourned *sine die*.

The epidemic of 1896 had already compelled the delegates to the International Sanitary Conference at Venice in the following year to take notice of the threat to Europe of an infected Persian Gulf. After much discussion it was agreed that a sanitary station ought to be established at the entrance to the Gulf, that the control of this station should be in Persian hands and not international, and that Persia should have the privilege both of choosing the site and paying for the upkeep. The control of the ports by the British medical officers was not disputed.

When the next meeting was held in Paris six years later Persia had still not chosen any site. The Conference then asked them to hasten their decision and recommended Hormuz as a suitable post. The Persian Government replied by choosing Henjam. The French urged the British Government to agree to this choice. But Great Britain, in addition to having special interests in Henjam, was not eager to yield up a controlling position to Persia in the Quarantine Service. It was pointed out that it was by no means sure that epidemics could in fact be carried into Europe from the Gulf. The road across the Great Syrian desert to the Mediterranean was in those days only taken by slow-moving Arab caravans. Moreover, Henjam was unsuitable for a permanent station of any sort both from the point of view of climate and from food and water conditions. In any case it would be easy for native craft, the type against which this foundation was chiefly aimed, to avoid Henjam. British opposition thus brought to naught this first attempt to form a Persian quarantine service.

Another and more satisfactory result of the Conference was the re-establishment of the Sanitary Council. By its constitution of 1904 all the doctors of the foreign legations became members by right. The duties of the Council were still purely advisory, but the Council, although under the aegis of the Ministry of Foreign Affairs claimed the right of direct approach to the other Ministries. Dr Schneider again took office as President.

Thereupon Sir Cecil Spring Rice, who had become British Minister, privately approached Dr Schneider and urged him to avoid any discussion by the Council of the Henjam question. Dr Schneider for his part was quite willing to allow the matter to drop, but considered that if Great Britain desired to have the sole responsibility for the health of the Gulf, it was her duty to render it secure by increasing the European personnel in the quarantine service and by supplying more disinfecting stoves.

In this supremacy of the British in the Gulf the Russians saw a threat to their own prestige. Though fully occupied with the control of an outbreak of plague in Seistan, they nevertheless did their utmost to prevent the smooth running of the British-manned Gulf Quarantine Service. At their instigation the Daryá Bégí, or Governor of the Persian Gulf, made the astonishing demand that not only all boats engaged in quarantine work but also all ships undergoing quarantine inspection should fly the Persian flag. In December a Russian vessel anchored off Bandar Abbas and joyfully refused to admit the quarantine officer on board because his launch was flying at the stern the Union Jack. The matter was referred to Teheran and the Sanitary Council persuaded the Daryá Bégí to withdraw his tiresome regulation.

It must not be thought that the Gulf was the only source of danger to public health in Persia. In 1897 a brisk outbreak of plague had occurred in Eastern Persia. To avoid any risk to Central Persia the Russians formed a sanitary cordon, known as the Turbat-i-Haydari cordon, extending from Karez to Turchiz. This was not withdrawn after the epidemic had died down. It soon became clear when another epidemic broke out in 1906 that they were about to form another quasi-permanent cordon which would completely cut off Seistan from Meshed and the north. There could, of course, be no objection to the Russians giving the same aid to the Persians in the north that the British were so readily supplying in the south. But when it was evident that the real object of the cordon was not to check disease but to strangle trade with the north-west of India, then the Government of India thought the time had come to take some steps in the matter of the quarantine service in general.

In January the Russian consulate reported plague. At once the local Russian authorities took steps to close the Duzdab-Meshed road. The Sanitary Council sent down a mixed commission of Russians, British and Persians to set up an effective sanitary barrier. They chose Bandan, a town 60 miles north-west of Nasratabad, as the sanitary post. So effective and so unpleasant was their method of isolation and disinfection that at the end of March the people of Nasratabad could stand it no longer, rose in a body and destroyed the isolation huts. At the same time they vented their wrath on the foreigner by destroying the British Consulate Dispensary and by a half-hearted attack on the Consulate itself. To maintain order a few armed sowars were moved up from Robat.

In the meantime plague spread. In April another sanitary post was formed at Birjand, a long way north of Nasratabad and others were formed to link up with the Turbat-i-Haydari cordon. Over the new line of defence the Russians had complete control. So complete and strict was this control that Persian land trade with India ceased.

In May the epidemic was still spreading. In June there were still no signs that the elaborate Russian precautions were of any avail. In July the inhabitants were heartily sick of sanitary law and a second attack was made upon the Consulate. The Persian Government was held responsible for these acts of violence, though the source was clearly elsewhere. A series of demands were put forward by the British Legation which were ultimately simplified into a demand for an apology from the deputy governor and the ringleaders of the attack and a permission to buy 10,000 *zars* of land at a nominal price for the extension of the dispensary and hospital. Honour was satisfied, said the Legation, thus lightly 'as a graceful concession to the new shah', Muḥammad 'Alí, who had just succeeded to the throne on the death of Muẓaffar-ul-Dín early in the year.

It was not until the middle of August that the last case was notified. Nevertheless, quarantine was not raised until February and the Russian cordon at Turbat-i-Haydari was not withdrawn until the end of the following year. The usual charges of grave incompetence were made against the Russians as a matter of course. A more interesting suggestion came from Captain Kelly, I.M.S., who, discussing the method by which infection had reached Seistan, suggested that wild fowl in their flight southwards from Astrakhan had carried with them plague-infected fleas.

All this time the British and Persian Governments were discussing the problems of the Quarantine Service in the Persian Gulf in the light of the suggestions from Paris and the proposals of Dr Schneider. Unfortunately another epidemic of plague broke out in the late spring of 1907 which showed only too clearly both the efficiency and the failings of the service. The Russians displayed keen interest that the British service should be competent and efficient and did not fail to point out every defect. Yet it was noticed that when cholera appeared in Astrakhan, the Persian Legation in St Petersburgh was not informed until a month had passed.

To a commission appointed by the Sanitary Council to report on any desirable changes in the Quarantine Service the Russian delegate made proposals which were intended to associate other nations with the British control. The British pointed out that international control was already guaranteed by the general control which the Sanitary Council at Teheran exercised over the whole service. Ultimately the British were obliged, through fear of less acceptable proposals being forced upon them, to accept Dr Schneider's original demands. Disinfecting stoves were therefore set up at Bandar Abbas, Lingah, Jask and Mohammerah. A Clayton Apparatus was also provided at Bushire. And Captain Williams, I.M.S., the Chief Quarantine Medical Officer, was given another British assistant. These improvements took the wind out of the Russian sails and for the moment there was peace. But it should not pass without remark that though in this instance international rivalry ended in a more efficient service for Persia, it was more usual for the Public Health and Sanitary Services to suffer from these diplomatic duels and obstructionist tactics. The objective of both Russians and British was security and supremacy for their own trade. In passing judgement upon the high-handed action of the Persians 20 years later when they ejected both Russian and British medical officers with small thanks, the political motives underlying the foreign sanitary intrusion into their country should not be forgotten.

The Quarantine Service did not enjoy a very long respite from attack. This time it came from a different quarter, though it is not difficult to believe that the inspiration came from the same. Dr Listemann, the German Consul at Bushire, now made a series of attacks upon the quarantine administration. His Legation in Teheran supported him and in the person of Dr Bussière found another ally. This gentleman had been in turn in the service of the Belgians and Russians; now he was physician to the French Legation. Some dead rats were found in Bahrein. Major Prideaux, the Political Resident, discovered that these rats had been caught in a trap and that there was no question of plague. He so informed the Chief Quarantine Officer. At the same time the Chief Quarantine Officer received a private letter from the Director of Customs at Bushire, telling him that Dr Bussière had asked him to telegraph the news confidentially to the Sanitary Council at Teheran. Dr Bussière had got his information from Dr Listeman who in his turn had received it from the agent of a German firm at Bahrein. Neither the Consul nor Dr Bussière acted as they should, which was to have informed the Chief Quarantine Officer. By going to the Sanitary Council behind his back they attempted to throw discredit upon the whole British administration.

In the course of this year 1907, Dr Schneider resigned the office of President of the Sanitary Council and Dr Coppin, a physician to the shah, took his place. During his temporary absence in Europe the office of president was assumed for the first time by a Persian physician when Dr Loqmán-ul-Mamálik, another royal physician, took his place. This last was a physician of the old school, but there was now in the land a small body of Persians who had received their training abroad. A certain number had seats on the Council. Their influence was to be seen by the greater interest in local affairs now shown and by the increased part that Persians now began to play in the debates of the Council. To make the Council more effective it was essential that it should possess its own budget. To raise funds they proposed that a tax should be levied on pilgrims and corpses on their way to the Holy Cities. Such a tax had long ago been made payable, but until then was retained by the local authorities. The tax was now fixed at seven krans a corpse and it was decided to spend the money thus raised in building a quarantine station somewhere between Kermanshah and Kerbela. The Council even succeeded in persuading the Government to allot to them a tenth of the tax on horses and carriages, which they decided to spend upon the support of a service for free public vaccination. They also drew up a scheme for a quarantine service in the Caspian ports similar to that existing in the Persian Gulf. The importation of cholera from Russia, which caused fatal cases at Ardebil, Hamadan and Kermanshah, made the matter of immediate importance and the Government was persuaded to allot some 20,000 tomans towards the provision of lazarets, doctors and drugs.

Dr Coppin now left Persia for good. His place as President was taken by Dr Georges, a Frenchman and Professor of Medicine in the University. Dr Feistmantel, an Austrian, was elected Vice-President. The number of European members of the Council was now very large and unfortunately the council hall became the arena for their quarrels. First the Germans attacked the British quarantine service. To strengthen their voting power Dr Ilberg, the physician to the German Legation, although there was another German member of the Council, claimed yet another vote by virtue of being representative also of Norway and Sweden. A most unseemly race to collect the right of representation of the smaller nations now began. In this game of 'Happy Families' Britain managed to secure Belgium and France got Greece. The only change in the constitution of the Council was that it was made into a department of the Ministry of Interior instead of being under the Ministry of Foreign Affairs. Nevertheless, the year 1911 was an important one in the annals of the Council, for, for the first time they had money of their own to spend upon public health works and they ceased to be a purely advisory body.

In April 1911 Dr Georges resigned the office of President in order to represent Persia at the International Sanitary Conference in Paris. Dr Neligan, who had been appointed to the British Legation in 1906 in place of Dr Oddling and had recently been elected Vice-President, became acting-President. The public vaccination service was once again revived. An attempt to make the vaccination lymph locally failed, but supplies from Europe soon arrived and during the last four months of the year nearly 15,000 people in Teheran and the surrounding villages applied for free vaccination.

It is obvious that the general outlook upon medicine had by now considerably changed. Fifty years of tuition by foreign professors had produced a generation in the towns whose outlook was entirely different from that of their fathers. This Westernization received a considerable impetus from the establishment of Christian medical missions in different parts of the country. The lion's share of the credit must be given to the Church Missionary Society. Not that this was the first in the field. The Jesuits and the Carmelites had been established and had retired again many years before the Protestant missions even began to think of evangelizing Persia. These early Catholic missions paid very little attention to the strictly medical side of their work and in fact their own views on medical questions differed so little from the current Persian views that their influence in effecting any change in native scientific thought was nil.

The first two men who may correctly be styled medical missionaries, in that they were primarily doctors and not missionaries who had acquired a smattering of medicine, were two Moravians named Hocker and Rueffer, who appeared in Persia in 1747 with the intention of working among the Parsees. They suffered repeated robberies and hardships. The lawless state of the country under Nádir Sháh was the greatest barrier to any spread of their faith and they departed unable to accomplish anything. In the early nineteenth century Protestant missionary work became more active. Henry Martyn reached Shiraz, the 'seat of Satan' he called it, on 9 June 1811. Dr Pfander of the Basle Society entered Tabriz in 1829 and Dr William Glen of the Scottish Missionary Society arrived in Persia in 1838. By then the American Congregational Mission was already established in the northern provinces, but this mission did not attempt any medical work until after its transference to the Presbyterian Board in 1871.

Dr Cochran was the physician in charge of the first American Mission Hospital to be opened in Persia. This was at Urumia. His life story is of extreme interest. In 1880 he began to build, and two years later he had two wards of twenty beds each, an operating theatre, and two medical students to help. His statement that it was 'the first hospital of any kind in Persia' is, of course, not quite accurate.[1]

1 Speer, *The Foreign Doctor: a biography of Joseph Plumb Cochran*, 1911, p. 23. New York: Revell.

To the Reverend Robert Bruce must be given the credit of building the first British Mission Hospital. Mr Bruce was a missionary in the Punjab from 1858 to 1868. Realizing the importance of a knowledge of Persian for social intercourse with educated Indians he obtained permission to spend a year in Persia learning the language. This year was prolonged to another year. The great famine of 1871 found him in charge of relief measures and he stayed on. Thus instead of staying for a holiday of one year he remained in Persia until the end of his working days.

The visit of the shah to England in 1873 was made the opportunity of presenting to him a memorial praying for religious liberty. Only a very limited amount was granted. But it was enough to make a start and in 1879 the Rev. E. F. Hoernle, an Edinburgh medical man, went out to join Mr Bruce and to establish a Medical Mission.

Work now began. The first hospital was opened in Julfa, an Armenian village two miles south of Ispahan. The resignation of Dr Hoernle left the hospital for three years without a qualified head. The advent of Dr D. W. Carr in 1894 meant the beginning of a new era and the beginning of successful missionary and medical work for which Ispahan and Persia as a whole cannot be too grateful. Two dispensaries were opened in different quarters of the city of Ispahan by that heroic worker Miss Mary Bird and were closed again by orders of the authorities. Another at Jubara was closed by force on two occasions, but being in the Jewish quarter permission was obtained for it to be reopened. In these few years from 1894 to 1897 no fewer than five dispensaries were forcibly shut up. Yet the Society persevered and in 1897 a separate hospital for women was opened in Julfa under the care of Dr Emmelina Stuart.

In 1902 there was made what proved to be the final attempt to open a dispensary in the Mohammedan quarter of Ispahan. Dr Carr rented a house in the city in which he resided. In this, his own private house, he opened a dispensary and the work went quietly on and without further difficulty. In the following year negotiations were opened with a wealthy Persian gentleman and through him a suitable piece of ground was obtained of about seven acres on the edge of the city where a hospital for men, a hospital for women, and houses for the doctors and nurses could be built. Nor was Ispahan the only city to benefit by the unselfish learning of these medical missionaries. They settled at Yezd in 1898, in Kerman in 1901 and in Shiraz in 1923. Their arrival in each of these towns was soon followed by the building of a hospital.

This work in the provinces was complimentary to the work that the Dár-ul-Fanún was performing in Teheran. In the Mission hospitals in a far humbler manner young Persians were receiving a grounding in anatomy and physiology. Their clinical teaching was at the least as good as others were receiving in Teheran. Ultimately these facts were acknowledged by the Persian Government and these hospitals were recognized by the central licensing body as the only method of graduation in medicine in the whole country outside Teheran. Being ostentatiously Christian the work met with the greatest opposition from the *mullás*, the Islamic clergy, with whom the old-fashioned practitioners allied themselves with a keenness which does no credit to their ethical code. Their hostility was, however, short-lived. In less than 20 years these same chief *mullás*, who at one time sent men to drive away the patients from the hospitals, now begged that they themselves be admitted and treated. The Persian practitioners followed this lead and began to ask the mission doctors to see cases in consultation. The upper classes, who at one time would not even come near a hospital, at length approached without hesitation. Finally, in 1914, the Persian Government made a grant of government funds to the hospital in Ispahan.

This changed outlook in the provinces was the reflection of what the Central Government was thinking. A series of laws regulating the practice of medicine and pharmacy, approved by the Sanitary Council and ratified by the *Majlis*, drove the last nail into the coffin which held the body of Greek and Arab medicine. By the law of 1911 a Medical Register was established. All practitioners had to apply for registration. All who had already been in practice for ten years or more were without further question inscribed. Others had to pass an examination or get a certificate of capacity. There was no Sinán in the land in those days and none of the incidents, so dear to the old Arab medical chroniclers, seem to have occurred. The number of applications for registration is said to have been just over five hundred. From that date it became illegal for anyone to practise as a physician within the frontiers of Persia who did not hold a diploma of the University of Teheran or of a University approved of by the Sanitary Council. The post of lecturer in Avicennan medicine was at the same time abolished. All these reforms meant that with the death of the practising exponents of the system of Rhazes, Haly Abbas and Avicenna, the system too would die. The time honoured custom of serving a medical apprenticeship was also killed. The *shaykhs* and native *ḥakíms* could no longer attract pupils to whom they could impart their empirical knowledge and practical experience. Just when advanced thinkers in Europe were beginning to grow dissatisfied with their system of medical education and to wish to revert to what was good in the old, Persia decided to be up-to-date and to imitate blindly the unsatisfactory system of her contemporaries.

The Persian Government were by no means content with having raised thus far the general medical standard. They determined to raise it still higher. For this purpose fresh professors were brought out to infuse new life and new ideas into the Dár-ul-Fanún. Among those attached to the medical faculty were Dr Gachet, a French naval surgeon, who was given a three-year contract as Professor of Physiology and was at once elected President of the Sanitary Council in the place of Dr Georges. With him came Dr Lattes as Professor of Chemistry and Dr Le Blanc as Professor of Natural History. Another newcomer was

Dr Stump who came to Persia as dentist to the shah and became the first lecturer in dentistry in the Medical School.

The internal situation of the country gave no great cause for alarm. The mutual antagonism of Russia and Great Britain had been temporarily settled by an agreement between the two. The renaissance of medicine had been followed by a renaissance of nationalism. The shah's position was as yet unshaken by the democratic movement, and no doubt with wise advisers he could have steered the new political creeds into safe channels. Medicine, public health and sanitary knowledge were all advancing rapidly under the wise and far-seeing policy of the later Qájárs. All these advances were abruptly checked by the politics of Europe in which Persia had no say, no concern and no interests at stake.

CHAPTER XIX

THE NATIONALIZATION OF THE MEDICAL SERVICES

IN order to understand the various moves in the medical politics of the years that immediately followed the War of 1914–18, it is necessary to know something of the internal history of Persia during the years of the war. For, though nominally a neutral power, Persia suffered relatively as much as any of the combatants, and medicine, being so linked to politics in that country, it was the final position on the political chess-board, when Europe had time to think of something beyond the manufacture of ammunition, that determined the solution of the various medical problems which arose in rapid succession.

For many years the Government of India held firmly to the idea that one day Russia would invade India by way of Persia. This was the mainspring of their foreign policy. St Petersburgh and the Press gallantly responded, so that at the dawn of the twentieth century Persia found herself still alternately flattered and threatened by the British and by the Russians. To a large extent Persia gained by this policy, for she could always play off one power against the other. But it was an humiliating position and galling to a certain section of the better educated and more patriotic Persians. The weakness and selfishness of Muẓaffar-ul-Dín S͟háh led to the so-called Persian Revolution, which opened with the Bakhtiari march on Teheran under the Sipah Sálár in 1906. The hospitality of the British Legation, albeit unwilling, to the odd 10,000 citizens who sat in *bast* within its gates, like an ancient Jewish city of refuge, lead directly to the destruction of the autocracy of the shah and to the granting of a charter of constitutional liberties and parliamentary institutions. For their share in this the British received an undue amount of credit.

However, the prestige thus gained was very largely lost again in the following year when the British Government entered into an agreement with the Russian to cease to set up altar against altar and to cease to proselytize except within a defined area. To the Russians was allotted the north of Persia; to the British the south-east. Between the two ran a small neutral sphere which included the whole of the Persian Gulf littoral. The patriotic party at once denounced the Agreement and both parties to it. But the howling patriots howled in vain. An infuriated parliament, still wrapped in the swaddling clothes of novelty and hardly yet articulate, was persuaded by the Royal Artillery to disperse. The shah again became an autocrat and a little later was once again forced to call a parliament. In the midst of the strife Muẓaffar-ul-Dín died and the young *Valí ʻAhd*, too young to ascend the throne, became the nominal ruler of Persia.

In 1914 Aḥmad was still uncrowned: he was still a minor. The Regent Náṣir-ul-Mulk was an old man and was anxious to lay down the burden of holding the balance between the activities of the two paramount foreign powers and of suppressing the bubbling enthusiasms of his patriotic countrymen. By a juggling with the calendar he succeeded in getting the *mujtahids* to proclaim that Aḥmad would be of the correct age by July to ascend the throne and to his intense relief on 21 July Aḥmad was indeed crowned and proclaimed *S͟háhins͟háh*.

By now, so well had the Russians used their privileges that England had granted them over Persian territory, that the northern provinces were filled with their troops. In the south the British had been somewhat less active; but there were regular troops stationed at Bushire and within the compounds of the Legation and the Consulates. Hence it is not surprising that when war broke out in Europe and the British and the Russians were found to be fighting as allies, the Persians were as a whole sympathetic with the powers that were opposing them. When Turkey, another great Mohammedan power the boundaries of whose empire were contiguous with the whole of the western frontier of Persia, also joined in with the Central Powers against the Russians and British, the Persians could scarcely be expected to conceal with which side their hopes and well-wishes lay.

Before the end of the year Persia was involved in the struggle; for the Turks, in order to forestall the flanking movement by the Russian Caucasian Army, violated Persian neutrality and entered the province of Azerbaijan. To meet this attack the Russians were unable to produce a sufficient force and in the first week of January 1915 the Turks occupied Tabriz.

In the following month it was British prestige which received the blow, for a party of Arabs attacked the pipe-line of the Anglo-Persian Oil Company and did considerable damage. Then the Teheranis, stirred up by pro-German agents and by Austrian prisoners who had escaped from the prison encampments of the Caucasus, rose up and attempted to destroy the Imperial Bank which was looked upon as a British institution. The small loans, bribes would be the more correct term, which the Russian and British Governments made to the Central Persian Government were useless and had no influence in the face of Turkish and pro-German successes. The Central Government was incapable of controlling even the populace of Teheran. The Swedish officers of the gendarmerie, who might have helped to maintain order, were withdrawn by their own government. The treasury was empty: the young king was without influence or power. Turkish troops were in occupation of Kermanshah and Tabriz: the Persian cabinet in despair resigned.

Active in the south was one of those uncanny, almost fabulous, German agents, whose power and influence was immense and who, like the Captain of the *Emden*, won as much respect from his foes as from his friends. This was Herr Wassmuss who, seeing the complete discomfiture in the north and the preoccupation of the British elsewhere, determined to complete the rout of the Allied cause. With this intention he organized an attack upon the British Residency in Bushire. The permanent Residency guard was too small to hold out for long. To defend the political resident the Government of India landed troops, and again Persian neutrality was violated. Bushire itself was held, but in the interior affairs did not go so well. In Shiraz the English Vice-Consul was killed by the populace. In Ispahan the Russian Consul was killed and the British Consul-General wounded. Finally in September the Allied consular staff was forced to evacuate Ispahan altogether and nearly all Persia fell into the hands of the pro-German party.

It was now that the shah received an offer of a loan from the Central European Powers. The temptation to accept must have been enormous. The Allies were not doing too well in the West; they were almost at the last ditch in Persia itself. But the shah vacillated, and in November Russian troops were hurriedly disembarked at Enzeli and pushed up to Kazvin with their outposts stationed at Keradj—only 25 miles from the walls of Teheran. This decided him and instead of accepting the German offer he attempted to come to some sort of agreement with the Allied forces. The all-but-victorious pro-German elements were not thus to be treated. The proximity of Russian troops to Teheran made it incumbent upon them to carry on their activities a little further away. Accordingly, the German, Austrian and Turkish diplomats transferred their Legations and staffs from Teheran to Ispahan and attempted to take the shah with them. The greater part of the Persian Government followed the foreign Legations, but the British minister was able to persuade the shah himself to remain in Teheran under the protection of the Russian and his own escorts.

With the exception of the sovereign the exodus was complete and the *Muḥájirín* set up a provisional government at Qum, some 90 miles south of Teheran. This did not long survive, for a threatened Russian attack upon the town forced the grandees and pro-German members of parliament to flee further south to Ispahan. Not unnaturally other parts of Persia received misleading reports about what was occurring in the capital. In Shiraz a rumour was circulated that the shah had left Teheran and declared war upon the Allies. The British Consul was promptly arrested and the Imperial Bank looted. All over Persia there were risings against the British and Russians and in November and December such widely distant places as Hamadan, Kerman and Yezd were evacuated by the nationals of the Allied nations. Only Bushire remained in British hands.

The Russians did their utmost to support the Allied cause. To threaten Ispahan they pushed beyond Teheran as far as Kashan. The result of this move was that on Christmas Day the Farmán Farmá became the theoretical head of the government. In the early part of 1916 the Russians met with an even greater success when they began to drive the Turks back towards the frontiers of Mesopotamia. Counting upon the services she was rendering to Persia by saving her from the Turks, the Russian Government now began to ask for certain concessions. The Farmán Farmá, who had no objections to the Turks and was not prepared to sell his country for these services, rather than yield resigned. His place was taken by that sturdy old patriot the Sipah Sálár, who though primarily a Nationalist was also a pro-Ally. With him in power an agreement was rapidly made, allowing a Russian and British control of the finances. But within a few days of its signature the paper upon which it was written became more valuable than the concession, for the Turks were reinforced and vigorously attacking drove back the Russians to the east of Hamadan and threatened Teheran itself. This time it was the Allied community which evacuated Teheran and all women and children were rapidly removed to Enzeli. So the year closed with governments rising and falling as Turks or Russians were reinforced and advanced or retreated.

The opening months of 1917 were scarcely a happy time for the supporters in Persia of the Allied cause. The Bolshevik rebellion, which broke out in Russia in March, did nothing to make it more hopeful. Many Persians who favoured the Allies, were murdered in different parts of the country. The Cabinet of the moment under Vossugh-ul-Doula, which sympathized with the Allies, resigned. A most unfortunate lack of rain, which caused a very poor harvest and a minor degree of famine, completed the discontent of the populace. By the end of the year Russian influence was at its lowest ebb. Discipline among such Russian troops as remained was almost non-existent: there was no co-ordination or union among the pro-Ally groups. Great Britain stood as the sole organized representative of the Allied cause. Thus it was that Great Britain alone received the curses of the Persians when the Allied cause was low and Great Britain alone who received the rewards of the ultimate Allied victory.

But if in this year the Russian defection is to be set against the Allied cause, the capture of Baghdad is certainly to be added to the credit side. Nevertheless, the effect was not so great on internal Persian politics as might have been expected. The effect was not an immediate crumpling up of the Turkish forces. In the following year they made another determined attack upon the province of Azerbaijan, and finding no Imperial Russian troops to bar their progress pushed on towards Kazvin. A small British mission, sent off to Enzeli to join up with the White Russian forces there, was foiled by the bandit Kuchik Khán and his horde of *jangalís*, and once again to save the capital Allied troops were hurried up. This time it was British forces which were sent from Baghdad and which joining the White Russian Colonel Bicharakoff occupied Resht and Enzeli. Teheran was saved. But the Persians were far from considering that Teheran had been saved for their sake. After a succession of cabinets the government at that moment was under Ṣamṣám-ul-Salṭana. Perversely, it seems, he now looked upon Soviet Russia as his friend. Always is the Persian fated to consider that party which is not in power or is even twice removed from power, as his greatest friend. Ṣamṣám-ul-Salṭana, holding that his country's salvation would come through Soviet hands now did his utmost to defeat the only power which was capable of keeping order in Persia. He induced the Kashgais to declare war upon the South Persia Rifles, a police force organized by Sir Percy Sykes and officered by British and

Indian officers. He took no steps to stop the brigandage around Ispahan which was a continual menace to the scattered British forces of law and order. In his political actions the same hostility was manifest, for he suppressed the Foreign Office tribunals and abolished all concessions granted to Imperial Russia. But his policy recoiled upon his own head, for disturbances broke out in Teheran and in August the shah, seeing which way the war was going in France, determined not to have a pro-German government in power and summarily dismissed him. Once again Vossugh-ul-Doula came into power, and, when the Allies were signing the armistice in the West, Persia was on the right side of the fence. The Central Cabinet was pro-British; Sirdár Jang of the pro-British Bakhtiari tribe was Governor-General in Ispahan; and in the south the South Persia Rifles under a British general held the land in moderate control. Only around Tabriz, where Turkish troops were still on Persian soil, was the Allied cause disputed.

It is not difficult to see that during these five years of incessant change, when no cabinet lasted for more than a few months, when the reverses on the Western Front were reflected in the varying opinions of Persian statesmen and people, no advances in the medical or sanitary situation of the country were possible. But with the signing of the Armistice in the West at once an important epoch of medical history in Persia began. It is important therefore to realize the position which Great Britain held and to see how that position was obtained. For it explains why the great wave of nationalism broke mainly upon Britain. It explains how it was that the Qájár dynasty fell, a dynasty which had done so little for the advancement and promotion of medicine, and how the Pahlaví dynasty came into being under a ruler who from his earliest days of power showed himself interested in the public health of the people of Persia.

The Cabinet of Vossugh-ul-Doula, which had come into power in the summer of 1918, remained in office longer than any of its predecessors. British prestige was now at its highest point.

The voice of the Turks was silent owing to their double defeat in Palestine and Mesopotamia. Not unnaturally the shah personally regarded the Soviet Republic with suspicion. Both the condition of Europe and the internal position of Persia warranted a closer relationship with England. Accordingly, in the August of the following year the famous Anglo-Persian Convention was drawn up and signed and the shah, having gained, as he thought, a breathing space, left his kingdom for Europe.

Of the terms of the Convention it is unnecessary to go into detail. Suffice it to say that the terms were not made known to the general public and that the *Majlis* was not called upon to ratify them, although the British Legation again and again urged Vossugh to adopt the normal legal procedure. Although not actually part of the Convention a subsidiary agreement was entered upon between Vossugh-ul-Doula and Sir Percy Cox, the British minister, by which the Imperial Persian Hospital was handed over to British control, to be conducted upon British lines, maintaining a Persian only as the nominal director. The story of the brief period of this rule illustrates the immense difficulties which Persia had to contend with in those times in all matters of medical reform. It also shows the sad effects of politics and nepotism upon science and public health.

Almost in the centre of the city of Teheran midway between the old and the new royal palaces stands a low old-fashioned building, lying back from the road. It is approached through an ornate gateway, decorated by glazed tiles bearing an inscription in elaborate Arabic lettering. Through the wide doors is to be seen a courtyard with a formal garden and tiled pond in the centre. At the back of this building lie the slums of the 'Arq quarter of the city. In front is the tramway, the big Artillery Square, in turn parade ground, polo ground, and public garden, and in the distance the snow-capped hills of Shimran. The hospital, as I have already mentioned, was founded in 1868 and for the first twelve years was directed by Persian graduates. It was then placed under the control of a German doctor who was lecturer in medicine in the Dár-ul-Fanún. In 1896 Muẕaffar-ul-Dín Sháh gave a new *firmán* to the physician of the German Legation to organize and direct the hospital upon modern lines. Under his guidance the hospital grew and a second German doctor came out as assistant. In 1914, both doctors being military officers, one of them was recalled and Dr Ilberg, the senior physician to the German Legation, remained in control.

In November 1915, the month when the Legations of the Central Powers left Teheran, Dr Ilberg was obliged to follow his chief, and the hospital, thus deprived of both its European physicians, again passed into Persian hands. The shah appointed to the vacant post of Director his own physician Loqmán-ul-Mamálik, but the clinical work was carried on by the two senior Persian assistants. In the following year their rule received a brief but violent interruption when the Russian General Baratov obtained permission to use part of the hospital for his troops. The uncertainties of the situation, the rough usage of the buildings by a people always in a state of war, frequently in a state of siege, led to a steady deterioration in personnel and equipment, so that by 1918 the hospital could deal with not more than thirty in-patients at a time. This fact, the long-felt want for a hospital under British administration, and the probability of the Germans returning led His Majesty's Minister when negotiating the Anglo-Persian Convention, to propose that an offer should be made to reorganize the hospital. The Persian Government were not slow in agreeing and gave its formal acceptance on 11 May 1919. According to the terms of the agreement Great Britain undertook to provide two medical officers and to give financial assistance for the purchase of material. The Persian Government undertook to raise the budget from Ts. 12,000 to Ts. 24,000 in view of the great rise of prices. Thereupon Dr A. R. Neligan, Physician to the British Legation, and Dr J. Scott, the Medical Superintendent of the Indo-European Telegraph Department, were appointed as the first medical officers. The British Government at once contributed £2500.

The medical administration of the hospital was formally taken over on 1 June. By the instructions of the Prime Minister the two British doctors were received at the main door of the hospital by Dr Ḥakím-ul-Doula, the Director and Physician to the shah. Their reception was cordial and they at once made an inspection of the hospital and its contents. The result was appalling; they found before them an Augean task. The number of beds was now forty-eight. But everything was hopelessly worn out and in a terrible state of dirt and decay. In his first official report Dr Neligan thus summed up the situation:

> The buildings were old, inconvenient, ill-ventilated, and badly lighted; sanitation and conservancy generally were very bad; repairs and cleaning were required everywhere; the material was absolutely insufficient; there was no separate section for women, no isolation wards, no rooms for special departments, no laundry, no proper baths, no laboratory, no mortuary; the nurses were untrained and were not of the class that could be trained. The hospital was badly thought of, was in debt, and had difficulty in obtaining payment of its budget. War conditions still prevailed, extravagant local prices, impossibility of finding at Teheran much that was urgently needed, slow transport from abroad. Dr Scott and I were in fact not a little dismayed at the prospect. We had, however, the goodwill of the Persian Government, of the staff, and of the Persians generally; the promise of a substantial increase in the budget and the certainty of a generous contribution from His Majesty's Government.

Within a month of the beginning of British control the Director Ḥakím-ul-Doula left with the shah for Europe and Dr Aalam-ul-Mulk was appointed to act in his place. Unfortunately both British officers also felt the need for home leave, having been virtual prisoners in Persia since their last leave before the war. Dr Scott was the first to go; in his place Dr Woollatt, also of the Telegraph Department, came on to the staff. In Dr Neligan's place came Col. A. Irvine Fortescue, a military doctor who had arrived in Persia with the British expeditionary forces. A British matron arrived in the spring and there seemed every possibility that with the return of the two regular physicians the hospital would take on a fresh lease of life.

But troubles, internal and external, soon developed. Even before Dr Neligan's departure on leave one of the assistant physicians sent in an application for an increase in salary, adding that he would resign if it was not granted. At the same time he absented himself from the hospital without permission or warning. He was summarily dismissed, an action which was quite unexpected and caused considerable stir among the native medical confraternity. His post for a short time being unfilled the Minister of Public Instruction without any consultation with the medical staff nominated his own family doctor to the vacant post. He was a man utterly unsuitable and in the words of Dr Neligan 'dangerously ignorant'. He left at the end of a month. The post was then formally advertised, and the two British doctors acting in consultation with the Director elected a well-qualified young Persian of the name of Ḥusayn Kh̲án Moqaddam.

This hospital should, of course, have been made the centre of clinical study for all medical students wishing to receive the diploma of the University. But unfortunately it was impossible to interest any of the Teherani physicians. In an attempt to do so three more Persians were elected to the staff, Dr Lessan Chams, the Lissán-ul-Ḥukamá, who was given charge of the department for diseases of the eyes, Dr Mirzá Muḥammad Kh̲án 'Alá'í, who was a graduate of the University College of London and an excellent general physician, and Dr Moussa Kh̲án, who had also received some training in London, having been clinical assistant in Moorfields Hospital. In the meantime progress had been made. The number of beds was raised to eighty-eight, and the out-patient attendances for the first year were only a few short of 4000.

In the first year of the British control the checks to the growth of the hospital were only slight. The work went on normally except for increasing money difficulties. This was due to the pressure of political events upon the Central Government. In

April 1920 a Bolshevik invasion was threatened. The British troops in North Persia were too few to withstand it and they withdrew to Manjil, a little village midway between Resht and Qazvin. Here they blew up the bridge over the Safid Rud and prepared to hold the pass which led up to Qazvin. The Bolsheviks landed at Enzeli without any opposition and advanced to Resht where they were joined by Kuchik Khán and the *jangalís*. In May the shah returned to find his country even more disturbed than when he had left in the previous August. His return synchronized with a rising anti-British feeling. The terms of the Anglo-Persian Convention had now become known. The star of the Bolsheviks appeared to be rising. The policy of the British Government at home was known to be one of non-interference in Asiatic affairs. Was this not evident from the hurried retreat to Manjil and the failure to send up reinforcements from Baghdad? Popular opposition grew, and in June Vossugh-ul-Doula resigned. He was succeeded by Mushír-ul-Doula, who feebly asked the *Majlis* to ratify the Anglo-Persian Convention. The English experts, lent to the Government by the terms of the Convention, were already on the spot and the *Majlis* felt in no mood to ratify contrary to popular opinion a *fait accompli*. In spite of some success against the Bolsheviks in Mazanderan and Azerbaijan the British were compelled in July to fall back from Manjil upon Qazvin. From that moment the Anglo-Persian Convention was a dead letter and without waiting to be formally expelled the British experts ceased work. The autumn was occupied in a pendulum-like movement of the Bolshevik and Persian troops and with the fall of the Mushír-ul-Doula cabinet. The startling event at the end of the year was an offer from Moscow to withdraw all Soviet troops from Persian territory on condition that the British were also withdrawn. This suited the Home Government excellently and England placed no difficulty in the way of Persian agreement. Accordingly, on 26 February 1921, the Russo-Persian Treaty was signed. By June all Russian forces were withdrawn.

It was now the financial situation that assumed the leading place in deciding how events were to shape themselves. The Persian Government had long ceased to pay the budget to the British hospital in advance and a return had been made to the hand-to-mouth existence with relatively heavy debts outside and arrears of pay within. The Persian administration was still bad. The director visited the hospital only at rare intervals. The frequent changes of cabinet provided the authorities with an excuse for not remedying matters and the alleged Bolshevik menace to Teheran supplied a further reason.

The Persian Government had towards the close of 1920 collected a large number of Bolshevik prisoners in a camp just outside Teheran. It was quite evident that this camp was disgracefully mismanaged. Typhus, small-pox, scurvy and dysentery broke out. The Government took fright, fearing complications with the Bolshevik minister who was due to arrive soon. They turned to the hospital as the only means of saving the situation. The medical and nursing staff had then a most unpleasant task for the next few weeks. The hospital was over-crowded and over-worked. At one time there were ninety in-patients. By March 1921 the worst was over, though the camp continued to send in its worst cases for some time longer. This episode caused a heavy drain upon the funds of the hospital and it was many months before they were refunded.

The political situation had by this time altered adversely towards the English and the change made itself felt even in the hospital. It now became known as 'The English Hospital', for the hospital arrangement was looked upon as a part of the Anglo-Persian Convention. Later on this feeling showed itself in some minor disturbances with the students. The Medical School authorities had not kept to their promise to make regular attendance at the hospital compulsory. Students came and went or did not come at all, just as they pleased. In July a young man was corrected for gross carelessness to a patient and ordered to leave the operating theatre. The students were seized upon by agitators and went on strike. A newspaper campaign against the English staff was started. At the same time indignation meetings were arranged for the local professors. The students formulated their complaints. The medical staff on their side also made some proposals for the regulation of clinical instruction and the teaching of the pre-medical subjects. But through the supineness of the School authorities none of these reforms was carried out. The prestige of the hospital sank rapidly; and finally its influence in the teaching of the University fell to vanishing point.

In the meantime an event of first-rate importance to Persia had occurred. On 19 January 1921 the Sipahdár-i-A'ẓam, who had succeeded Mushír-ul-Doula as Prime Minister in the November of the previous year, resigned. The shah could find no one to take his place and on 16 February reinstated him. But the treasury was empty; the Cossack forces, which had once been the trained and disciplined escort of the sovereign, were demoralized; the British forces by the terms of the Russo-Persian Treaty were about to leave the country; discontent was general; there was nothing between the shah and a pro-Bolshevik rising. On the night of 21 February there rode over the empty moat of the city of Teheran, through the Qazvin Gate and up the rough Khiábán-i-Aḥmadiyya a party of 3000 Cossacks with one Riẓá Khán in command. A colonel about whom not very much was known but who was reputed to be firm and resolute came into the city to protect the throne, as he said, and to eject an inefficient government. The Sipahdár at once disappeared and the shah under the guidance of Colonel Riẓá Khán appointed Sayyid Ẓiyá'-ul-Dín as Prime Minister. The director of the Government Hospital, Ḥakím-ul-Doula, obtained a seat in the new Ministry and became the first Minister of Public Health. Dr Seif-ul-Atibba was appointed Director of the Hospital in his place. The new Cabinet promptly denounced the Anglo-Persian Convention, and reforms of a far-reaching character were declared to be the object of the *coup d'état*.

But their excellent programme was too drastic for the Teheranis. Popular acclamation died down when it was found that Riẓá

Khán was determined to carry out his word. All classes were dissatisfied, above all the nobility, and within three months the Sayyid was in flight. The Ministry of Health was closed and Ḥakím-ul-Doula returned to the hospital. For his services the shah conferred upon Riẓá Khán the title of Sirdár Sipah.

The short-lived ministry of Ẓiyá'-ul-Dín was followed by that of Qawám-ul-Salṭana and the Fourth *Majlis* was summoned. But the political situation was too tense for anyone except one man to carry out any reforms. All departments of state were moribund, except one, his, and that the army. The financial situation grew steadily worse. In October and November things at the hospital were so bad that the British doctors wrote to the Minister of Public Instruction on the subject. The Director seldom came inside the hospital, the subordinate staff was unpaid and was with difficulty prevented from leaving. The patients were not properly fed, the buildings had not been repaired since the previous winter, no stocks of wood or fuel had been laid in for the coming winter. In November a number of beds were closed and it was decided to accept only urgent cases. Over and over again it was said that money would be forthcoming. The position of the British doctors was acute. The hospital was not only unable to fulfil its duties to the public, but it was also obliged to admit an unduly large proportion of severe cases, although there were no funds to ensure proper dieting, warming of the wards and theatres, disinfection and protection of the medical and nursing staffs. A large number of patients arrived in the last stages of surgical sepsis. The admission list included typhoid and typhus fevers, anthrax, glanders, leprosy, erysipelas, tetanus, dysentery and many cases of surgical tuberculosis. The most regrettable feature of all was the non-payment of the subordinate and menial staffs for nearly five months in an administration for which they regarded the British as responsible. In the circumstances it was not surprising that a great deal of pilfering went on or that window panes began to disappear at an alarming rate in view of the very high price of glass at the time. By December the number of in-patients had been reduced to twenty-five. About this time the Shaykh Hádí Hospital of thirty beds, which was opened in June for the French professors in the School of Medicine, was closed.

The activities of the hospital having been reduced to a minimum, it dragged on a bare existence for weeks on fees from paying patients, many presents from friends, an occasional gift of game and such like. Lady Cox's Fund kept it in coal and tree prunings in firewood. The municipality lent some money; the American Mission Church had a special collection. Thus they managed to avoid putting the remaining patients into the street and closing the doors (a method which had been used more than once in the past history of the hospital for solving similar situations) and on 13 February 1922 the Persian Government paid the budget for the previous five months and for the moment saved the situation. By now Qawám-ul-Salṭana had quarrelled with the Sirdár Sipah, the Cabinet had become the most hostile to England of modern times, the shah had again left for Europe, and the Director of the hospital had with a great sigh of relief left Persia in the suite of his royal master.

The year 1922 was indescribably bad for the hospital. Anti-British feeling running so strong and the work of the hospital being of such very little use either to the British community or to the poor of the town, the British Government refused to continue their annual allowance. Lest the closing down of the hospital should be attributed to poverty of the British Government or to British unwillingness to offer a helping hand to Persia or even given a political twist, the Anglo-Persian Oil Company were asked if they would be willing to continue to subsidize it. The Oil Company, though not without some misgivings, conceived it to be to their interests to take over the obligation of the British Treasury and agreed to continue the subsidy on condition that the British association with the hospital should be maintained. The Persian Government, who now scarcely attempted to conceal the fact that their object was to oust the British doctors and replace them by Persians, refused to accept the money on these conditions. An inefficient service under Persian control or even no hospital at all seemed better to them than a capable administration under British control. However, they were willing to let matters remain for the moment in *statu quo*, and agreed that the Oil Company should have the right to cease the subsidy without previous notice. These terms the Company found sufficient, and for a while the hospital was enabled to carry on under the British doctors.

The internal condition of the country remained in the same chaotic condition. Riẓá Khán, now Commander-in-Chief, was the only minister to hold office continuously throughout the year. The shah, when he returned in December, now found that it was neither the English nor the Russian peril which was to cause him sleepless nights. The *Majlis* had met and during the session passed into law a proposal that was ultimately to be used as a lever to drive out the British from all the medical posts in the country. It provided that no foreigner should remain in, or be appointed to, any post under the Persian Government unless he possessed a contract approved of by the *Majlis*. This, though obviously aimed at the prevention of the recurrence of any secret agreement, like the Anglo-Persian Convention, also in theory deprived Drs Neligan and Scott of their positions in the Imperial Hospital. For the moment no steps were taken. It appeared that the activities of the hospital would collapse from sheer inertia. In April the British matron left and no successor was appointed. When Dr Scott went on leave, a Persian took his place. Dr Neligan delegated part of his duties to Dr Ḥabíb Adlé, a French-trained Persian physician.

But these concessions were not enough. In the spring of 1923 it became evident that the status of the British doctors was going to be challenged, using as an excuse their inability to produce a contract ratified by the *Majlis*. Sir Percy Loraine, who had now succeeded Sir Percy Cox as Minister, contended that they were in a special position, as they were British Government servants, whose position in the hospital was regulated by the arrangement recorded in the exchange of notes in 1919, pointing out that it would be irregular and inconvenient for them to have contracts with a government other than that of their own. This question of a double contract had already arisen in the case of Major Stokes, once military attaché to the Legation, when he wished to work at the same time in the Persian gendarmerie, and was to arise again in the case of the officers of the Indian Medical Service who were serving in the Quarantine Service in the Persian Gulf. Such objections were brushed aside by the Persian authorities and in the late summer, Dr Scott being at the moment on leave, Dr Neligan was notified by Ḥakím-ul-Doula, who had again become Minister of Public Instruction, that he should cease attendance at the hospital, as he had refused to sign the contract. Loraine, as soon as he was shown this letter, took the strongest exception to the proceeding and had the letter returned. Thereupon an exhausting series of discussions took place with the Persian Government, who professed ignorance of the previous formal discussions, maintained that the arrangement of 1919 had in fact lapsed, owing to the withdrawal of the Treasury's annual subvention, that the law must be applied, and that the doctors could not serve in the hospital until the new *Majlis* had met and regularized the situation.

The Minister strongly suspected—and, as was afterwards shown, correctly—an intrigue by Ḥakím-ul-Doula to secure the positions in the hospital of Drs Neligan and Scott for his own relations, several of whom were members of the Persian medical faculty. He therefore insisted upon being told whether it was the intention of the Persian Government to rid themselves of the British doctors or merely to regularize the position. In the former case he would be compelled to take a very stiff line; in the latter he would do what he could to arrange matters in consultation with his Home Government. He was assured officially by the Persian Ministry of Foreign Affairs on several occasions that the sole desire of the Persian Government was to regularize the situation and harmonize it with the new law. The Minister therefore asked that the doctors should be invited to resume their duties at the hospital in the capacity of indispensable technical experts, for which there was a loop-hole left by the law and that pending the assembly of the new *Majlis* he should ascertain from London whether the doctors would be allowed to sign the contracts and, if so, of what nature. Time and time again it appeared that the Persian Government, who fully admitted the complete reasonableness of the Minister's attitude, were about to consent to this or to some similar arrangement; but the most constant pressure failed to extract a decision from them.

During all this year the position of Aḥmad Sháh was becoming more and more uncomfortable. He was terrified of his Commander-in-Chief, but hesitated to lose his kingdom by a secret flight. At last he determined to assure his own personal safety by yet another State visit to Europe. In Persia it is unconstitutional for the shah to announce in person his own departure to some foreign capital. Such an announcement had always to be made through the mouth of the Prime Minister. Unfortunately, at that moment there was no Prime Minister. The shah was reluctant to give that office to the one obvious man. In the autumn he could bear the strain no longer. Fears for his own physical safety took the upper hand and in return for a guarantee of safe conduct to the frontier he offered the Prime Ministership to the Sirdár Sipah. On 27 October the Sirdár accepted both the office and the conditions and in a due constitutional manner announced the impending departure of the reigning shah on a visit to Europe. On 4 November Aḥmad left Persia on the grounds of ill-health and the need for medical treatment and to Persia he never returned. Just two years later Riẓá Khán, Sirdár Sipah, Prime Minister, became Sháh Pahlaví, the *Sháhin-sháh* of Persia.

But to revert to the hospital. At the British Minister's first interview with the new Prime Minister in November, the Sirdár Sipah told Sir Percy Loraine that he wanted to settle this question.

He agreed that the doctors had been very badly treated and that their prestige ought to be vindicated. But he pleaded that it would be difficult for him to reinstate them in the Imperial Hospital, as this would involve the cancellation of appointments in their places of Persian doctors which the previous government had made just before their resignation. The Minister expressed his deep indignation at this treacherous violation of the official and repeated assurances given to him by the previous Ministry of Foreign Affairs which these appointments involved. It was afterwards found out that the Ministry were not so two-faced as it at first appeared and that neither the former Prime Minister nor Foreign Secretary were privy to the matter. Presumably the appointments were made by Ḥakím-ul-Doula on his own authority as Minister of Public Instruction for the profit of his relatives. Sir Percy Loraine added that the only adequate satisfaction was reinstatement. The Sirdár Sipah said that this was too difficult in the circumstances and suggested as an alternative that the two doctors should be appointed inspectors-general of all military and sanitary establishments. Sir Percy Loraine after further consideration made a final appeal for reinstatement in the hospital, saying that the doctors wished to do serious, practical and beneficial work for which the hospital alone offered both opportunities and facilities. The reply was most conciliatory and friendly in tone; it regretted that the question as regards the hospital could not be suitably reconsidered and put forward a new suggestion that the two doctors should be attached in some capacity to a new school of health which was to be founded in Teheran and in which it was believed that the doctors would be able to do much the same sort of work as in the hospital. The Minister was authorized to assent to these proposals, but such an authorization was never required. No new school of health was founded in Teheran in the days of Dr Neligan or Dr Scott. When the last of these two left the country for good, a stroller down the Khiábán-i-Sipah would have seen, as in the good old days before the English hustle, a sentry with a washed-out, much patched, blue tunic leaning up against the main gate of the Imperial Hospital. Within, an old man will be peaceably smoking his *qaliyán*, some dirty urchins will be playing in the corner, a butterfly floats lazily over the tank in the courtyard where the mosquitoes hum and rear their young, only occasionally is the peace broken by the arrival or departure of a sick man, a bearded doctor, or a mourning relative.

The signal success of the Persians in asserting their rights in the case of the Imperial Hospital stimulated them to yet further efforts in other directions. Leaving aside the questions of consular guards, capitulations and oil concessions which do not concern us here, the most important is the question of the quarantine in the Persian Gulf. It was only with the advent to power of the Sirdár Sipah that any policy could be both definite and continuous. It is not surprising then that it was in the year 1921 that the question of the British control of the Persian Gulf ports was reopened.

The first shot was fired by the Ministry of Foreign Affairs, who, in December of that year, politely requested from the Legation information about the right of the British to control the quarantine service in the Persian Gulf; 'for', they said, 'the Persian Government considers that the administration of quarantine, when necessary, is the duty of the sanitary officers of the Persian Government'.

No satisfactory reply being given, satisfactory that is in Persian eyes, the Cabinet followed up their letter by issuing an order to the local customs administration not to pay the quarantine expenses which they had been accustomed to do. They bade them inform the quarantine authorities that they should negotiate for their expenses directly with the Central Government. Unfortunately, by the time these orders reached the quarantine officials the cabinet had fallen and there was no constitutional central government. And more unfortunately still, plague had broken out at Basra and Mohammerah. The Sirdár Sipah was therefore only too glad, when approached on the subject by the

British Minister, to counter-order these instructions and to command that the payments should be continued as heretofore.

But the advance was not thus easily repulsed. The same line of attack was adopted by more subtle methods when the routine accounts of the Customs Department were submitted to the Treasury. In these accounts was included the payment to the quarantine officers. The Ministry of Public Instruction was asked to verify this item and, not wishing to have the responsibility of approving an item of expenditure which the late government had directly forbidden, passed the papers on to the Sanitary Council. The President of the Sanitary Council was equally unwilling to bless the accounts lest the Sirdár Sipah for any reason go back on his word. He therefore passed them on to the Ministry of Foreign Affairs who were in his opinion the only body competent to deal with the quarantine officers who were foreign subjects. The Ministry also was not thus to be caught and, unable to think of anywhere else to send the accounts, returned them to the Sanitary Council with the minute that they had no information to give. The Sanitary Council in despair turned the matter over to the Commission d'Hygiène, whose members being young and enthusiastic asked the Ministry of Finance for an explanation and called for a detailed report on the sanitary conditions in the Gulf and the quarantine arrangements in the Gulf ports.

At this time quarantine stations were being maintained and staffed by British medical officers at Mohammerah, Bushire, Bandar Abbas, Lingah and Jask. The Government of India supplied the medical officers. It paid their salaries, which, with the exception of the salaries of the Residency Surgeon at Bushire and of his two assistants, were recovered from the Persian Government. This item together with the ordinary expenses involved in the working and upkeep of the services, cost the Persian Government an annual sum of about £4500. This sum was not sufficient to meet repairs, new buildings or renewal of apparatus. In 1907 the Imperial and Indian exchequers had found it necessary to incur additional expenditure on various improvements, and again in this year the Chief Quarantine Medical Officer was compelled to ask for additional funds, pointing out to his Government that 'although the quarantine service operates primarily in the interests of Persia, it is also of real importance for the sanitary defence of adjacent countries, notably Iraq and India, and it is still of interest in checking the infiltration of plague, cholera, etc., from the East of Europe'.

There is no denying that the British authorities were bound to put their hands in their pockets and pay out something. The original plea of the Government of India had been one of danger from epidemics. To assure their own safety they had presented the Persian Government with a number of disinfecting apparatuses. That at Lingah had fallen into disrepair in 1914; those at Bandar Abbas and Jask during the following year. The Clayton Apparatus at Bushire was commandeered by the Mesopotamian Field Force in 1916, used, worn out and scrapped in 1918. The continuance of the Quarantine Service in British hands could only be justified if the disinfecting apparatus was maintained. The control of the Quarantine Service, as the Persians knew full well, offered the British a large measure of political and commercial prestige. If the service was to be found inefficient, the Persian Government would be well within their rights in taking it out of British hands and placing it under international control. To prevent any excuse for such action the Home and Indian Governments were prepared both to pay and to fight. A sum of £800 was sufficient for the moment, as the Sanitary Council on receipt of the report from the Chief Quarantine Medical Officer voted Ts. 2000 for unforeseen expenditure and Ts. 5000 for repairs and new work. The question of the repair of the Clayton Apparatus dragged on for several more months.

The year 1923 passed relatively quietly, but signs were not wanting that the Persian Government were mobilizing their forces for a yet more furious attack upon the Quarantine Service with a determined effort to replace the British by Persian doctors.

When the battle opened it was found that exactly the same methods were to be used as were successful in making untenable the position of the British doctors in the Imperial Hospital. The question of contracts was again raised. The British medical officers entered the Gulf at the request of the Persian Government. They were never offered contracts. When, then, the Ministry of Foreign Affairs asked the Legation for papers to show how British officers came to be employed in the Persian Gulf, they knew perfectly well what the answer would have to be. They then went a step further and announced that the question of payments to these unauthorized officers would be raised when the budget came to be voted upon by the *Majlis*. So important did the Government of India at that time think the retention of the British Quarantine Service that they were even willing to regularize the position and remove this opportunity of Persian attack by allowing their officers to sign contracts under the Persian Government. But the threatened attack in the *Majlis* was not made; the British service was not this year a subject of debate. The only change in the routine procedure was that Dr Millspaugh, the new American financial adviser, ordained that the salaries of the personnel of the service should be paid directly by the Treasury and not through the intermediary of the Customs Administration.

The Government of India was still fearful that an attempt would be made at the International Sanitary Conference in Paris in 1926, to show that they were not carrying out efficiently their obligations towards the shipping of all nations in the Gulf and that Persia, winning to its side nations unfriendly to Great Britain, would secure the transfer of the Quarantine Service to an international commission. They determined therefore, to strengthen their position by every possible means. They again raised the question of the desirability of establishing a sentinel sanitary station at Henjam. Any epidemic on the Arab side of the Gulf would cause a great flight of natives across to the Persian coast. In their opinion there should be a British quarantine officer at every port. Above all Henjam and Charbar should be protected, where at present there was no resident medical officer. The proposal for the use of Henjam was, however, again dropped, as it was pointed out that if the suggested quarantine station was part of a scheme for the prevention of the spread of epidemics outside the Gulf, the already existing station at Bandar Abbas was equally convenient. If, on the other hand, the object of the new station at Henjam was only to prevent the spread of disease within the Gulf, then such a station was quite unnecessary, because the island of Henjam is very small and very few passengers tranship there.

During all these troubled years the Sanitary Council had continued its chequered career. Dr Gachet, the President, was recalled to France in the opening months of the war and his place was taken by Dr Amir Aalam, a competent, single-minded physician, who had received a French training, spoke English and French moderately well, and was a relation by marriage with Vossugh-ul-Doula. During the troubled days of the war the Council did very little except meet with laudable regularity. Unfortunately, all the money which had been collected from the pilgrim and horse taxes disappeared and again it became an impotent, though principal, sanitary authority in the country.

After the *coup d'état* of Riẓá Kh̲án the Council was absorbed into the Ministry of Health in the Cabinet of Sayyid Ẓiyá'-ul-Dín. Dr Moadebod Dowleh, son of the famous Dr Náẓim-ul-Aṭibbá, was nominated as first Minister of Health and *ex-officio* became President of the Council. The Sayyid's Cabinet lasted only a few months. When it fell, Moadebod Dowleh retired into private practice again and Ḥakím-ul-Doula took his place. Again the Cabinet thought fit to change the Sanitary Council. A new set of rules governing both the constitution and the procedure were drawn up. Instead of being attached to the Ministry of the Interior as before, its transference to the Ministry of Health (Ministère de l'Hygiène et de l'Assistance publique) was confirmed. Its title received a corresponding change. It now became known as the Supreme Council of the Ministry of Health (Conseil Supérieur du Ministère de l'Hygiène). Its composition remained unchanged: the representatives of the foreign legations retained their seats. Its duties, chiefly advisory before, now became completely so. No budget was allotted. Amir Aalam resumed the office of President.

Very soon, however, it became clear that the Council, probably because of the large foreign representation upon it, was regarded by certain members of the Government with no favourable eye. Its ancient model, the Constantinople Board of Health, had already disappeared. It seemed to be the policy of the Government to let the Persian Council follow suit. This could easily be brought about by the simple expedient of paying no attention to its recommendations, a method used with success before. At the April meeting of 1923 the President informed the members that the Minister of Public Instruction, to whom he was responsible, had informed him that in future all communications were to be transmitted through that ministry and not sent direct either to other ministries or to the foreign legations. This was an order in direct defiance of the *Règlement Intérieur*, approved of by the Government. Dr Amir Aalam was not slow in pointing out that their constitution of two years previous gave the Council the right of direct access, that such access assisted rapidity of action; and that the peculiar composition of the Council was greatly appreciated by the Persians in general and gave it great authority. In these circumstances he proposed to disregard the ministry's instructions until the cabinet as a whole took the same line. In this he was supported by the vote of the whole Council excepting the representative of the Ministry of Public Instruction.

A less direct attack was then made by the formation of a health section within the Ministry of Public Instruction. Through this health section the Minister could at any time take action without consulting the Council. This called forth a protest from Dr Mesnard, the Director of the Pasteur Institute, who was now the Vice-President of the Council.

It was clear that the Council was on its death-bed. To stave off dissolution Dr Amir Aalam appealed to the Sirdár Sipah. He first attempted to get the Council transferred from the aegis of the hostile Ministry of Public Instruction back to the Ministry of the Interior. In this he was unsuccessful. But he succeeded in persuading the Sirdár to abolish the health section of the Ministry of Public Instruction and to form a new department of State, which he called the Public Health Department. This was practically independent and had the authority of the Sanitary Council behind it. Dr Amir Aalam was appointed the first Director of this new department and Dr Khalil Shafaghi Alam-ul-Doula took his post of President of the Sanitary Council.

In his final address to the Council Dr Amir Aalam made a bold and frank exposure of the fearful state of the public health of the country. Personal rivalries, political disturbances and national bankruptcy had completely destroyed the organization which Dr Tholozan and Dr Schneider had spent so much time in building up. His position gave him such a unique knowledge and his nationality so surely removes all fears of exaggeration that I am inclined to quote this speech in full. He said:

Before leaving you I would like to give you some detailed information on the general condition of the Public Health Services.

For the last two years the general sanitary situation of the country has left much to be desired. Provincial Medical Officers of Health, having failed to receive for several months their salaries, have for the most part abandoned their posts. That is especially true of Khorasan. An indifference, a *laissez aller* truly regrettable reigns with regard to all questions of public health. Our plans, our schemes, our cries have had no chance of finding an echo in governmental or parliamentary circles. The Minister of Public Instruction in spite of his formal promises has done almost nothing for us during the two long years which have just passed. Forgetful of the written assurances which he gave to us, that Minister in one of his latest replies admits that he has been unable to fulfil his pledges and seems to me to insinuate that if nothing has been done, it is my fault, because during the two and a half months when I occupied the post of Minister of Public Instruction, no plans were put forward. It was, I regret to say, H. E. Ḥakím-ul-Doula who signed that letter.

To avoid all misunderstanding you will kindly allow me to quote the history of the three months when I was Minister in order to show you that your President has always done his duty.

The Cabinet, which two years ago entrusted to me the portfolio of Minister of Public Instruction, to which was attached that of Public Health, from the very beginning found itself in a financial crisis of the most severe and unfortunate kind the details of which you will allow me to pass over. The affairs of the Sanitary Council were no more satisfactory than those of the Ministry of Public Instruction. The provincial Medical Officers of Health had received no salary for seven, eight or even nine months. The personnel of the sanitary stations at Astara and Enzeli had not only not been paid for more than a year, but their salaries had been suppressed in the budget on the grounds that the Caspian Ports were in revolt. The sanitary personnel, who, contrary to the action of the functionaries of other administrations, had not deserted their posts, were punished instead of being rewarded. No warning had been given to them that they would not be paid.

It is not the Ministries of Public Instruction and Public Health alone which suffered. All ministries, all government departments found themselves in a similar state. In addition to these difficulties and an equally disquietening poverty the Government found itself faced with troubles and almost universal uprisings, the most serious being those in Khorasan, Gilan, Azerbaijan, Luristan and Kurdistan. During the three months of the life of our Cabinet the Ministers were occupied almost continuously with questions of prime importance and urgency. Expeditions had to be sent out on every side and means found to cover their expenses. The solution of troubles and the putting down of insurrections necessarily absorbed all our time and all the activities and efforts of the Government. Thanks to our young and valiant army with a commander of such courage at its head as H. H. the Sirdár Sipah, our renowned Minister of War, we were sure of success in the end. But still, money had to be found. Everything had to be sacrificed for the Army.

This does honour to our country, for it is a story of success after success in spite of all, of quietening of troubles and of suppressing of insurrections. In spite of its watch over this general grave situation, the Government did not fail to occupy itself with financial reforms. To be able to give the necessary development to public health I proposed a budget of Ts. 2,000,000. This sum well employed would have assured to us the means of ameliorating our public education and sanitary condition and was not disproportionate to our finances and the other expenses of the Treasury General.

I think that Persia could and ought to make great sacrifices in order to teach her people and assure her health. Money spent on education and physical health is money set out at interest, not money spent. Education and public health are the fundamental source of the riches and greatness of a country. This has been and always will be my principle.

In brief, on the days when I was due to explain to the Chamber the budget which I had drawn up, unfortunate quarrels arose among the deputies. The Budget Commission opposed my plans. And some days later the Cabinet fell and the financial crisis was over.

Although obliged to put a limit to our ambitions in sanitary matters, we are now forced to claim our arrears. We prepared and presented to the Minister of Public Instruction a restrained budget and in return we were promised marvels. But two long years have slowly passed during which we have been put off by promises and official assurances. When all the departmental budgets have been passed by Parliament, ours, which we had presented the first, has not even reached the committee stage owing to the dictates of the deputies or it has been forgotten by the committee at the command of the Minister of Public Instruction. In the closing days of the fourth session of the *Majlis* we see that we have been passed over. In all haste H. E. Ḥakím-ul-Doula has taken immense trouble to get approved a budget of cooked figures.

In 1925 Major Nicholson succeeded to the post of Chief Quarantine Medical Officer. In his initial report he did not attempt to conceal either from the British or from the Persian authorities the defects of the service. He found that payment by the Persian Government was in arrears. A sum of Rs. 25,700 for salaries and pensions for the twelve months July 1923 to June 1924 was still unpaid by the Persian Government. The Persian personnel who should have received their pay direct from the Persian Treasury, not through the Government of India, were threatening to strike. Against a routine annual expenditure of about Ts. 218,000 only Ts. 184,000 were allotted. In all these matters Major Nicholson found himself tied and helpless. He had no hand in the preparation of the budget, which was left to whatever official in Teheran happened to be in charge of the medical and sanitary affairs of the country. He reported to the Sanitary Council that there were no funds available for the hire of boats, for routine telegrams, and for emergencies. To the Legation in Teheran he reported that there was urgent need for new buildings and repairs to old ones, extra hospitals, extra equipment such as transport and jetties, and finally he begged the Minister to urge upon the Persian Government the need for payment of their past dues.

These reports received a very sympathetic hearing from Dr Amir Aalam, who was then still head of the newly founded Health Department. Again he drew up an ambitious programme. He proposed to construct quarantine stations at Pahlevi and Astara, Qasr-i-Shirin, Julfa, Lutfabad and Bandar-i-Gaz. The sanitary condition of Teheran was to be improved by the construction of a tuberculosis sanatorium and by improvements in the Women's Hospital. And, finally, Ts. 20,000 were to be allotted to repairs in the quarantine buildings in the Persian Gulf and Ts. 8000 were to be spent on the purchase of a new Clayton Apparatus. His programme was rejected *in toto* by the finance department.

In April 1926 Dr Neligan left the Legation after twenty years of service, devoted whole-heartedly to the welfare of Persia, and it fell to my lot to fight the battle of the Quarantine Service in the capital. In his final speech to the Sanitary Council, when bidding them farewell, he spoke very freely of the defects of the Persian public medical services. Dr Neligan never held a very high opinion of their methods or their men. His speech was listened to with a mixture of respect and relief. The loss to Persia which his departure meant was so completely overshadowed by the rejoicings of the coronation of Riẓá Khán, who in the same month was crowned Shah of Persia under the title of Riẓá Sháh

Pahlaví. With the exception of a few personal friends scarcely a Persian noticed the departure of a man who had been an outstanding figure in the Persian medical world from the first days of the Revolution until the accession of the Pahlaví dynasty. A small reception in the School of Medicine was hardly the reward which might be expected by a man who had been President of the Sanitary Council, founder of the Vaccination Service, personal physician to all the leading families of the realm, and a willing adviser at all times on all matters connected with medical education.

In May the International Sanitary Conference opened in Paris. It seemed to be passing off as smoothly as such conferences usually do. The Persian delegate appeared to be ignorant of the defects in the Gulf Quarantine Service; at least, he showed no signs of attacking the British Government for any failures in this respect. Quite suddenly, on 16 June a few days before the new Convention was to be signed, he refused to re-indorse Article 83 of the 1912 Convention, which had been incorporated in the new Convention and up to that moment had been passed without debate. He claimed that 'it consecrated a system which was humiliating for Persia and unjustifiable on technical grounds' and that the Persians were now quite capable of managing their own affairs. The article in question ran as follows:

> Le régime sanitaire du Titre 1er de la présente Convention sera appliqué, en ce qui concerne la navigation dans le Golfe Persique, par les authorités sanitaires des ports tant au départ qu'à l'arrivée.

In vain the President of the Conference pointed out that the issue so raised was a political and not a sanitary question. The Persian stood to his guns; he was determined to make a gesture for Persian independence before the whole world. The scene in the Council Chamber was the most dramatic of the session. A vote on the retention of the article in its old form was made by a show of hands. There were many abstentions and the total count showed an equal vote.

The British delegate then spoke at great length on the question. He pointed out the danger to shipping, to India and to Europe, that it had certainly grown no less since the Quarantine Service was established, but rather the reverse. The advent of aeroplanes, the establishment of a trans-desert motor service and the opening of the Basra-Baghdad-Aleppo railway had brought the Levant and Eastern Europe to within the incubation period for plague and cholera, if a passenger was infected in the Gulf. Persian medical training had not yet reached the stage necessary for entrusting such responsibility to the Persians. But the delegate would not compromise. It was then put to a secret vote. This time the Persian objection was overruled. Unwillingly he signed the Convention, but added a reservation, to which the British, when they in turn signed, added the following reply:

> La délégation britannique tient à faire constater que la réserve persane ne peut en aucun façon modifier le *statu quo* actuel en attendant un accord à intervenir entre les gouvernements persan et britannique.

It was now perfectly clear that it was only a matter of time before the Persian Government assumed the complete control of the Quarantine Service in the Gulf. In fact, in January 1927 the Ministry of Foreign Affairs without any concealment or veiling of their aim asked the Legation when the Quarantine Service was to be transferred to them.

Such was the state of affairs when Sir Robert Clive arrived in Teheran as British Minister. He was apparently instructed to set the whole service upon a permanent and legal footing. The position of the British officers had to be regularized according to the latest laws of the *Majlis*. He tried to make certain that the Persian Government would meet with regularity the financial needs of the service and that at no time should they be able to exercise pressure upon the Government of India by a threat to withhold salaries and pensions. And, finally, he had to make sure that the Persian Government accepted the service as a whole and would leave the individual appointments to the discretion of the Government of India. The foundations upon which he could build were the articles of the International Convention of 1912. The Convention of 1926, although reaffirmed with a reservation by both English and Persian delegates, was not ratified by the *Majlis* and left the Quarantine Service in *statu quo*. It was only upon the earlier Convention that diplomatic conversations could be based.

But the Persians would have none of this. On their side were two strong men—Taimur Tash, Minister of Court, and Bahrami, Head of the Health Department. The former, who had been a simple provincial deputy, had risen by skill and hard work to be the shah's right-hand man. The shah himself dealt with the army, Taimur Tash with everything else. Bahrami, although his critics were not slow to speak scathingly of his medical knowledge, was a man of fixed purpose. Neither he nor Taimur Tash were violently anti-English. Both meant to secure the immediate cession of the Quarantine Service to the Persians and steadily they pursued their course. Step after step was taken slowly and deliberately. Expostulations were in vain: Bahrami never withdrew.

In the spring of 1927 Dr Bahrami visited the Persian Gulf ports in person. On his return to Teheran he sought an interview with Mr Havard, then Oriental Secretary to the Legation, and explained to him what his scheme for a newly constituted quarantine service was. He had no desire to replace the British officers by doctors of his own nation, although he was careful to point out that he had already deprived all the Russian doctors in the Caspian ports of any power of interference in quarantine work. All he desired, he said, was that the service should remain as it was, but that the Persian Health Department should supervise and direct it. As the Quarantine Service had always worked under the direction of the Sanitary Council to whom the Chief Quarantine Medical Officer had held himself responsible, this did not seem a very important modification. It was accepted without demur.

On 28 May, a few days after Dr Bahrami's return, I received an invitation to a party at the house of Dr Hakim Aazam, the doctor who had represented Persia at the Sanitary Conference in Paris in the previous year and had created the storm in the teacup. There I found that Jawad Khan Sineke of the Foreign Office and I were the only guests. In the conversation that followed Hakim Aazam advanced the Persian demands a stage further than Dr Bahrami had told Mr Havard. Hakim Aazam declared himself perfectly satisfied with the present arrangements in the Gulf and maintained that all that he desired was that the position should be regularized. He suggested as a modification that the whole staff should be Persian and that the British medical officers should be appointed in the same way that the American financial advisers were, that is to say, supernumerary to the regular staff but with executive powers. Finally he said that the pay of the British medical officers was included in the budget of this year, but would not be included next year unless some satisfactory arrangement was made in the meantime.

This conversation I reported to the Minister who thought the demands reasonable.

Dr Bahrami then took a most audacious and far-reaching step; he appointed a Persian doctor as Chief Quarantine Officer in the place of Major Macgregor. The letter of appointment is on record:

To Dr Sayyid Abdul Ali Khan Tayyibi, Director of the Southern Health Department, Shiraz.

Farvardin 17th 1306.

On the authority of this letter you should bring all the quarantine stations of the Gulf Ports under your supervision, making inquiry into their precedence and giving necessary instructions regarding their personnel, budget, financial and professional affairs. Submit necessary reports to the Capital.

The newly appointed Chief Quarantine Officer thereupon wrote to Major Macgregor as follows:

Farvardin 23rd 1306.

In forwarding a copy of an order issued by the Director of General Health Department, I beg to state that it is necessary that you should in future submit your reports to the Southern Health Department direct concerning your actions connected with quarantine matters in the southern ports. You should ask from this Department for instruction in all professional matters as well as in questions of personnel, budget, appointments and dismissals of members and employees, and of finance. As was told to you verbally, you should send to the Southern Health Department as early as possible two copies of last year's budget and the budget prepared by you and Major Hall for this year. Also please send a nominal roll of Medical Officers and Staff together with a list of furniture and other articles of the Quarantine Service of the Southern Ports.

Major Macgregor briefly replied that he took his orders from Teheran and refused to obey. At once Dr Bahrami was informed by Mr Havard that he had acted *ultra vires* and that the whole subject was not to be thus prejudiced but would be settled by normal diplomatic action in due course.

A serious outbreak of cholera in the Persian Gulf in July put a stop for the moment to further quarrelling. Dr Tayyibi was only too glad to leave Major Macgregor in undisputed charge. The action of the Sanitary Council was prompt, even if somewhat melodramatic. An Anti-Cholera Commission was formed in Teheran with Dr Bahrami as chairman: vaccine was bought in Berlin and sent south by aeroplane: the Iraqo-Persian frontier was closed and all movement between Shiraz and the south was forbidden.

In view of the Persian claim to manage their own quarantine affairs it is well to enlarge a little on these last two measures. Basra had a single case of cholera on 26 July. Quarantine was promptly established at Qasr-i-Shirin, a frontier village on the Baghdad-Kermanshah road, although there was still no cholera within 500 miles of this frontier. At the same time passports were refused to any Persian wishing to travel to Iraq. One is almost forced to hold that these measures were actuated not by medical prudence at all, but by a desire to cause trouble to Iraqis coming to Persia and to hold up the pilgrim traffic which carried much Persian wealth into Iraq. For at that time political relations between Iraq and Persia were not at all friendly.

The quarantine camp at Qasr-i-Shirin was so disgracefully mismanaged that the British Minister was forced to protest and a commission of Persian doctors went down to examine the state of affairs. Their report was never made public. At the same time it was reported that inoculation certificates were unheeded and that immune travellers were compelled to undergo the full quarantine. The official legation mail also was detained. The report of an actual *détenu* is not pleasant reading:

> The camp is situated below the town on the edge of the river. A large double-fly tent is provided for First Class travellers. Iron bedsteads and bedding are provided, but the sheets and pillow cases are very dirty. One long table, covered with oil cloth, and a few rickety chairs are also provided. Food is obtainable from the cook attached to the Quarantine Station. It is filthy and expensive. During the daytime the tent is full of flies; the food and table are covered with them. There is a filter provided for drinking water, which is not boiled. This is brought direct from the river which has previously passed the town. Sanitary conditions are appalling. There is a deep water-course passing the camp. Over this two boards with a space in-between have been placed across the ditch. This platform is enclosed with reeds. While I was in quarantine, this water-course was being cleaned and the stench was appalling.
>
> It would be hard to conceive any better breeding ground for germs of every sort than in the quarantine station. No medical attention is given that I saw. Should a case of cholera ever develop there, it would spread like wild-fire throughout the camp.
>
> A separate single-fly tent is provided for European ladies, but it is quite uninhabitable during the day.

The official reply to the protest came from the Health Department, who countered the British charge of Persian inefficiency by stating that cholera had only appeared in Persian ports owing to the incompetency of the British quarantine officers at Basra and Mohammerah; that the closing of the frontier was entirely the fault of the Iraq Government who kept the Persian Government uninformed of any precautionary measures that were being taken; and that the frontier medical authorities had no confidence in some of the certificates of injection produced by travellers and that they were therefore compelled to reject them all.

These quarantine arrangements were not only inefficient, but also were hopelessly inadequate. To guard hundreds of miles of desert frontier is a gigantic task. Chauffeurs, camel-drivers and others who knew the by-paths or the guards passed backwards and forwards without molestation.

Conditions in the quarantine station at Shiraz were very little better. An English doctor, who was interned there, thus described it:

> The only drinking water available was from a water-channel. No steps were taken to protect it or to render the water for drinking sterile....No latrine accommodation or urinals of any kind existed... nor were there any soakage pits to dispose of the fluid refuse from the place....The Medical Officer in charge...had no cholera apparatus and no drugs...save calomel and quinine.

It was not until 20 November that the country was declared free of cholera. Officially the number of cases which occurred was 829 with 700 deaths; but this must certainly be an under-statement.

I have already said that there was a third party interested in this dispute. This was the Company formerly known as the Anglo-Persian Oil Company. This Company has been established in South Persia since the beginning of the century. The Company have constructed their own port of Abadan, which is the termination of the pipe line. The health of the whole territory involved in the concession, including the port of Abadan, is supervised by their own medical officers. Just above Abadan lies the Persian port of Mohammerah and only a few hours above Mohammerah lies the Iraqi port of Basra. Thus within a few miles are three ports under three different controls. After the defeat of the Turks until the present dispute arose, all these ports were under British management, which assured a certain amount of unanimity of plan and action. Should the port officer at Mohammerah be replaced by a Persian, there would be grave risk of friction with his Iraqi colleague above stream and his British colleague below.

Clive now reopened negotiations in the face of Bahrami's high-handed action in the appointment of Dr Tayyibi. He suggested that the Chief Quarantine Officer should be a Persian with British medical officers serving under him, that the service should be a Persian Government service, responsible to and controlled by the Health Department of Teheran, and that the British medical officers should have contracts granted to them by the *Majlis* not terminable before five full years had passed. In this way he hoped to ensure that the passage of executive control into Persian hands should be gradual and not abrupt. At the same time all arrears of pay owing to the Government of India by the Persian Government were to be paid in full.

Whilst these notes were passing between the Legation and the Ministry of Foreign Affairs, Bahrami had not let the grass grow under his feet. In January of 1928 he informed the Minister that the Budget Commission had definitely refused to contribute another halfpenny towards the pay of the British medical officers and that they were to be dismissed on 20 March, that is, the last day of the Persian year. To protests at this abrupt dismissal while the matter was still under negotiation, Taimur Tash sent a written reply. He regretted the whole affair, but explained that it was part of the policy of his government to 'engage in their service no citizen of a limitrophe country and that moreover no foreigner could be engaged in any capacity without his contract first being approved by the *Majlis*'. He himself was powerless to help the English doctors, because their salaries had been omitted from the new budget and there could be no question of contracts being granted to them by the *Majlis*. He assured the Minister that Bahrami could lay hands upon a sufficiency of trained and competent doctors and that in order to make doubly sure the *Majlis* had just passed an Act authorizing the employment of a French or German doctor as technical councillor to the Health Department. There was therefore not a vestige of reason for the retention of the British doctors in the Persian ports.

The British Government could now do nothing except point out the selfish attitude that the Persian Government had adopted, their ingratitude to a body of men who had served Persian interests for nearly half a century, and attempt to save British prestige by receiving some public acknowledgement of these services. This last Taimur Tash agreed to do. Accordingly, on 21 May the official thanks of the Persian Government were thus conveyed to the British Government over the signature of the Minister of Foreign Affairs.

Ordibihasht 1307.

My dear Minister,

At a time when Persian doctors are engaged in taking over the quarantine service in the southern ports I am glad to express in the name of my Government the appreciation of the philanthropic and humane services rendered there in the past by English doctors. I beg you to convey to these doctors the thanks of the Persian Government.

Yours etc.,

Fatoullah Khan Pakrevan.

The whole incident seems strangely similar *mutatis mutandis* to the abrupt dismissal of the British doctors from the Imperial Hospital five years previously.

The transfer being thus accomplished the Persian Government expected the British quarantine officers to give up their posts in March. No foreign technical adviser was even approached until May. It is not untrue to say that the Government of India was seriously alarmed at the possibility of a fresh outbreak of cholera during that summer. They even offered to finance the whole quarantine service for another six months in order that the transfer might be more gradual and Persian control commence during a less dangerous season. At the same time they offered to train a Persian doctor in the duties of Port officer in one of their own ports.

The Persian reply was the appointment of doctors to Bushire, Mohammerah, Bundar Abbas, Jask and Lingah. On 17 July they arrived in Bushire. In the meantime the acting quarantine officers had received no instructions from the Government of

India to hand over their duties and at first they declined to do so. Within a week they received orders by telegram to comply with the Persian demands. The Chief Quarantine Medical Officer handed over the keys of office on 28 July and the more distant ports surrendered one by one as their Persian successors arrived. On 4 August British control came to an end.

The new Chief Quarantine Medical Officer was a nephew of the Head of the Health Department and was also of the name of Bahrami. Scarcely had he taken over his new and difficult post when his chief resigned and was succeeded by Dr Sayyid Malek Loqmán-ul-Mulk, a surgeon rather than an administrator, but a man trained in Western methods. About the same time Sir Lionel Haworth was succeeded by Sir Frederick Johnston as Consul-General in Bushire. The younger Bahrami was keen and energetic. Had he had any special training in Port Administration he would have made a good quarantine officer. He owed his knowledge of bacteriology largely to Dr Mesnard of the Pasteur Institute, Teheran, where he had served a long apprenticeship. He was a friend of Dr Neligan, spoke French well, and understood a little English. But his job was bound to bring him into conflict with the English in the south. No sooner had he entered into office than he was ordered to demand the further surrender of the Charitable Hospital at Bushire which had remained in British hands.

Until 1916 the poor of Bushire were treated gratuitously in the Charitable Dispensary attached to the Residency. In that year the suggestion was made that a voluntary hospital should also be founded and for this object both English and Persians subscribed. The merchants of the place voluntarily agreed to the imposition of a small tax upon all packages passing through the port. The new hospital was placed under the direction of the Surgeon to the Residency. Because he was also Chief Quarantine Officer he often found it more convenient to remove sick cases from ships in the harbour to this hospital rather than to the quarantine hospital which lay on an island out in the bay. It is quite clear that the hospital was a benevolent, voluntary institution, essentially Anglo-Persian in character, built by British and Persian charity and maintained mainly by joint British and Persian money. It was intended from the beginning—by the Persian as well as the British founders (neither party of whom would otherwise have felt safe in contributing)—to be used by the Residency Surgeon in conjunction with the Residency Dispensary. The management of it was legally confided by the founders to a committee of two Persian and two British members. It is clear that it was not a Persian official or government hospital, because the Persian Government contributed nothing towards construction or annual upkeep. It had nothing to do with the Quarantine Service. On the contrary, it had an official British connection, because the British Government had a partial proprietary right in the hospital as it stood, which the Persian Government had not. And it was the British Government that worked up the scheme, superintended the building, provided the medical apparatus, and paid the salaries of the superior staff.

In spite of their inability to support their claim in January of the following year the Persian Government were informed that the hospital would be handed over to them. A new, though smaller hospital, was constructed within the Residency walls, all the equipment was transferred from the old building to the new, the Consul-General and Colonel Dickson resigned from the Committee of Management and Dr Bahrami Junior proudly took possession of his empty shell. Once again Persia had succeeded and Nationalism triumphed over the foreigner.

With the exception of the trouble over the Charitable Hospital, some minor disputes concerned with the landing of shore-leave men off H.M.S. *Lupin* and H.M.S. *Triad*, and a small difficulty in arranging the status of Dr Lincoln of Mohammerah who was both Quarantine Officer and British Vice-consul in that port, the first year of Persian control of the ports passed without friction. Neither cholera nor plague appeared which might worry the peace of mind of the new Chief Medical Officer. In the spring of 1930 I had the good fortune to be able to visit Bushire and see for myself how the new system was working. I found that Dr Bahrami Junior had established his office in Bushire and was assisted by Dr Amidi, who had been trained in Beirut and Cairo. He was an excellent and willing worker, even though his salary was somewhat in arrears. The Persian Government was still unable to meet the calls of Public Health upon its purse. The subordinate personnel had not received their salaries for four months. The Charitable Hospital was closed owing to the inability of Dr Bahrami to pay the drug bill. The emergency quarantine hospital in the bay was closed for similar reasons.

Numerous petty complaints were, of course, to be heard. As might be expected, the new doctors observed the letter of the law rather than the spirit. They were taking no risks. Occasionally, political jealousies were at the bottom of the trouble. Thus, the Oil Company's ship *Khuzistan*, which carried petrol and oil round the Gulf ports, became the centre of a squabble. International law requires all ships to be deratted once every six months. The *Khuzistan* used to go twice a year to Basra for this purpose. Suddenly the Persian authorities discovered that Basra had been omitted—clearly in error—from the list of ports approved of by the International Bureau in Paris as capable of issuing International Deratization Certificates. They were therefore within their rights in refusing to recognize the validity of such certificates issued in Basra. They demanded that the ship come down to Bushire twice a year for disinfection. The Oil Company replied that they were unable to go to the expense of sending the vessel to Bushire and back empty and that it was too dangerous to carry out the operation with the ship loaded. It is probable that in this matter it was not only a desire to stand upon their rights and to belittle the port of Basra that animated the Persian authorities. They also wished to pocket the fees which they would be entitled to charge. The deratting apparatus had yet to pay its way. The matter was easily settled by the placing of the name of the port of Basra on the roll of authorized ports.

A more serious complaint was that brought by the Government of India against the Quarantine Officer at Mohammerah for his failure to discover several cases of small-pox on board a vessel bound for Bombay. On 23 November ninety-three Irani gipsies embarked on the *Varela*. On arrival at Bombay no report of any infectious disease on board was made by the master. In consequence the ship was neither suspected nor quarantined. That night a child of one of the gipsies died and though they attempted to conceal the fact, the cause of death was found to be haemorrhagic small-pox. On the next day four more cases appeared. A close examination of the whole gang revealed that there was a boy of five among them who was convalescent from small-pox. On the following day three more cases occurred, all proving fatal within a few hours.

The Government of India put the blame upon the Persian Quarantine Officer who signed the clean bill of health at Mohammerah. The Persian Board of Health defended him and pointed out that the ship's doctor (an Indian assistant-surgeon) had also certified at Bushire (the next port of call after Mohammerah) that there was no infectious case on board. In the subsequent investigation the Indian doctor admitted that he suspected some disease among the gang, but failed to warn the port health authorities. He was dismissed from his ship and, I think, the honours in this case lie with the Persians.

During the year 1931 the bickering continued. This time it was the Persian authorities who laid complaints against the Iraqi Health Board. Unnecessary quarantine restrictions, they claimed, were being imposed upon Persian subjects in Fao. The facts are these. There was a mild outbreak of cholera in the Rafsindjan area, a district north of Bandar Abbas, in May of that year. The port of Bandar Abbas was not, however, declared infected. There had been no case of cholera in Basra or all Iraq since 1927. Three cases occurred at Basra on 27 July on board a vessel which had embarked several third class passengers at Bushire. As it was clear that the infection had been brought from a Persian port, the

Iraq authorities held that the Persian Gulf was infected. At the same time it was noted that the port of Bombay was reporting several cases of cholera with a serious epidemic in the province, a condition which was always associated with a spread of the disease into Persia and the Gulf ports. For this reason Iraq on 29 July applied the usual quarantine restrictions to all arrivals in the port of Basra from the Persian Gulf by land, sea and air. The Persian Government was immediately informed.

The geography of these parts is very complicated. All ships which enter the river, here known as the Shatt-ul-Arab, at Fao, also enter at the same time the port of Basra, because the limits of the port embrace all the waters of the Shatt-ul-Arab. The large Persian towns of Abadan and Mohammerah are 40 miles up the river from the sea; the Iraq town of Basra is 70 miles. Consequently ships passing to Persian ports are compelled to pass through Iraqi territorial waters to reach them. Large ships go straight to these towns and are dealt with by ordinary port and quarantine measures on arrival. Small coasting vessels which come from the western Indian ports, touch at various small uncontrolled ports *en route* and, when cholera is present in the Bombay Presidency, form a particular source of danger in the slow spread of the disease. Large numbers arrive at the Shatt-ul-Arab in the late summer and autumn to take cargoes of dates back along the Gulf.

On arrival at Fao these boats have to travel some 40 or 50 miles of river within Iraq territory to reach the Persian towns of Abadan or Mohammerah, a journey which usually involves one night's anchorage during a tide and in which the crew or passengers may land without much chance of interference at small villages on both the Persian and the Iraq sides of the river. They may thus carry infection to the shore. Port statistics of arrivals show that some passengers or crew almost invariably desert coasting vessels between Fao and the Persian towns.

Owing to these strange geographical limits a cholera epidemic was started this year which became very severe in Basra. The imposition of strict quarantine kept the southern part of the province from Abul Khassib to Fao free except for an occasional imported case. Nevertheless, the strictness of the regulations gave considerable annoyance to the Persian authorities. Their case was that small boats were only coast traffic, passing through territorial waters at sea on their way to a port of their own nation. By imposing quarantine on these the port of Basra was contravening the International Sanitary Convention. The Basra authorities retaliated by claiming that *de facto* they were dealing with shipping touching at foreign ports. Their measures were abundantly justified, for not only was Fao kept free from disease but the corresponding area of Persia on the opposite bank of the river was also unvisited by cholera.

In May 1931 arrived the long expected Dr Coulognier, a General in the French Army and the sanitary expert lent to Persia. Dr Loqmán-ul-Mulk resigned his post as Director of the Health Department, having performed a difficult task for four years with considerable success.

On arrival the General found himself in charge of a sanitary service which, although subject to very severe criticism at times, had considerably improved during the past few years. It is true that no epidemic had arisen since 1927 to test it. It is true that lack of funds still militated against an efficient service. But the Persians had in these last few years acted with unwonted energy. The problem of contacts and carriers had been met by wholesale inoculations. Road frontier conditions had been improved. The Indian system of quarantine in the Gulf had been adopted in its entirety. The weak point was, as always, domestic as much as scientific. An outbreak of cholera at Quetta, for instance, revealed that at Mirjawa, the frontier station on the Duzdab (Zahidan)-Quetta line, there was no isolation house provided and that the local quarantine doctor could only apply for some unused railway huts for this purpose. At Mohammerah passengers undergoing isolation were confined in some army barracks, a quarter of a century old. In none of the quarantine houses could the cooking, the sanitary or sleeping arrangements be considered satisfactory. In March 1932 the state of affairs was made the subject of an official protest by Sir George Buchanan at the Sanitary Conference in Paris. In his reply M. Rais, the Persian delegate, admitted that the state of affairs left much to be desired, but he claimed that already the Public Health Services were vastly improved and he hoped that under the aegis of General Coulognier this progress would be maintained. The British delegate was satisfied with this reply. The recognition of the Government of Iraq by the Persian Government removed another cause of friction. In fact, after a very stormy decade Persian medical affairs at last began to settle in a satisfactory and progressive manner.

CHAPTER XX

ARABIC RESEARCH AND MEDICINE

WHEN concluding his Fitzpatrick Lectures before the Royal College of Physicians in 1920 Professor Browne propounded two questions to his audience. The first was: How far can the fuller study of Arabian Medicine be regarded as likely to repay the labour that it involves? In this question there are two uncertainies. What meaning must be given to the word 'repay'? What does the student of Arabian Medicine expect to get as the result of his studies? And secondly, the beginner will very properly ask how much labour is involved. Upon that will depend what sort of reward he will expect. A full-time study demands a full-time salary.

Professor Browne certainly hoped that his lectures would inspire someone to make a study of this branch of Medicine, to specialize, as it were, in oriental historical Medicine. This is the first great difficulty, the first 'labour involved'. The student of Arabian Medicine must be well read in the theory, and very desirably also in the practice, of Medicine in general. Now this virtually demands that the research student be a qualified medical practitioner. This means at least seven years of concentrated study.

The student of Arabian Medicine must also know Arabic and be conversant with written Arabic as it has varied in the thousand years that have elapsed between the death of Muḥammad and to-day. He must be conversant with the variations of Arabic that occur between that written by the Moors in Spain and that written by the Indians in Delhi. And in between these people are all the variations of North Africa, Egypt, Syria, Iraq and Persia. But a knowledge of Arabic even thus wide is not sufficient. The Arabs came in contact with the Copts in Egypt, with the Sabaeans in Syria, with the Christians in South Persia, with Zoroastrians all over Persia, with Hindus in India and Jews everywhere. Each of these had its own language and had built up a native Medicine inscribed in the native tongue. And each of these people added to and modified considerably that corpus that we now call Arabian Medicine.

Nor was Arabian Medicine stagnant. It is not as though the Arabs in their spread East and West carried with them a scientific system which, snowball-like, grew by adding foreign systems to their own native system. The conquering Arabs had no system of indigenous Medicine other than the crude folk Medicine of an uncultured people. They built up that system of Medicine which we now call Arabian Medicine by harmonizing and inter-moulding the various native systems with which they came into contact, just as a woman might knead into one compact mass various lumps of dough. It is therefore an obvious requirement for the student of Arabian Medicine that he be capable of studying the foundations from which that system grew.

Unfortunately this does not conclude the preliminary difficulties. Long before Islam was preached, a system of Medicine had evolved and almost expired, a system into which Arab genius infused new life. This system is now known as Greek or Hippocratic Medicine. Second only in importance to a knowledge of Arabic is a knowledge of Greek. It is quite impossible to study Arabian Medicine without the ability to recognize the Greek factors which underlie it and to be able to read at first hand the texts of Hippocrates and Galen. It would be equivalent to studying the architecture of St Paul's cathedral with no knowledge of the Parthenon.

As the Arab Empire broke up and the Eastern Caliphate disappeared, Persian became the vehicle in which Arabian Medicine was transmitted. When the Western Caliphate disappeared before the attacks of the Christians, Latin, the language of the victorious Church, became the medium in that part of the world over which the Cross rather than the Crescent reigned. Where the Crescent did survive, Arabic still remained the main language of medical literature. But just as it would be insufficient to attempt to study Arabic medical literature of Turkey without some knowledge of Turkish, so the student of Arabian Medicine who wishes to embrace in his studies the whole period during which it flourished, must add to his attainments as well as Turkish a knowledge of Latin and Persian.

This sounds a very alarming list and may well make an aspirant to this line of research halt and reconsider his decision. But let him reflect that so little has been attempted as yet that there is a great deal of elementary and fundamental work still to be done which calls for considerable skill, it is true, but not for quite the same catholicity of knowledge.

The first thing required is more texts and more translations. So few are the published texts of writers of the Arabian School of Medicine, whether printed or lithographed, that I have been able to refer in the foregoing chapters of this book to the majority of them. There are still scores and scores of manuscripts scattered throughout the libraries of mosques, palaces, and museums which are quite unknown. Of many to publish the text is valueless, to translate them a waste of time. But so very few are available for students that many which ultimately will prove of no value should now be rendered accessible without the task being looked upon as a waste of labour. It is impossible to say dogmatically what is and what is not worthy of study until a larger number of authorities have had the opportunity to see and study them. I myself have for many years worked upon a medieval Persian manuscript. I completed the translation some years ago. When I looked at this work again in the light of greater knowledge, I came to the conclusion that the translation was almost valueless as a piece of historical or scientific research. The most that can be said is that no one else need follow the same line. The difficulty is to prevent anyone else from setting out on the same fruitless errand. I therefore had my work typed and bound and in that form offered it to the Royal College of Physicians of London. In that form it now rests in their Library.

Now, though any piece of work may prove valueless to another research worker, to me the labour involved in this research was far from valueless. First it taught me to read with ease the crabbed hand of the medieval copyist. Next it caused me to delve into and find out the correct equivalent of innumerable technical terms, botanical, medical and philosophical. Thirdly it taught me to recognize the ancient writers who were the source of the medical views of the fifteenth-century Persian authors. And finally, I learnt to love the intricate ramifications of the mind of an almost unknown medieval physician of Ispahan.

It is clearly not financially practicable to urge the publication of a large number of Arabic and Persian texts which may never be required, or if they are consulted, will be consulted but rarely. Nevertheless, I would counsel any young man or woman who is about to set out on this very enthralling line of research that he or she commence by studying one manuscript, any one hitherto not known, and that this study be concluded by translating into English, French or German that manuscript. Could not these translations, even if they do not get beyond the typewritten stage, be bound and placed upon the shelf of the Library of the Royal College beside my virgin effort? In this way there would be a gradual accumulation of texts which would act like the rungs of a ladder for each succeeding generation of students. There are so many manuscripts available and unknown, some of which must contain matter essential for a complete study of the growth and extent of Arabian Medicine. No man has time to read them all; and to skim an Arabic manuscript as one skims a printed text, well, it just cannot be done. There is a crying need for more texts and more translations, more especially of those works which were composed after the Mongol invasion of Persia and Baghdad.

Another great difficulty which the student of Arabian Medicine will meet is the absence of a scientific and accurate dictionary. There are glossaries attached to most of the few published translations. The less modern are these translations, the less accurate are the glossaries. Even the most modern are either inaccurate or give only the local meanings attached to technical terms. The eighteenth- and nineteenth-century glossaries are practically valueless. Medical nomenclature recently has so much changed that it is impossible that it should be otherwise. This would seem to be a very suitable moment to publish a large and up-to-date scientific dictionary after the model of Liddell and Scott's *Greek Lexicon*. The Royal College of Physicians has lately revised all technical terms (see *The Nomenclature of Diseases*, 6th ed., H. M. Stationery Office, 1931) and on this basis the translation of Persian and Arabic medical terms could also be standardized by anyone with sufficient knowledge of the subject. I have begun such a work.

In the face of such a formidable preparation it would be reasonable for the student to expect a large 'repayment'. If this is to be interpreted in terms of money or fame, I doubt if he will consider the return satisfactory. Scattered among the various pharmacopœias and the therapeutic sections of Arabic and Persian medical works there may be some excellent remedies once discovered and now lost. But I doubt it. It must be rare for a good and proved remedy to drop out of man's knowledge. I have suggested in the previous pages that there may have been some form of anaesthesia of which we are now ignorant. But it is highly improbable that it was more satisfactory than are our modern methods.

A few vegetable or animal drugs may have been employed and gained an empirical success and then forgotten. Ephedrin would seem to be one such. It grows wild in Persia, but it was recently introduced into Europe from China.

A few clinical oddities may have been remarked and incorporated into manuscripts no longer read and now await fresh discovery. Such were the heart involvement in Grave's Disease, the infectivity of whooping-cough, and the hay-fever which roses can produce in some people. These I have already noted in their proper places. There may be others still concealed, but they are not so important that they will bring wealth or fame to whoever re-discovers them.

It is not upon such grounds that further study of Arabian Medicine is justified. This is what may be termed the narrow scientist's point of view. Nor can it be justified, I think, upon the narrow orientalist's point of view. That scientific literature is a definite branch of oriental letters cannot be denied. But it is a dry and dusty path. 'Science is twofold: Theology and Medicine,' said the Prophet. And the study of an outworn medical creed is as sterile as the study of an outworn theology. No: not from such a point of view can further study be recommended.

It is only when these two aspects are united, when the objective is no longer of immediate practical application, when the health of neither the body nor the soul is the supreme quest that there is found abundant justification for a further and more intense research. A study of Arabian Medicine demanding, as it does, a study of its Greek ancestry, is in reality a study of the embryo of modern science. It is more than that: it is a study of the conception of that Medicine to which more and more modern thinkers are turning. Medicine is moving, as it were, in a great circle and is approaching the point once more at which the Persians and the Arabs picked it up. Names indeed have changed: yet even here there is less change than one would credit. Modern discoveries, such as the microscope, X-rays, electrical measuring devices have guaranteed that the circumference of the circle upon which we move will never quite coincide with the circumference of the Persians of old. But the basic ideas of the Persians, that Man is a distinct individual, that no two men are exactly alike, that a disease is a disease of the whole of man and not of a part, these views are also the views of the modern thinking man. Gone are the days when man was 'an uninteresting vehicle of a fascinating disease process'.

Far too long has the scientific Medicine of the nineteenth century distracted the attention from the patient to the disease. An extreme illustration is that of the unfortunate patient who was bandied about between medical and surgical wards and submitted to a number of exhausting examinations. All this because he had in addition to an unusually low blood pressure multiple tuberculous lesions and a very low sodium content in his blood. The physician in charge of the case ended his report without any suggestion of surprise by remarking that 'the patient seemed to withdraw markedly from his surroundings and to sink into a definite depression'.

Is our modern Medicine suffering from delusions of grandeur? All is not well in the relationship between patient and doctor. Perhaps the orthodox physician has always been inclined to give himself pontifical airs and to disregard the individuality of the patient. The result of such an attitude has always been the growth of quackery. The theosophy of to-day represents the charlatanism of medieval Baghdad.

The best that can be said for this domineering attitude is that it does at times effect a cure just because of the truth of the dictum that the patient is primarily an individual and not a case. For it makes possible the exercise of the healing influence of a strong personality over a weak and ailing one. Sir William Gull was once descanting at dinner upon his favourite topic that the successful medical man must be a bit of a quack. It is the old story, he said; *plebs vult decipi*. Dr Martin, a fellow-guest, promptly translated this as 'the public likes to be gulled'.

Underlying our conception of the sick man must first be our study of the healthy man. This is the science of physiology. Their physiological system the Persians borrowed from the Greeks. It is in consequence known as the Hippocratic System and, because it is based upon the four humours of the body, it is also known as the Humoural System. They held that upon the maintaining of an equilibrium between the humours depends a man's bodily health. To explain the operation of these non-existent humours an entirely erroneous physiological view of the functions of the arteries, veins, and nerves was invented. A completely false explanation of disease and its causes, and hence of its treatment, followed the acceptance of the Humoural Theory.

But the truth or falsity of the theory is of no importance. It served the Arabs and the Persians for five hundred years. It had served the Greeks and the Romans for a thousand years before that. For it expresses a fundamental psychological truth. The physicians of all these peoples had found it necessary in their approach to disease to classify first their patients into various types before they could attempt to recognize the maladies from which they were suffering. Only then could they give the appropriate treatment. Modern physicians, more especially modern psychiatrists, have the same need. Only the technical terms have changed. It is as important to us as it was to them.

The Persians pushed this theory a stage further. To them these humours represented both a physiological and a metaphysical conception. They were conceived of as corresponding closely to the four elements. Just as everything in Nature is composed of the four elements—air, fire, earth and water—so the personality of man, his ego, is the resultant of the four humours. And these correspond to the elements. Perhaps it is not too inexact to express the idea in Aristotelian language. The substance of Man is formed by the elements, the accidents of Man by the humours. From this arose the further doctrine that Man represents in himself a microcosm, that he is the World in miniature. The humours are therefore sometimes called the Daughters of the Elements. And it is not difficult to see that this theory of the temperament of the humours links up the humoural theory with the homeo- and allopathic theory of disease and hence is fundamental to one of the great unorthodox systems of Medicine of to-day.

The supreme importance of this intricate system of physiology is that it converted Medicine from a mere magical cult to an art with rules of its own which encouraged clinical observation. As such it survived throughout almost the whole of the period with which I have dealt in this book. It was shaken by Harvey when he published his discovery of the circulation of the blood and very slowly the Humoural System gave way to the Circulatory Theory. But so insufficient was Harvey's theory to explain disease that the underlying conception of the Arabian System survived until the materialists attacked it in the eighteenth and nineteenth centuries. It was left to Virchov to declare that 'there is no such thing as a sick body that is disordered in all its parts. I maintain that no doctor can systematically think of a morbid process unless he is able to assign to it a place in the body.' The wheel had moved the full half circle away from the Persian conception.

But such gross materialism did not last long. First came the role of the central nervous system with its glandular control; then came the breakdown of the dualism of mind and body under the assaults of psychologically-minded physicians, when disease and unhappiness alike were seen as the resultant of forces in the individual and his environment. Finally, when Berthold found that the implantation of testicular grafts into castrated cocks restored their appearance to that of normal birds and thus demonstrated that the testicles must pass some substance into the blood which reacts on the organism as a whole, the proof was complete. The Neo-Hippocratic or Neo-Humoural System was born. The turn of the wheel was complete.

The Neo-Humoural Theory, just like the old, not only considers the relation of the organs to the medium surrounding them, but also that of the individual to his usual environment. It is known that the vitality of living beings varies with changes wrought in their surrounding media. Differences in hydrogen-ion concentration influence osmotic pressure and thus the cellular function of organisms. Potassium, calcium and other inorganic ions have wide effect on cellular pathology, influencing structure, permeability and resistance of cell membranes. A minute portion of calcium chloride injected into the brain of a dog causes him to go to sleep: potassium chloride under the same conditions may cause epilepsy. An acid diathesis is said to predispose an individual to juvenile ailments, while an alkaline diathesis leads to disorders of old age. The astonishing foundations upon which this theory rests have been admirably set out in the *Revue Médicale de la Suisse Romande* of 25 April 1933. They make very interesting reading if an Avicenna lies open on the table at the same time.

Is there any need to justify at greater length a further study of Arabian Medicine? Is there any need to point out that a nation or profession which abandons its traditions and ceases to know the course of those traditions is by that very act convicted of decay? Is there any need to justify historical research into any branch of history? It there any need to call attention to the fact that only by taking the broadest possible view can a just perspective be gained of the age and epoch in which we live?

But there is a second question that Professor Browne put to his audience. Supposing that the fuller study is justified, he said, then how should that study be pursued in the future and what parts of the subject most merit attention? The first part of the question has, I think, already been answered. Clearly for many years the best way to pursue this study is to make more facts available. The expert in Arabic must give to others less expert in that language more and more of the early texts together with translations, if possible, at least with commentaries. The Syriac expert, the Hebrewist, the Old Persian scholar will have even more to give, for very very few know sufficient to be able to compare the Persian of pre-Islamic days with the written Persian of medieval times.

For the present the need is for all parts of the Arabian medical system to be made accessible. The time will come when certain portions of the medical manuscripts can safely be neglected. I imagine that the first of these will be the sections on drugs. Already one is beginning to feel that too much time has been spent on fruitless attempts to identify botanical names. Names must have varied from place to place and it is idle to expect consistency. Confusion must always have existed owing to the wide variations in one and the same species produced by the extremes of climate within which Arabian Medicine held sway. I feel sure that the Arab and Persian writers themselves must often have made the grossest errors through ignorance and lack of care in checking their descriptions.

Next I feel that the therapeutic parts of medical manuscripts will safely be neglected. Research into major and minor surgical proceedings will repay the time involved for many years. So will further elucidation of chemical technical works. Medical astrology, too, has been completely neglected. But the sections of the manuscripts on general medicine that deal with the administration of drugs can, I am sure, go into the limbo in which already lie the drugs themselves.

Clinical observations will always be of interest. They may not add to medical knowledge, but they usually portray the physician's character and frequently have a bearing on some historical aspect of the nation or the period. Medical anecdotes never weary.

But far more important than these is the philosophy and psychology that underlie all these works. Here is to be found a return to the first principles which are still in dispute. What is Disease? Fashion influences this fundamental conception. The reality of diseases as independent entities has been supported, challenged, reasserted within living memory. Is Disease a metaphysical abstraction, as Broussais asserted? Can it be defined and classified like a plant, as Sydenham essayed? Is the last word with the histologist, the bio-chemist or the bacteriologist? Until these and similar questions are finally answered, the thoughts of the great Arab and Persian scientists will continue to be worthy of study. Who would dream of studying moral philosophy without reading Aristotle and Plato? Arab and Persian views are worth as much as our own on these great fundamental questions. 'It is unwise', wrote the late Dr James Collier, 'to sneer at what the past has done, unwise to extol what your own generation has performed, and most unwise of all to denounce too quickly what a succeeding generation is doing.'

Though the methods differ, the objective is the same. Harvey placed the experimental method of approach to medical problems on a level which makes it almost sacrilege for anyone to attack. As far as clinical medicine is concerned the last word will always rest with the experimentalist. But even in clinical medicine problems arise which are out of reach of experiment. Man is so much more than flesh and blood. In such realms the Arab and the

Persian can speak with an authority equal to that of the German and the Frenchman. He puts forward opinions which should be set beside those of Greek and Roman philosophers. Did Avicenna approach nearer to what we now believe to be the true aspect of disease than did Galen? Did Rhazes give to clinical symptoms a juster appreciation than did Hippocrates? This, surely, is a fundamental question which only a study of the Arabian School of Medicine can answer. And this, surely, is what Professor Browne meant when he questioned whether a further study of the subject was worth while.

Medicine is international and recognizes frontiers neither of Time nor Age. National Medicine is a contribution to Medicine as a whole and must never degenerate into Nationalist Medicine. Galen, Avicenna, and Sydenham are heroes first of Medicine and only secondarily of the nations that begat them. The medical historian recognizes a spiritual kinship between all men who face the same problems of health and disease. To neglect any part of that family is to weaken the whole Tree. This is why further study of Arabian Medicine repays the student. He is completing a picture which is still far from complete. He is fitting into the puzzle those bits which have for so long lain neglected although so close at hand. And just as the picture of the jigsaw often lies hidden until the last few pieces are added, so it may be that Arabian thought with its synthesis of Indian and Chinese philosophy, may throw light on some of the dark problems which elude solution to-day.

That way
Over the mountain, which who stands upon
Is apt to doubt if it's indeed a road;
While if he views it from the waste itself,
Up goes the line there, plain from base to brow,
Not vague, mistakable.

GENEALOGICAL TREE OF THE QURRA FAMILY

Qurra
|
Ṣábit I
(Physician to al-Muʿtazid, 825–901)

Ibráhím I

Sinán
(Physician to al-Rází, d. 942)

Ṣábit II
(Director of the ʿAẓudí Hospital, 907–73)

Ibráhím II
(President of Board of Examiners, 908–47)

Isḥá-q

GENEALOGICAL TREE OF THE BU<u>KH</u>T YI<u>SH</u>Úʿ FAMILY
(after Browne's *Chahár Maqála*, p. 145)

1. Bu<u>kh</u>t Yi<u>sh</u>úʿ I
|
2. Jurjís I
(physician to al-Manṣúr, d. 152/769)
|
3. Bu<u>kh</u>t Yi<u>sh</u>úʿ II
(physician to al-Mahdí, al-Hádí, and Hárún-ul-Ra<u>sh</u>íd, d. 185/801)

4. Jibráʾíl I
(physician to Hárún-ul-Ra<u>sh</u>íd,
al-Amín and al-Maʾmún,
d. 213/828)

5. Jurjís II

6. Bu<u>kh</u>t Yi<u>sh</u>úʿ III
(physician to al-Muʿtazz,
d. 256/870)

Miká'íl

7. ʿUbayd-Ulláh I
(physician to al-Muttaqí)

8. Yaḥyá or Yúḥanná

9. Jibráʾíl II
(physician to ʿAzud-ul-Doula,
d. 397/1005)

10. Bu<u>kh</u>t Yi<u>sh</u>úʿ IV
(physician to al-Muqtadir,
d. 329/940)

11. Abu Saʿíd ʿUbayd-Ulláh II
(d. 450/1058)

NOTE. Wustenfeld, following Ibn abi Uṣaybiʿa, inserts a Jibráʾíl between Jurjís (2) and Bu<u>kh</u>t Yi<u>sh</u>úʿ (1). But al-Qifṭí represents Jurjís I as the son, not the grandson of Bu<u>kh</u>t Yi<u>sh</u>úʿ I.

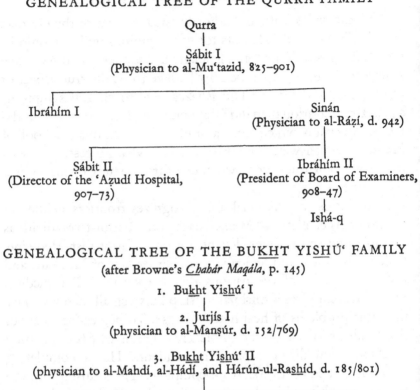

INDEX

In the following index the prefixes 'abu' ('father of...') and 'ibn' ('son of...') are disregarded in the arrangement of Muhammadan names into which they enter: thus, for example, such names as Abu Tahir and Ibn Sina are to be sought under 'T' and 'S' respectively. Similarly the Arabic definite article 'al-' is to be disregarded. So the title al-Muktafi will be found listed under 'M'. The letter 'b.' between two names stands for 'bin' or 'ibn' ('son of').

For typographical reasons it has been found necessary to omit in the index the accents indicating the long vowels and the dots and dashes that distinguish different forms of the same letter. The correct transliteration of such words must therefore be sought in the text.

INDEX

INDEX

INDEX

al-Musta'sim, 37th 'Abbasid Caliph, 233, 305
Mustaufi, 'Aziz-ul-Din, benefactor, 172, 175
Mustaufi al-Qazvini, writer, *see* al-Qazvini
al-Mustazhir, 28th 'Abbasid Caliph, 164, 224, 225
al-Mustazi, 33rd 'Abbasid Caliph, 227
al-Mu'tabar, of Abu ul-Barkat, 168
Mutabiqat bayn Qol-il-Inbiya wa il-Falasifat, of Bukht Yishu', ii, 159
al-Mu'tamid, 15th 'Abbasid Caliph, 109, 122, 270
Mu'tamid-ul-Doula, a Regent, 513
al-Mu'tasim, 8th 'Abbasid Caliph, 91, 107, 117, 118, 257, 328
al-Mutawakkil, 10th 'Abbasid Caliph, 89, 107, 108, 116, 118–22, 130, 270
al-Mu'tazid, 16th 'Abbasid Caliph, 74, 115, 122, 123, 124, 127, 128, 133, 231, 241
al-Mu'tazz, 13th 'Abbasid Caliph, 121, 122
al-Muti', 23rd 'Abbasid Caliph, 210
al-Muttaqi, 21st 'Abbasid Caliph, 149, 152, 158
al-Muwaffaq, father of al-Mu'tazid Caliph, 123
Muwaffaq-ul-Din Samarri, a writer, 309
Muzaffar-ul-Din Shah, 538, 539, 546

Naban, a village, 425
al-Nabigha of Zubyan, a poet, 63
Nadir Shah, viii, 273, 368, 374, 390, 391, 413–17, 419, 420, 423, 424, 437, 438, 533
Naficy, Dr Abbas, 218
Nafis b. 'Iwaz of Kerman, 156, 304, 336
Ibn Nafis, 309, 327, 333, 335, 336, 375
Nafsa, Shaykh, of Karrack, 490
Nafzawi, Shaykh, 296, 297
Najam-ul-Din Qazvini, an ophthalmologist, 143
Najib-ul-Din Samarqandi, a writer, 304, 336
Nakhchivan, a town, 452
Naples, 395
Napoleon I, emperor of France, 370, 439, 440, 441, 448
Ibn ul-Naqah, a surgeon, 161, 162
al-Nasir, 34th 'Abbasid Caliph, 227, 229, 230, 290
Nasir-ul-Din Shah, 457, 481, 494, 498, 500, 504, 518, 521
Nasir-ul-Doula, governor of Damascus, 213
Nasir-ul-Mulk, a Regent, 539
Abu Nasr, physician to al-Nasir Caliph, 228, 229
Abu Nasr b. ul-Duhali, 161
Abu Nasr Gilani, physician to Haydar Mirza, 358, 359
Abu Nasr-i-'Arraq, a physician and artist, 188
Abu-Nasr-ul-Din Tusi al-Muhaqqiq, 158, 305, 306, 379
al-Natali, a physician and logician, 185
Nathan the Jew, 142
al-Nazar, cousin of Muhammad the Prophet, 68
al-Nazar 'Ali, an *hakimbashi*, 488
Nazif al-Rumi, a physician and priest, 155, 161
Nazim-ul-Atibba, a doctor, 562
Nazuk, a general, 129, 130
Neligan, Dr A. R., 532, 546, 547, 548, 554, 555, 557, 567, 577
Nestorius, Patriarch of Constantinople, 46, 55
Neuburger, 94n., 202
New Account, of Fryer, 243
New Testament, tr. into Persian by Walton, 367
Nicholson, Prof. A., 180n., 219, 262n., 329
Nicholson, I. M. S., Major, 566, 567
Nidana, an Indian physician, 372
Nigar Khanum, Princess, 192
Nihavend, battle of, 61
al-Nili abu Sahl, 239
Nili Muhammad, a physician, 312
Nisibis, 38, 45, 46
Nizam-ul-Mulk, a *wazir*, 51n., 211, 212, 230, 232, 317
Nizami 'Aruzi Samarqandi, a poet, viin., 111, 124, 125n., 188, 195, 204, 216, 360
Nobakht, an astrologist, 366
Noeldeke, 52, 53
al-No'man, a general, 60, 61
Nonus Almansuris, see *Liber Nonus ad Almansorem*
Note-book of the Oculists of Jesu Haly, tr. by Casey Wood, see *Tazkirat-ul-Kahhalin*
Nuh b. Mansur Samani, 186, 192, 193
Nuh b. Nasr Samani, 102
Nur-ul-'Ayun, of Zarrindast, 142
Nur-ul-Din, physician to Shah Tahmasp, 358
Nur-Ullah 'Ala'-ul-Din, a pharmacologist, 365, 381
Nurses employed in hospitals, 132, 170, 173
Nurshirvan (also called Anusharwan), 38, 40, 49, 50, 51, 53, 54, 55, 58, 66, 98
abu Nuwas, a poet, 127
Nuzhat-ul-Ashab fi M'ashurat-il-Ahabab, of Samu'l b. Yahya, 295

Printed in the United States
By Bookmasters